ELIZABETH H. HOLT, M.D
3410 EXECUTIVE DRIVE
SUITE 205
RALEIGH, NC 27609

D1058923

Vitamin D

Guest Editor

SOL EPSTEIN, MD

ENDOCRINOLOGY AND METABOLISM CLINICS OF NORTH AMERICA

www.endo.theclinics.com

Consulting Editor
DEREK LEROITH, MD, PhD

June 2010 • Volume 39 • Number 2

SAUNDERS an imprint of ELSEVIER, Inc.

W.B. SAUNDERS COMPANY
A Division of Elsevier Inc.

1600 John F. Kennedy Boulevard • Suite 1800 • Philadelphia, Pennsylvania 19103-2899

http://www.theclinics.com

ENDOCRINOLOGY AND METABOLISM CLINICS OF NORTH AMERICA Volume 39, Number 2
June 2010 ISSN 0889-8529, ISBN-13: 978-1-4377-1817-1

Editor: Rachel Glover
Developmental Editor: Donald Mumford

© **2010 Elsevier Inc. All rights reserved.**

This journal and the individual contributions contained in it are protected under copyright by Elsevier, and the following terms and conditions apply to their use:

Photocopying
Single photocopies of single articles may be made for personal use as allowed by national copyright laws. Permission of the Publisher and payment of a fee is required for all other photocopying, including multiple or systematic copying, copying for advertising or promotional purposes, resale, and all forms of document delivery. Special rates are available for educational institutions that wish to make photocopies for non-profit educational classroom use. For information on how to seek permission visit www.elsevier.com/permissions or call: (+44) 1865 843830 (UK)/(+1) 215 239 3804 (USA).

Derivative Works
Subscribers may reproduce tables of contents or prepare lists of articles including abstracts for internal circulation within their institutions. Permission of the Publisher is required for resale or distribution outside the institution. Permission of the Publisher is required for all other derivative works, including compilations and translations (please consult www.elsevier.com/permissions).

Electronic Storage or Usage
Permission of the Publisher is required to store or use electronically any material contained in this journal, including any article or part of an article (please consult www.elsevier.com/permissions). Except as outlined above, no part of this publication may be reproduced, stored in a retrieval system or transmitted in any form or by any means, electronic, mechanical, photocopying, recording or otherwise, without prior written permission of the Publisher.

Notice
No responsibility is assumed by the Publisher for any injury and/or damage to persons or property as a matter of products liability, negligence or otherwise, or from any use or operation of any methods, products, instructions or ideas contained in the material herein. Because of rapid advances in the medical sciences, in particular, independent verification of diagnoses and drug dosages should be made.

Although all advertising material is expected to conform to ethical (medical) standards, inclusion in this publication does not constitute a guarantee or endorsement of the quality or value of such product or of the claims made of it by its manufacturer.

Endocrinology and Metabolism Clinics of North America (ISSN 0889-8529) is published quarterly by Elsevier Inc., 360 Park Avenue South, New York, NY 10010-1710. Months of issue are March, June, September, and December. Periodicals postage paid at New York, NY and additional mailing offices. Subscription prices are USD 271.00 per year for US individuals, USD 457.00 per year for US institutions, USD 139.00 per year for US students and residents, USD 340.00 per year for Canadian individuals, USD 560.00 per year for Canadian institutions, USD 394.00 per year for international individuals, USD 560.00 per year for international institutions, and USD 206.00 per year for international and Canadian and foreign students/residents. To receive student/resident rate, orders must be accompanied by name of affiliated institution, date of term, and the signature of program/residency coordinator on institution letterhead. Orders will be billed at individual rate until proof of status is received. Foreign air speed delivery is included in all *Clinics* subscription prices. All prices are subject to change without notice. **POSTMASTER:** Send address changes to *Endocrinology and Metabolism Clinics of North America*, Elsevier Health Sciences Division, Subscription Customer Service, 3251 Riverport Lane, Maryland Heights, MO 63043. **Customer Service: Telephone: 1-800-654-2452** (U.S. and Canada); **1-314-447-8871** (outside U.S. and Canada). **Fax: 1-314-447-8029. E-mail: journalscustomerservice-usa@elsevier.com** (for print support); **journalsonlinesupport-usa@elsevier.com** (for online support).

Reprints. For copies of 100 or more, of articles in this publication, please contact the Commercial Rights Department, Elsevier Inc., 360 Park Avenue South, New York, NY 10010-1710; phone: (+1) 212-633-3813; fax: (+1) 212-462-1935; e-mail: reprints@elsevier.com.

Endocrinology and Metabolism Clinics of North America is covered in *MEDLINE/PubMed (Index Medicus), EMBASE/Excerpta Medica, Current Contents/Clinical Medicine, Current Contents/Life Sciences, Science Citation Index, ISI/BIOMED, BIOSIS,* and *Chemical Abstracts.*

Printed in the United States of America.

Contributors

CONSULTING EDITOR

DEREK LEROITH, MD, PhD
Chief, Division of Endocrinology, Metabolism, and Bone Diseases, Mount Sinai School of Medicine, New York, New York

GUEST EDITOR

SOL EPSTEIN, MD, FRCP, FACP
Professor of Medicine and Geriatrics, Mount Sinai School of Medicine, New York, New York

AUTHORS

DARE V. AJIBADE, BA
MD/PhD Student, Department of Biochemistry and Molecular Biology, New Jersey Medical School, University of Medicine and Dentistry of New Jersey, Newark, New Jersey

ARTI BHAN, MBBS
Senior Staff Physician, Division of Endocrinology, Diabetes and Bone and Mineral Disorders, Henry Ford Hospital, Detroit, Michigan

NEIL BINKLEY, MD
University of Wisconsin-Madison Osteoporosis Clinical Center and Research Program, Madison, Wisconsin

HEIKE A. BISCHOFF-FERRARI, MD, DrPH
Director, Centre on Aging and Mobility, University of Zurich; Swiss National Foundations Professor, Department of Rheumatology and Institute of Physical Medicine, University Hospital Zurich, Zurich, Switzerland

ROGER BOUILLON, MD, PhD
Emeritus Professor of Medicine, Laboratory for Experimental Medicine and Endocrinology (LEGENDO), Katholieke Universiteit Leuven, UZ Gasthuisberg, Leuven, Belgium

SYLVIA CHRISTAKOS, PhD
Professor, Department of Biochemistry and Molecular Biology, New Jersey Medical School, University of Medicine and Dentistry of New Jersey, Newark, New Jersey

PUNEET DHAWAN, PhD
Assistant Professor, Department of Biochemistry and Molecular Biology, New Jersey Medical School, University of Medicine and Dentistry of New Jersey, Newark, New Jersey

ADAM J. FECHNER, MD
Post Doctoral Fellow, Department of Obstetrics and Gynecology and Women's Health, New Jersey Medical School, University of Medicine and Dentistry of New Jersey, Newark, New Jersey

DAVID FELDMAN, MD
Professor of Medicine, Department of Medicine, Division of Endocrinology, Gerontology and Metabolism, Stanford University School of Medicine, Stanford, California

CONNY GYSEMANS, PhD
Researcher, Laboratory for Experimental Medicine and Endocrinology (LEGENDO), Katholieke Universiteit Leuven, UZ Gasthuisberg, Leuven, Belgium

MARTIN HEWISON, PhD
Professor in Residence, Department of Orthopaedic Surgery and Molecular Biology Institute, David Geffen School of Medicine at UCLA, Los Angeles, California

MICHAEL F. HOLICK, MD, PhD
Professor of Medicine, Physiology, and Biophysics, Section of Endocrinology, Nutrition, and Diabetes, Department of Medicine, Vitamin D, Skin and Bone Research Laboratory, Boston University School of Medicine, Boston University Medical Center, Boston, Massachusetts

BRUCE W. HOLLIS, PhD
Professor of Pediatrics; Director of Pediatric Nutritional Sciences, Departments of Biochemistry and Molecular Biology, and Pediatrics, Children's Research Institute, Medical University of South Carolina, Charleston, South Carolina

CANDACE S. JOHNSON, PhD
Professor of Oncology and Chair, Department of Pharmacology and Therapeutics; Deputy Director, Roswell Park Cancer Institute, Buffalo, New York

GLENVILLE JONES, PhD
Craine Professor and Head, Department of Biochemistry; Professor of Medicine, Queen's University, Kingston, Ontario, Canada

ARUNA V. KRISHNAN, PhD
Senior Research Scientist, Department of Medicine, Division of Endocrinology, Stanford University School of Medicine, Stanford, California

DIANE KRUEGER, BS
University of Wisconsin-Madison Osteoporosis Clinical Center and Research Program, Madison, Wisconsin

LEILA J. MADY, BA
MD/PhD Student, Department of Biochemistry and Molecular Biology, New Jersey Medical School, University of Medicine and Dentistry of New Jersey, Newark, New Jersey

PETER J. MALLOY, PhD
Senior Scientist, Division of Endocrinology, Gerontology and Metabolism, Stanford University School of Medicine, Stanford, California

KEVIN J. MARTIN, MB, BCh, FACP
Professor of Medicine and Director, Division of Nephrology, Saint Louis University, Saint Louis, Missouri

CHANTAL MATHIEU, MD, PhD
Professor of Medicine, Laboratory for Experimental Medicine and Endocrinology (LEGENDO), Katholieke Universiteit Leuven, UZ Gasthuisberg, Leuven, Belgium

MARK B. MEYER, PhD
Assistant Scientist, Department of Biochemistry, University of Wisconsin-Madison, Madison, Wisconsin

JOHN M. PETTIFOR, MBBCh, FCPaed(SA), PhD(Med)
Professor of Pediatrics; Director, MRC Mineral Metabolism Research Unit, Department of Pediatrics, Chris Hani Baragwanath Hospital, Johannesburg, South Africa

J. WESLEY PIKE, PhD
Professor of Biochemistry, Department of Biochemistry, University of Wisconsin-Madison, Madison, Wisconsin

RIZWAN A. QAZI, MD
Assistant Professor of Internal Medicine, Division of Nephrology, Saint Louis University, Saint Louis, Missouri

REKHA RAMAMURTHY, MD
University of Wisconsin-Madison Osteoporosis Clinical Center and Research Program, Madison, Wisconsin

AJAY D. RAO, MD
Clinical Research Fellow, Division of Endocrinology, Diabetes, and Hypertension, Brigham and Women's Hospital, Boston, Massachusetts

D. SUDHAKER RAO, MBBS, FACP, FACE
Director, Bone and Mineral Research Laboratory, Henry Ford Hospital, Detroit, Michigan

TATIANA TAKIISHI, MSc
Researcher, Laboratory for Experimental Medicine and Endocrinology (LEGENDO), Katholieke Universiteit Leuven, UZ Gasthuisberg, Leuven, Belgium

KEBASHNI THANDRAYEN, MBBCh, FCPaed(SA), MMed(Paeds)
Pediatrician, MRC Mineral Metabolism Research Unit, Department of Pediatrics, Chris Hani Baragwanath Hospital, Johannesburg, South Africa

DONALD L. TRUMP, MD
Professor of Oncology, Department of Medicine; President and CEO, Roswell Park Cancer Institute, Buffalo, New York

Contents

The biologically active metabolite of vitamin D, 1,25(OH)$_2$D$_3$, affects mineral homeostasis and has numerous other diverse physiologic functions including effects on growth of cancer cells and protection against certain immune disorders. This article reviews the role of vitamin D hydroxylases in providing a tightly regulated supply of 1,25(OH)$_2$D$_3$. The role of extrarenal 1α(OH)ase in placenta and macrophages is also discussed, as well as regulation of vitamin D hydroxylases in aging and chronic kidney disease. Understanding specific factors involved in regulating the hydroxylases may lead to the design of drugs that can selectively modulate the hydroxylases. The ability to alter levels of these enzymes would have therapeutic potential for the treatment of various diseases, including bone loss disorders and certain immune diseases.

The actions of the vitamin D hormone 1,25-dihydroxyvitamin D$_3$ (1,25(OH)$_2$D$_3$) are mediated by the vitamin D receptor (VDR), a ligand-activated transcription factor that functions to control gene expression. After ligand activation, the VDR binds directly to specific sequences located near promoters and recruits a variety of coregulatory complexes that perform the additional functions required to modify transcriptional output. Recent advances in transcriptional regulation, which permit the unbiased identification of the regulatory regions of genes, are providing new insight into how genes are regulated. Surprisingly, gene regulation requires the orchestrated efforts of multiple modular enhancers often located many kilobases upstream, downstream, or within the transcription units themselves. These studies are transforming our understanding of how 1,25(OH)$_2$D$_3$ regulates gene transcription.

The unique *cis*-triene structure of vitamin D and related metabolites makes it susceptible to oxidation, ultraviolet (UV) light-induced conformational changes, heat-induced conformational changes, and attacks by free radicals. Vitamin D_2 is much less bioactive than vitamin D_3 in humans. Metabolic activation and inactivation of vitamin D are well characterized and result in a plethora of metabolites, of which only 25-hydroxyvitamin D (25(OH)D) and 1,25-dihydroxyvitamin D (1,25(OH)$_2$D) provide any clinically relevant information. 25(OH)D_2 and 25(OH)D_3 are commonly known as calcifediol and the 1,25(OH)$_2$D metabolites as calcitriol. In this review the current state of the science on the clinical assessment of circulating 25(OH)D and 1,25(OH)$_2$D is described.

Low Vitamin D Status: Definition, Prevalence, Consequences, and Correction

Neil Binkley, Rekha Ramamurthy, and Diane Krueger

Vitamin D is obtained from cutaneous production when 7-dehydrocholesterol is converted to vitamin D_3 (cholecalciferol) by ultraviolet B radiation or by oral intake of vitamin D_2 (ergocalciferol) and D_3. An individual's vitamin D status is best evaluated by measuring the circulating 25-hydroxyvitamin D (25(OH)D) concentration. Although controversy surrounds the definition of low vitamin D status, there is increasing agreement that the optimal circulating 25(OH)D level should be approximately 30 to 32 ng/mL or above. Using this definition, it has been estimated that approximately three-quarters of all adults in the United States have low levels. Low vitamin D status classically has skeletal consequences such as osteomalacia/rickets. More recently, associations between low vitamin D status and increased risk for various nonskeletal morbidities have been recognized; whether all of these associations are causally related to low vitamin D status remains to be determined. To achieve optimal vitamin D status, daily intakes of at least 1000 IU or more of vitamin D are required. The risk of toxicity with "high" amounts of vitamin D intake is low. Substantial between-individual variability exists in response to the same administered vitamin D dose. When to monitor 25(OH)D levels has received little attention. Supplementation with vitamin D_3 may be preferable to vitamin D_2.

Maternal Vitamin D Status: Implications for the Development of Infantile Nutritional Rickets

Kebashni Thandrayen and John M. Pettifor

The mother is the major source of circulating 25-hydroxyvitamin D concentration in the young infant. Maternal vitamin D status is an important factor in determining the vitamin D status of the infant and their risk of developing vitamin D deficiency and infantile nutritional rickets. There is evidence that the current supplementation recommendations, particularly for pregnant and lactating women, are inadequate to ensure vitamin D sufficiency in these groups. A widespread and concerted effort is needed to ensure daily supplementation of breastfed and other infants at high risk with vitamin D 400 IU from birth and of pregnant women in high-risk communities with 2000 IU. Future studies are required to determine the optimal doses of vitamin D supplementation in pregnancy and during lactation, and for normalizing vitamin D stores in infancy to reduce the prevalence of infantile nutritional rickets. Operational research studies are needed to understand the best methods of implementing supplementation programs and the factors that are likely to impede their success.

Osteomalacia is an end-stage bone disease of chronic and severe vitamin D or phosphate depletion of any cause. Its importance has increased because of the rising incidence of vitamin D deficiency. Yet, not all cases of osteomalacia are cured by vitamin D replacement, and furthermore, not all individuals with vitamin D deficiency develop osteomalacia. Although in the past osteomalacia was commonly caused by malabsorption, nutritional deficiency now is more common. In addition, recent literature suggests that nutritional vitamin D deficiency osteomalacia follows various bariatric surgeries for morbid obesity. Bone pain, tenderness, muscle weakness, and difficulty walking are all common clinical manifestations of osteomalacia. Diagnostic work-up involves biochemical assessment of vitamin D status and may also include a transiliac bone biopsy. Treatment is based on aggressive vitamin D repletion in most cases with follow-up biopsies if patients are started on antiresorptive or anabolic agents.

Two rare genetic diseases can cause rickets in children. The critical enzyme to synthesize calcitriol from 25-hydroxyvitamin D, the circulating hormone precursor, is 25-hydroxyvitamin D-1α-hydroxylase (1α-hydroxylase). When this enzyme is defective and calcitriol can no longer be synthesized, the disease 1α-hydroxylase deficiency develops. The disease is also known as vitamin D–dependent rickets type 1 or pseudovitamin D deficiency rickets. When the VDR is defective, the disease hereditary vitamin D–resistant rickets, also known as vitamin D–dependent rickets type 2, develops. Both diseases are rare autosomal recessive disorders characterized by hypocalcemia, secondary hyperparathyroidism, and early onset severe rickets. In this article, these 2 genetic childhood diseases, which present similarly with hypocalcemia and rickets in infancy, are discussed and compared.

This article discusses the amount of vitamin D supplementation needed and the desirable 25-hydroxyvitamin D level to be achieved for optimal fracture prevention.

Vitamin D physiology has gained more importance and publicity than any of its counterparts in the water- and fat-soluble vitamin groups combined. This is partly because vitamin D deficiency is still widely prevalent in the developed world and the beneficial effects are thought to extend beyond the regulation of calcium and phosphorus homeostasis alone. Vitamin D deficiency becomes even more important in the various stages of chronic kidney disease (CKD); CKD itself is also on the increase. How vitamin D physiology is altered in CKD and how the various treatment modalities can alter the morbidity and mortality associated with CKD is the topic of discussion for this article.

Martin Hewison

Interaction with the immune system is one of the most well-established nonclassic effects of vitamin D. For many years this was considered to be a manifestation of granulomatous diseases such sarcoidosis, in which synthesis of active 1,25-dihydroxyvitamin D_3 ($1,25(OH)_2D_3$) is known to be dysregulated. However, recent reports have supported a role for $1,25(OH)_2D_3$ in mediating normal function of the innate and adaptive immune systems. Crucially, these effects seem to be mediated via localized autocrine or paracrine synthesis of $1,25(OH)_2D_3$ from precursor 25-hydroxyvitamin D_3, the main circulating metabolite of vitamin D. The ability of vitamin D to influence normal human immunity is highly dependent on the vitamin D status of individuals, and may lead to aberrant response to infection or autoimmunity in those who are lacking vitamin D. The potential health significance of this has been underlined by increasing awareness of impaired vitamin D status in populations across the globe. This article describes some of the recent developments with respect to vitamin D and the immune system, and possible clinical implications.

Michael F. Holick

Vitamin D deficiency is the most common nutritional deficiency and likely the most common medical condition in the world. The major cause of vitamin D deficiency has been the lack of appreciation that the body requires 5- to 10-fold higher intakes than is currently recommended by health agencies. There is now overwhelming and compelling scientific and epidemiologic data suggesting that the human body requires a blood level of 25(OH)D above 30 ng/mL for maximum health. To increase the blood level to the minimum 30 ng/mL requires the ingestion of at least 1000 IU of vitamin D per day for adults. In general, there is no downside to increasing either a child's or adult's vitamin D intake.

Aruna V. Krishnan, Donald L. Trump, Candace S. Johnson, and David Feldman

Calcitriol (1,25-dihydroxyvitamin D_3), the hormonally active form of vitamin D, exerts growth inhibitory and prodifferentiating effects on many malignant cells and retards tumor growth in animal models. Calcitriol is being evaluated as an anticancer agent in several human cancers. The mechanisms underlying the anticancer effects of calcitriol include inhibition of cell proliferation, stimulation of apoptosis, suppression of inflammation, and inhibition of tumor angiogenesis, invasion, and metastasis. This review discusses some of the molecular pathways mediating these anticancer actions of calcitriol and the preclinical data in cell culture and animal models. The clinical trials evaluating the use of calcitriol and its analogues in the treatment of patients with cancer are described. The reasons for the lack of impressive beneficial effects in clinical trials compared with the substantial efficacy seen in preclinical models are discussed.

Type 1 (T1D) and type 2 (T2D) diabetes are considered multifactorial diseases in which both genetic predisposition and environmental factors participate in their development. Many cellular, preclinical, and observational studies support a role for vitamin D in the pathogenesis of both types of diabetes including: (1) T1D and T2D patients have a higher incidence of hypovitaminosis D; (2) pancreatic tissue (more specifically the insulin-producing β-cells) as well as numerous cell types of the immune system express the vitamin D receptor (VDR) and vitamin D-binding protein (DBP); and (3) some allelic variations in genes involved in vitamin D metabolism and VDR are associated with glucose (in)tolerance, insulin secretion, and sensitivity, as well as inflammation. Moreover, pharmacologic doses of 1,25-dihydroxyvitamin D (1,25(OH)$_2$D), the active form of vitamin D, prevent insulitis and T1D in nonobese diabetic (NOD) mice and other models of T1D, possibly by immune modulation as well as by direct effects on β-cell function. In T2D, vitamin D supplementation can increase insulin sensitivity and decrease inflammation. This article reviews the role of vitamin D in the pathogenesis of T1D and T2D, focusing on the therapeutic potential for vitamin D in the prevention/intervention of T1D and T2D as well as its complications.

Vitamin D has gone through a renaissance with the association of vitamin D deficiency with a wide array of common diseases including breast, colorectal and prostate cancers, cardio-vascular disease, autoimmune conditions and infections. Vitamin D analogs constitute a valuable group of compounds which can be used to regulate gene expression in functions as varied as calcium and phosphate homeostasis, as well as cell growth regulation and cell differentiation of a wide spectrum of cell types. This review will discuss the full range of vitamin D compounds currently available, some of their possible uses, and potential mechanisms of action.

THE CLINICS ARE NOW AVAILABLE ONLINE!

Access your subscription at:
www.theclinics.com

Foreword

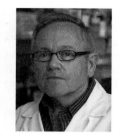

Derek LeRoith, MD, PhD
Consulting Editor

Drs Christakos, Ajibade, Dhawan, Fechner, and Mady review the metabolism of vitamin D. Hydroxylases are involved in converting the parent molecule to 25-OH vitamin D and then to 1,25-OH vitamin D, the active form. The regulation of these hydroxylases is still not well defined, and this area of research may be of value in considering new therapeutic possibilities, especially the possibility that vitamin D may be involved in many nonclassical functions, as described in this issue.

Drs Pike and Meyer describe new information on the vitamin D receptor. The receptor is expressed in cell types, including those of the immune system, skin, pancreas, and bone. This may explain the widespread effects of vitamin D that have recently become known and spurred a large amount of research. When 1,25-OH vitamin D binds its receptor, it activates the receptor that in turn affects varied gene expression in multiple cells and tissues. As the authors outline, new technologies have been instrumental in these new discoveries.

Measurement of vitamin D is important in metabolic bone disease and, we now realize, in many other diseases; this is becoming increasingly clear and is a theme developed in this issue. As described by Dr Hollis, 25-OH vitamin D is the most important indicator of nutritional adequacy, and 1,25-OH vitamin D2 as the active form, which is of concern. Both have stability issues; however, currently available methods for measuring these are reasonably accurate. The methodology to measure circulating levels of the 2 vitamin Ds are discussed, as are currently accepted levels.

In the United States today, it is estimated that almost two-thirds of adults have a level of circulating of 25-OH vitamin below the accepted normal level of 30 ng/mL. The consequences of low levels of vitamin D are under intensive investigation, because many different systems may be affected, including bone, muscle, and cancer. Although the effect on bone has been well established for many decades, the effect on other systems is still poorly defined. It has been advised that the current recommended supplementation of 400 IU per day is far too low and that 800 IU per day is preferable. This dose has raised concerns of hypercalciuria and hypercalcemia occurring, but Drs Binkley, Ramamurthy, and Krueger correctly suggest that vitamin D toxicity from supplementation is uncommon and supplementation is, therefore, essential.

Endocrinol Metab Clin N Am 39 (2010) xiii–xv
doi:10.1016/j.ecl.2010.02.015
0889-8529/10/$ – see front matter © 2010 Elsevier Inc. All rights reserved.

Infantile nutritional rickets was thought to be eradicated in developed countries due to vitamin D supplementation but for several reasons has re-emerged. In underdeveloped countries, breastfeeding is common and continues for many months post partum; this continued widespread practice in immigrants with darker skins in developed countries can result in the appearance of nutritional rickets in offspring, because the mother's vitamin levels determines the levels in infants. Drs Thandrayen and Pettifor discuss the importance of vitamin supplementation during pregnancy and during lactation to avoid this problem. To maintain normal circulating 25-OH vitamin D levels in high-risk individuals, they recommend 400 IU daily for breastfed infants and 2000 IU per day for pregnant women.

Osteomalacia is usually secondary to vitamin D deficiency. Classically, it was seen in poor countries due to malnutrition or in countries where dark skin pigmentation or lack of sunlight prevented adequate vitamin D synthesis in the skin. With supplementation, the disorder may be prevented or readily treated. As discussed in the article by Drs Bhan, Rao, and Rao, the disorder still exists for many reasons. One cause seen in developed countries is secondary to malabsorption syndromes. More recently, the increase in bariatric surgery may be associated with an increased incidence. Fortunately, diagnosis is still standard and treatment with vitamin D is effective.

There are two rare genetic disorders of vitamin D–related rickets; in one, named vitamin D–dependent rickets type 1, calcitriol can no longer be synthesized, and in the second, hereditary vitamin D–resistant rickets, the vitamin D receptor is defective. Both disorders present with early-onset rickets and hypocalcemia; however, the former has low 1,25-OH vitamin D levels whereas the latter has elevated levels, but the vitamin D receptor mutation prevents it from functioning normally. Drs Malloy and Feldman have been instrumental in characterizing these disorders in humans and animal models.

Dr Bischoff-Ferrari describes the importance of vitamin D supplementation particularly as related to falls and fracture incidence. Clinical trials have demonstrated the efficacy of vitamin D supplementation in preventing falls and fractures at hip and vertebral sites. Given this evidence, it is appropriate to consider 700 to 1000 IU daily as a minimally adequate dose.

Vitamin D metabolism and renal disease are intimately related. Chronic kidney disease (CKD) is commonly associated with low vitamin D levels, leading to secondary hyperparathyroidism and metabolic bone disease. As discussed in the article by Drs Qazi and Martin, CKD is a major risk factor for vitamin D deficiency, and the mechanisms are well studied. Vitamin D therapy at various stages of kidney disease is important to reverse the associated hyperparathyroidism and subsequent renal osteodystrophy, with observational studies suggesting improved survival.

Dr Hewison discusses an interesting topic relating vitamin D to the immune system. Vitamin D, or the active form 1,25-OH, not only is associated with sarcoidosis but also is involved in the normal regulation of innate and adaptive immunity. As described in this article, this effect is mediated by local 1,25-OH vitamin D, derived from the circulation and acting in a local paracrine or autocrine fashion. Therefore, low circulating 25-OH vitamin D, commonly seen as a manifestation of nutritional lack, can perhaps lead to alterations in immune function. The clinical implications are numerous, including infections, such as tuberculosis, and autoimmune disorders, such as type 1 diabetes mellitus.

Dr Holick presents a historical perspective regarding vitamin D, its metabolites, and importance, initially for bone metabolism and more recently for extraskeletal effects. Cancer prevention and even a reduction of metastatic disease, as in the case of prostatic cancer, have been correlated with vitamin D intake. Inhibition of keratinocyte proliferation makes vitamin D a candidate therapeutic approach for psoriasis. Involvement in the autoimmune process suggested a role in type 1 diabetes mellitus, multiple sclerosis, and autoimmune encephalitis. In addition, possible benefits may be seen for patients with hypertension and patients with type 2 diabetes mellitus. Although its role is still being defined, replacement with vitamin D to achieve normal circulating levels is advised.

Is vitamin D, specifically calcitriol, useful in cancer prevention and cancer therapy? As discussed by Krishnan, Trump, Johnson, and Feldman, 1,25-OH vitamin D has been shown in preclinical studies to inhibit cell proliferation, stimulate apoptosis, and inhibit tumor angiogenesis, invasion, and metastasis. This review discusses some of the molecular pathways. The trials currently conducted in human cancer patients have not been completed, however, and its potential has not been fully tested.

The relationship between vitamin D and diabetes is complicated, as described in the article by Drs Takiishi, Gysemans, Bouillon, and Mathieu. Patients with type 1 diabetes mellitus have lower circulating vitamin levels, and vitamin D treatment may reduce insulitis in NOD mice that develop type 1 diabetes; whether or not this will be effective in humans remains to be proved. Treatment of patients with type 2 diabetes mellitus (who also have low circulating 25-OH vitamin D levels) can improve insulin sensitivity and reduce inflammatory processes, most likely due to effects on immune and pancreatic beta cells that express the vitamin D receptor. Thus, the relationship of vitamin D and diabetes is under intense study in preclinical models and in humans.

Vitamin D and its metabolites (25-hydroxyvitamin D_3 [calcidiol] and $1\alpha,25$-dihydroxyvitamin D_3 [calcitriol]) have always been important for treating vitamin D deficiency and disorders related to abnormal calcium homeostasis. More recently, as discussed by Dr Jones, the idea of using metabolites that have minimal effects on calcium but are useful for treating unrelated disorders (see the articles by Hewison, Holick, Krishnan and colleagues, and Takiishi and colleagues, elsewhere in this issue for further exploration of this topic) has led to the discovery of calcipotriol, oxacalcitriol, 19-nor-1α, 25-$(OH)_2D_2$, and 1α-OH-D_2. These and future metabolites, such as those that block the vitamin D receptor and others that inhibit CYP24 that catabolizes the vitamin D receptor, may prove useful in these nonclassic situations.

Derek LeRoith, MD, PhD
Division of Endocrinology, Metabolism, and Bone Diseases
Mount Sinai School of Medicine
One Gustave L. Levy Place
Box 1055, Altran 4-36
New York, NY 10029, USA

E-mail address:
derek.leroith@mssm.edu

Preface

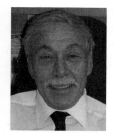

Sol Epstein, MD, FRCP
Guest Editor

It is with great pleasure that I am afforded the opportunity to act as Guest Editor of this issue of *Endocrinology and Metabolism Clinics of North America*, entitled "Vitamin D." This issue features internationally renowned experts who have graciously provided their expertise on a variety of topics related to the importance of vitamin D. Vitamin D initially was considered an essential nutrient that prevented rickets and osteomalacia. It was not until feedback loops were identified, between its production and parathyroid hormone, phosphate, and so forth, that it earned its place as a true endocrine hormone. Its importance, however, seemed to be forgotten until current social and economic conditions brought it back into the limelight with outbreaks of rickets and osteomalacia, even in developed countries. Its complex regulation, however, together with the identification and characterization of the vitamin D receptor and its role in influencing multiple genetic pathways and function, has heralded a new era highlighting its importance in health and disease. Low vitamin D has been implicated in association with autoimmune diseases, such as multiple sclerosis, diabetes mellitus, and cancer (especially breast and prostate); skin, neurologic, and cognitive disorders; and infectious diseases, such as tuberculosis. We now know that adequate levels of vitamin D are important in preventing falls and fracture. Adequate circulating levels have been revised (ie, above 30 ng/mL [75–80 nmol/L]), and the definition of this value has also been facilitated by the availability of more accurate methods to measure circulating levels of vitamin D and metabolites. The need for supplementation and the amount recommended have also changed considerably from what were previously considered sufficient. The ongoing development of selective active analogs of vitamin D targeted to specific organs and function leads to the exciting possibility of improving outcomes of diseases associated with vitamin D regulation. Finally, I

Endocrinol Metab Clin N Am 39 (2010) xvii–xviii
doi:10.1016/j.ecl.2010.02.014
0889-8529/10/$ – see front matter © 2010 Elsevier Inc. All rights reserved.

would like to thank all the authors for their time and effort in contributing to this issue, which will be of considerable benefit to readers in all disciplines.

Sol Epstein, MD, FRCP
231 Jeffery Lane
Newtown Square, PA 19073, USA

E-mail address:
bonedocsol@aol.com

Vitamin D: Metabolism

Sylvia Christakos, PhD[a,*], Dare V. Ajibade, BA[a],
Puneet Dhawan, PhD[a], Adam J. Fechner, MD[b], Leila J. Mady, BA[a]

KEYWORDS

- Vitamin D metabolites • Vitamin D hydroxylases
- Vitamin D binding protein • FGF23 • Kidney • Placenta

SYNTHESIS OF 1,25(OH)$_2$D$_3$ FROM VITAMIN D$_3$

Vitamin D$_3$ (cholecalciferol) is taken in the diet (from fortified dairy products and fish oils) or is synthesized in the skin from 7-dehydrocholesterol by ultraviolet irradiation. The vitamin D produced by 7-dehydrocholesterol depends on the intensity of UV irradiation, which varies with season and latitude.[1] Sunscreen and clothing have been reported to prevent the conversion of 7-dehydrocholesterol to vitamin D$_3$.[2,3] To be biologically active and affect mineral metabolism, and to have effects on numerous other diverse physiologic functions including inhibition of growth of cancer cells and protection against certain immune mediated disorders, vitamin D most be converted to its active form.[4,5] Vitamin D is transported in the blood by the vitamin D binding protein (DBP, a specific binding protein for vitamin D and its metabolites in serum) to the liver. In the liver vitamin D is hydroxylated at C-25 by one or more cytochrome P450 vitamin D 25-hydroxylases (including CYP2R1, CYP2D11, and CYP2D25), resulting in the formation of 25-hydroxyvitamin D$_3$ (25(OH)D$_3$). It has been suggested that CYP2R1 is the key enzyme required for 25-hydroxylation of vitamin D since a homozygous mutation of the CYP2R1 gene was found in a patient with low circulating levels of 25(OH)D$_3$ and classic symptoms of vitamin D deficiency.[6] 25(OH)D$_3$, the major circulating form of vitamin D, is transported by the DBP to the kidney. In the kidney, magalin, a member of the low-density lipoprotein receptor superfamily, plays an essential role in endocytic internalization of 25(OH)D$_3$.[7] In the proximal renal tubule 25(OH)D$_3$ is hydroxylated at the position of carbon 1 of the A ring, resulting in the hormonally active

Studies referenced from the laboratory of S.C. were supported in part by NIH grant DK-38961-21.

[a] Department of Biochemistry and Molecular Biology, New Jersey Medical School, University of Medicine and Dentistry of New Jersey, 185 South Orange Avenue E609, Newark, NJ 07103, USA
[b] Department of Obstetrics and Gynecology and Women's Health, New Jersey Medical School, University of Medicine and Dentistry of New Jersey, 185 South Orange Avenue E609, Newark, NJ 07103, USA
* Corresponding author.
E-mail address: christak@umdnj.edu

Endocrinol Metab Clin N Am 39 (2010) 243–253
doi:10.1016/j.ecl.2010.02.002
endo.theclinics.com
0889-8529/10/$ – see front matter © 2010 Elsevier Inc. All rights reserved.

from of vitamin D, 1,25-dihydroxyvitamin D_3 (1,25(OH)$_2D_3$), which is responsible for most, if not all of the biologic actions of vitamin D (**Fig. 1**). The cytochrome P450 mono-oxygenase 25(OH)D 1α hydroxylase (CYP27B1; 1α(OH)ase), which metabolizes 25(OH)D_3 to 1,25(OH)$_2D_3$, is present predominantly in kidney. This enzyme is also found in extrarenal sites including placenta, monocytes, and macrophages.[8–11] As with all mitochondrial P450 containing enzymes, during the 1α(OH)ase reaction electrons are transferred from reduced nicotinamide adenine dinucleotide phosphate (NADPH) to NADPH-ferrodoxin reductase through ferrodoxin. Inactivating mutations in the 1α(OH)ase gene result in vitamin D dependency rickets (VDDR) type 1 despite normal intake of vitamin D, indicating the importance of the 1α(OH)ase enzyme.[12] Type 1 VDDR is characterized by growth failure, hypocalcemia, elevated parathyroid hormone (PTH), muscle weakness, and radiologic findings typical of rickets.[12] The 1α(OH)ase null mutant mouse has provided a mouse model of VDDR type 1.[13,14] It is of interest that in these mice, in addition to rickets, reproductive and immune defects have been noted.[13] Further studies are needed to test the role of 1α(OH)ase in extrarenal sites, which has been a matter of debate.

ROLE OF THE VITAMIN D BINDING PROTEIN IN VITAMIN D METABOLISM AND ACTION

Studies using mice deficient in DBP have resulted in new insight into the role of DBP in vitamin D metabolism and action. Although DBP null (−/−) mice have markedly lower total serum levels of 25(OH)D and 1,25(OH)$_2D_3$ than wild-type (WT) mice, the levels of serum calcium and PTH are normal in the DBP −/− mice.[15] In patients with reduced levels of circulating DBP, serum calcium levels have also been reported to be normal.[16] More recent studies using DBP null mice have shown that DBP is important for total circulating 1,25(OH)$_2D_3$ but DBP does not influence the pool of 1,25(OH)$_2D_3$ that enters cells and affects the synthesis of vitamin D target proteins.[17] Thus direct

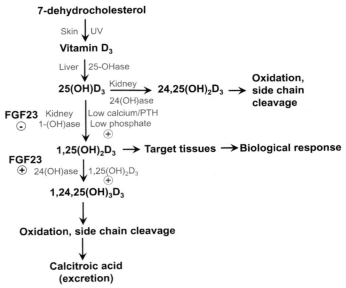

Fig. 1. The metabolic pathway for vitamin D.

measurement of $1,25(OH)_2D_3$ may not, in all cases, reflect the biologically active $1,25(OH)_2D_3$.[16] This may be, in part, why $25(OH)D_3$, which is also more stable than $1,25(OH)_2D_3$, is used to assess clinical vitamin D status. It has been suggested that the maintenance of normal serum calcium levels in the DBP null mice may be caused by the ability of the vitamin D receptor to concentrate $1,25(OH)_2D_3$ in tissues due to its high affinity for $1,25(OH)_2D_3$, resulting in transcriptional regulation of genes involved in maintenance of calcium homeostasis.[17]

24-HYDROXYLASE (24(OH)ASE)

In addition to $1,25(OH)_2D_3$, the kidney can also produce 24,25-dihydroxyvitamin D3 $(24,25(OH)_2D_3)$, a relatively inactive metabolite compared with $1,25(OH)_2D_3$. 25-Hydroxyvitamin D_3 24-hydroxylase (CYP24), also a mitochondrial P450 enzyme, can hydroxylate both $25(OH)D_3$ and $1,25(OH)_2D_3$.[5] It has been suggested that the preferred substrate for 24(OH)ase is $1,25(OH)_2D_3$.[18] Thus, 24(OH)ase limits the amount of $1,25(OH)_2D_3$ in target tissues by accelerating the catabolism of $1,25(OH)_2D_3$ to $1,24,25(OH)_3D_3$, resulting in calcitroic acid, or by producing $24,25(OH)_2D_3$, thus decreasing the pool of $25(OH)D_3$ available for 1-hydroxylation (see **Fig. 1**). Studies using 24(OH)ase null mutant mice provided the first direct evidence for a role for 24(OH)ase in the catabolism of $1,25(OH)_2D_3$. 24(OH)ase null mutant mice are unable to clear $1,25(OH)_2D_3$ from the bloodstream after both chronic and acute treatment with $1,25(OH)_2D_3$.[19] Lack of 24(OH)ase resulted in impaired mineralization in intramembranous bones. This defect was normalized by crossing 24(OH)ase deficient mice to vitamin D receptor (VDR) ablated mice, indicating that elevated $1,25(OH)_2D_3$ levels, and not the absence of $24,25(OH)_2D_3$, was responsible for the abnormalities in bone. Thus, the main function of 24(OH)ase is vitamin D inactivation.

REGULATION OF RENAL VITAMIN D HYDROXYLASES
By Calcium, Phosphate, PTH, and 1,25(OH)₂D₃

The widespread effects of $1,25(OH)_2D_3$ necessitate a tight regulation of its bioavailability and a process of activation and deactivation that occurs through a series of negative and positive feedbacks, resulting in changes in the expression of the hydroxylase enzymes depending on the physiologic state.[20,21] Regarding regulation of vitamin D metabolism, low dietary calcium and phosphate result in enhanced activity of $1\alpha(OH)ase$ (see **Fig. 1**).[5] Elevated PTH resulting from hypocalcemia is a primary signal mediating the induction of $1,25(OH)_2D_3$ synthesis in the kidney.[22–24] PTH stimulates the transcription of $1\alpha(OH)ase$.[25–27] Recent studies have shown that the nuclear receptor 4A2 (NR4A2) is a key factor involved in the induction of $1\alpha(OH)ase$ transcription by PTH.[26] $1,25(OH)_2D_3$ in turn suppresses PTH production at the level of transcription.[28] The $1\alpha(OH)ase$ gene is also negatively regulated by $1,25(OH)_2D_3$.[29,30] When compared with the regulation of $1\alpha(OH)ase$, 24(OH)ase is reciprocally regulated (stimulated by $1,25(OH)_2D_3$ and inhibited by low calcium and PTH).[5] The marked induction of 24(OH)ase by $1,25(OH)_2D_3$ results in an autoregulatory suppression of $1,25(OH)_2D_3$ when gene transcriptional effects of $1,25(OH)_2D_3$ need to be attenuated to protect against hypercalcemia. Various factors that cooperate with the VDR in the transcriptional regulation of 24(OH)ase have been identified, including the transcription factor C/EBPβ, SWI/SNF (complexes that remodel chromatin using the energy of adenosine triphosphate hydrolysis), and histone methyltransferases (CARM1 and G9).[31–33] Recent studies have suggested a synergy between acetylated and methylated histones to disrupt histone/DNA binding, resulting in enhanced VDR activation of 24(OH)ase transcription.[33]

By FGF23

In addition to calcium, phosphate, PTH, and $1,25(OH)_2D_3$, fibroblast growth factor 23 (FGF23), a phosphaturic factor that promotes renal phosphate excretion by decreasing its reabsorption in the proximal tubule, is also a physiologic regulator of vitamin D metabolism.[34] Unlike classic FGFs that function via paracrine mechanisms, FGF23 belongs to the FGF19 subfamily that acts in an endocrine fashion.[35] From its identification as a causative factor in autosomal dominant hypophosphatemic rickets, X-linked hypophosphatemic rickets, and tumor-induced osteomalacia, FGF23 has been shown to be a significant regulator of phosphate homeostasis and vitamin D biosynthesis.[36–39] $1,25(OH)_2D_3$ stimulates the production of FGF23 in bone.[40] Administration of $1,25(OH)_2D_3$ to mice results in increased serum levels of FGF23 prior to elevations in serum phosphate, suggesting that $1,25(OH)_2D_3$ induces FGF23 expression independent of changes in serum phosphate.[40] Increased FGF23 in turn suppresses the expression of $1\alpha(OH)$ase and induces $24(OH)$ase in kidney (see **Fig. 1**; **Fig. 2**).[41] By inhibiting synthesis and promoting catabolism of $1,25(OH)_2D_3$, FGF23 functions to reduce levels of $1,25(OH)_2D_3$, which in turn decreases FGF23 expression in bone, forming a negative feedback circuit between the FGF23 and the vitamin D endocrine system.[41] Overactivity of FGF23 has been suggested to be a common pathogenic mechanism of phosphate wasting disorders that may explain their shared clinical characteristics, including hypophosphatemia, low serum $1,25(OH)_2D_3$, and rickets/osteomalacia.[41]

It has been reported that FGF23 requires klotho (a multifunctional protein involved in phosphate and calcium homeostasis) as a cofactor for FGF signaling.[42] Expressed predominantly in the kidney and also in parathyroid gland and choroid plexus,[43] the klotho gene was first identified when mice homozygous for the gene mutation developed a syndrome resembling human premature aging, including a short life span, infertility, arteriosclerosis, skin atrophy, osteoporosis, and emphysema.[44] $1,25(OH)_2D_3$ up-regulates klotho gene expression in kidney and the loss of klotho results in induction of $1\alpha(OH)$ase, suggesting that klotho participates in $1,25(OH)_2D_3$ autoregulatory suppression.[45] Klotho can bind to several FGF receptor isoforms and can convert the canonical FGF receptor to a receptor specific for FGF23.[46] The cooperation of klotho and FGF23 in a common signal transduction pathway (see **Fig. 2**) may explain why klotho-deficient mice and FGF23-deficient mice exhibit identical phenotypes, including premature aging and metabolic disturbances such as hyperphosphatemia and increased synthesis of $1,25(OH)_2D_3$.[41,45,47]

By Other Hormones (Sex Hormones, Calcitonin, Prolactin)

In avian species, estrogens alone or when combined with androgens or progesterone have been reported to stimulate $1,25(OH)_2D_3$ production.[48,49] In addition, estrogens have been reported to suppress $24,25(OH)_2D_3$ synthesis.[48] However, whether this relationship exists in mammalian species has been a matter of debate.[50]

Although calcitonin is known to have a role in shrinking osteoclasts under high calcium conditions, under conditions whereby serum calcium levels are normal calcitonin has been reported to stimulate $1,25(OH)_2D_3$ production.[51–53] The stimulation of $1,25(OH)_2D_3$ production by calcitonin may have physiologic significance during lactation when calcitonin levels as well as $1,25(OH)_2D_3$ levels are elevated and when the need for calcium is increased.[54,55] Recent studies have shown a direct effect of calcitonin on renal $1\alpha(OH)$ase transcription.[56] The transcription factor C/EBPβ and the SWI/SNF chromatin remodeling complex were found to mediate the calcitonin regulation of $1\alpha(OH)$ase transcription, indicating a mechanism responsible, at least in part, for the

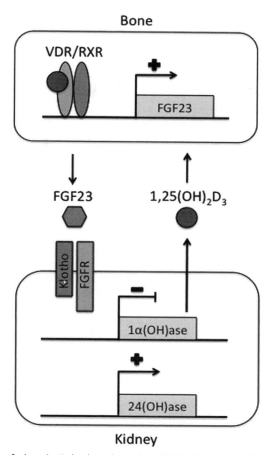

Fig. 2. Regulation of vitamin D hydroxylases by FGF23-Klotho. 1,25(OH)$_2$D$_3$ binds to VDR. The ligand-bound VDR forms a heterodimer with nuclear retinoid X receptor (RXR) resulting in increased expression of FGF23 in osteocytes. Secreted FGF23 activates FGF receptor (FGFR) bound by Klotho in renal tubular cells. FGF signaling suppresses expression of 1α(OH)ase and induces 24(OH)ase, thereby inhibiting synthesis and promoting catabolism of 1,25(OH)$_2$D$_3$. Thus, the FGF23-Klotho results in decreased levels of 1,25(OH)$_2$D$_3$. (*Adapted from* Kuro-o M. Endocrine FGFs and Klothos: emerging concepts. Trends Endocrinol Metab 2008;19:239–45; with permission.)

increase in plasma 1,25(OH)$_2$D$_3$ during these times of increased calcium requirement.[56]

It has been suggested that prolactin, which is also elevated during lactation, can stimulate 1,25(OH)$_2$D$_3$ production. Bromocriptine, which inhibits pituitary prolactin secretion, has been reported to significantly reduce plasma 1,25(OH)$_2$D$_3$ levels in lactating animals, and recent studies have shown that prolactin also has a direct effect on the transcription of the 1α(OH)ase gene.[57,58] Clinical studies have also suggested that factors besides PTH stimulate 1α(OH)ase during lactation. For example, lactating hypoparathyroid women treated with the usual dose of calcitriol have been reported to develop hypercalcemia. In the absence of treatment, serum 1,25(OH)$_2$D$_3$ levels in the hypoparathyroid women remain within the normal range during lactation.[59,60] Thus, it is likely that prolactin and calcitonin have a physiologic function to increase $1,25(OH)_2D_3$ levels during lactation to protect the maternal skeleton.

EXTRARENAL 1-HYDROXYLASE (1α(OH)ASE)
Placenta

In pregnancy, the placenta regulates communication and transport between mother and fetus, with the placental trophoblasts and maternal decidua serving as the functional interface for exchange. 1α(OH)ase is expressed in both fetal trophoblast and maternal decidual cells beginning early in gestation.[61] 1α(OH)ase is most abundant in decidua.[61] Synthesis of 1α(OH)ase is eightfold higher in first trimester decidual cells than in third trimester cells.[62] This trend indicates an important role for $1,25(OH)_2D_3$ in early pregnancy. It has been suggested that the immunosuppressive effects of $1,25(OH)_2D_3$ are crucial for allowing proper trophoblast invasion of the uterus without triggering a maternal immune response.[61] Decidual natural killer cells isolated from the first trimester decidua show decreased synthesis of cytokines such as tumor necrosis factor and interleukin-6 in response to $1,25(OH)_2D_3$.[62] A role of $1,25(OH)_2D_3$ as an activator of innate immunity in the placenta has also been suggested. It has been shown that in trophoblasts $1,25(OH)_2D_3$ increases the expression of cathelicidin, an antimicrobial peptide.[63] In addition to up-regulation of 1α(OH)ase expression, recent findings indicate that the increased bioavailability of $1,25(OH)_2D_3$ at the fetomaternal interface may also be partially attributed to a decrease in activity of the catabolic 24(OH)ase enzyme in placenta.[64] Taken together, these findings suggest the importance of the local production of $1,25(OH)_2D_3$ in the placenta to regulate both acquired and innate immune responses, and a possible role for $1,25(OH)_2D_3$ in the immunoregulation of implantation.

Monocytes/Macrophages

Monocytes and macrophages express 1α(OH)ase and produce $1,25(OH)_2D_3$. However, monocyte/macrophage 1α(OH)ase is regulated differently to renal 1α(OH)ase.[10,11] Clinical evidence for a different regulation of macrophage 1α(OH)ase is observed in patients with sarcoidosis. In sarcoidosis patients there is increased production of $1,25(OH)_2D_3$ despite hypercalcemia.[65] The disordered calcium homeostasis in sarcoidosis is caused by dysregulated production of $1,25(OH)_2D_3$ by activated macrophages.[65] Unlike renal 1α(OH)ase, 1α(OH)ase produced by macrophages is not suppressed by elevated calcium or $1,25(OH)_2D_3$, and is up-regulated by immune stimuli such as interferon-γ and lipopolysaccharide.[10,11] Multiple pathways have been reported to be involved in this up-regulation, including JAK/STAT, MAPK, and NFκB.[10] Activation of 1α(OH)ase transcription by immune stimuli also requires the binding of C/EBPβ to its recognition sites in the 1α(OH)ase promoter region.[10,11] These findings suggest mechanisms responsible for the hypercalcemia of granulomatous disorders in which activated macrophages constitutively express 1α(OH)ase in the presence of elevated calcium and $1,25(OH)_2D_3$.

VITAMIN D P450S IN AGING AND CHRONIC KIDNEY DISEASE

The capacity of the kidney to convert $25(OH)D_3$ to $1,25(OH)_2D_3$ has been reported to decline with age. An increase in 24(OH)ase gene expression and an increase in clearance of $1,25(OH)_2D_3$ with aging have been reported.[66–68] These findings suggest that the combined effect of a decline in the ability of the kidney to synthesize $1,25(OH)_2D_3$ and an increase in renal metabolism of $1,25(OH)_2D_3$ may contribute to age-related bone loss.

Chronic kidney disease (CKD) has been shown to result in decreased vitamin D metabolism through multiple mechanisms.[69] The loss of functional renal mass leads to decreased production of $1\alpha(OH)$ase, specifically in the later stages of CKD.[69] However, studies have also shown a suppression of enzyme activity due to associated aspects of the disease, including metabolic acidosis,[70] hyperphosphatemia,[71] and uremic toxins that accumulate in CKD.[72] Elevated levels of FGF23 have also been shown in early CKD, resulting in decreased activity of $1\alpha(OH)$ase.[73]

In summary, understanding vitamin D metabolism is of fundamental importance in understanding mechanisms involved in the maintenance of calcium homeostasis. The vitamin D hydroxylases have an important role in providing a tightly regulated supply of $1,25(OH)_2D_3$. Understanding specific factors involved in regulating the hydroxylases may lead to the design of drugs that can selectively modulate the hydroxylases. The ability to alter levels of these enzymes would have therapeutic potential for the treatment of various diseases, including bone loss disorders and certain immune diseases.

REFERENCES

1. Webb AR, Kline L, Holick MF. Influence of season and latitude on the cutaneous synthesis of vitamin D3: exposure to winter sunlight in Boston and Edmonton will not promote vitamin D3 synthesis in human skin. J Clin Endocrinol Metab 1988; 67:373–8.
2. Matsuoka LY, Ide L, Wortsman J, et al. Sunscreens suppress cutaneous vitamin D3 synthesis. J Clin Endocrinol Metab 1987;64:1165–8.
3. Matsuoka LY, Wortsman J, Dannenberg MJ, et al. Clothing prevents ultraviolet-B radiation-dependent photosynthesis of vitamin D3. J Clin Endocrinol Metab 1992; 75:1099–103.
4. Prosser DE, Jones G. Enzymes involved in the activation and inactivation of vitamin D. Trends Biochem Sci 2004;29:664–73.
5. Omdahl JL, Morris HA, May BK. Hydroxylase enzymes of the vitamin D pathway: expression, function, and regulation. Annu Rev Nutr 2002;22:139–66.
6. Cheng JB, Levine MA, Bell NH, et al. Genetic evidence that the human CYP2R1 enzyme is a key vitamin D 25-hydroxylase. Proc Natl Acad Sci U S A 2004;101: 7711–5.
7. Nykjaer A, Dragun D, Walther D, et al. An endocytic pathway essential for renal uptake and activation of the steroid 25-(OH) vitamin D3. Cell 1999;96:507–15.
8. Weisman Y, Harell A, Edelstein S, et al. 1 alpha, 25-dihydroxyvitamin D3 and 24,25-dihydroxyvitamin D3 in vitro synthesis by human decidua and placenta. Nature 1979;281:317–9.
9. Gray TK, Lester GE, Lorenc RS. Evidence for extra-renal 1 alpha-hydroxylation of 25-hydroxyvitamin D3 in pregnancy. Science 1979;204:1311–3.
10. Stoffels K, Overbergh L, Bouillon R, et al. Immune regulation of 1alpha-hydroxylase in murine peritoneal macrophages: unravelling the IFNgamma pathway. J Steroid Biochem Mol Biol 2007;103:567–71.
11. Esteban L, Vidal M, Dusso A. 1alpha-Hydroxylase transactivation by gamma-interferon in murine macrophages requires enhanced C/EBPbeta expression and activation. J Steroid Biochem Mol Biol 2004;89-90:131–7.
12. Kitanaka S, Takeyama K, Murayama A, et al. Inactivating mutations in the 25-hydroxyvitamin D3 1alpha-hydroxylase gene in patients with pseudovitamin D-deficiency rickets. N Engl J Med 1998;338:653–61.

13. Panda DK, Miao D, Tremblay ML, et al. Targeted ablation of the 25-hydroxyvitamin D 1alpha -hydroxylase enzyme: evidence for skeletal, reproductive, and immune dysfunction. Proc Natl Acad Sci U S A 2001;98:7498–503.

14. Dardenne O, Prud'homme J, Arabian A, et al. Targeted inactivation of the 25-hydroxyvitamin D(3)-1(alpha)-hydroxylase gene (CYP27B1) creates an animal model of pseudovitamin D-deficiency rickets. Endocrinology 2001;142:3135–41.

15. Safadi FF, Thornton P, Magiera H, et al. Osteopathy and resistance to vitamin D toxicity in mice null for vitamin D binding protein. J Clin Invest 1999;103:239–51.

16. Bikle DD, Siiteri PK, Ryzen E, et al. Serum protein binding of 1,25-dihydroxyvitamin D: a reevaluation by direct measurement of free metabolite levels. J Clin Endocrinol Metab 1985;61:969–75.

17. Zella LA, Shevde NK, Hollis BW, et al. Vitamin D-binding protein influences total circulating levels of 1,25-dihydroxyvitamin D3 but does not directly modulate the bioactive levels of the hormone in vivo. Endocrinology 2008;149:3656–67.

18. Shinki T, Jin CH, Nishimura A, et al. Parathyroid hormone inhibits 25-hydroxyvitamin D3-24-hydroxylase mRNA expression stimulated by 1 alpha,25-dihydroxyvitamin D3 in rat kidney but not in intestine. J Biol Chem 1992;267:13757–62.

19. St-Arnaud R, Arabian A, Travers R, et al. Deficient mineralization of intramembranous bone in vitamin D-24-hydroxylase-ablated mice is due to elevated 1,25-dihydroxyvitamin D and not to the absence of 24,25-dihydroxyvitamin D. Endocrinology 2000;141:2658–66.

20. Henry HL, Norman AW. Vitamin D: metabolism and biological actions. Annu Rev Nutr 1984;4:493–520.

21. DeLuca HF. Evolution of our understanding of vitamin D. Nutr Rev 2008;66:S73–87.

22. Boyle IT, Gray RW, DeLuca HF. Regulation by calcium of in vivo synthesis of 1,25-dihydroxycholecalciferol and 24,25-dihydroxycholecalciferol. Proc Natl Acad Sci U S A 1971;68:2131–4.

23. Henry HL. Parathyroid hormone modulation of 25-hydroxyvitamin D3 metabolism by cultured chick kidney cells is mimicked and enhanced by forskolin. Endocrinology 1985;116:503–10.

24. Murayama A, Takeyama K, Kitanaka S, et al. Positive and negative regulations of the renal 25-hydroxyvitamin D3 1alpha-hydroxylase gene by parathyroid hormone, calcitonin, and 1alpha,25(OH)2D3 in intact animals. Endocrinology 1999;140:2224–31.

25. Brenza HL, Kimmel-Jehan C, Jehan F, et al. Parathyroid hormone activation of the 25-hydroxyvitamin D3-1alpha-hydroxylase gene promoter. Proc Natl Acad Sci U S A 1998;95:1387–91.

26. Zierold C, Nehring JA, DeLuca HF. Nuclear receptor 4A2 and C/EBPbeta regulate the parathyroid hormone-mediated transcriptional regulation of the 25-hydroxyvitamin D3-1alpha-hydroxylase. Arch Biochem Biophys 2007;460:233–9.

27. Murayama A, Takeyama K, Kitanaka S, et al. The promoter of the human 25-hydroxyvitamin D3 1 alpha-hydroxylase gene confers positive and negative responsiveness to PTH, calcitonin, and 1 alpha,25(OH)2D3. Biochem Biophys Res Commun 1998;249:11–6.

28. Kim MS, Fujiki R, Murayama A, et al. 1Alpha,25(OH)2D3-induced transrepression by vitamin D receptor through E-box-type elements in the human parathyroid hormone gene promoter. Mol Endocrinol 2007;21:334–42.

29. Brenza HL, DeLuca HF. Regulation of 25-hydroxyvitamin D3 1alpha-hydroxylase gene expression by parathyroid hormone and 1,25-dihydroxyvitamin D3. Arch Biochem Biophys 2000;381:143–52.

30. Murayama A, Kim MS, Yanagisawa J, et al. 2004 Transrepression by a liganded nuclear receptor via a bHLH activator through co-regulator switching. EMBO J 2000;23:1598–608.

31. Dhawan P, Peng X, Sutton AL, et al. Functional cooperation between CCAAT/enhancer-binding proteins and the vitamin D receptor in regulation of 25-hydroxyvitamin D3 24-hydroxylase. Mol Cell Biol 2005;25:472–87.

32. Christakos S, Dhawan P, Shen Q, et al. New insights into the mechanisms involved in the pleiotropic actions of 1,25dihydroxyvitamin D3. Ann N Y Acad Sci 2006;1068:194–203.

33. Zhong Y, Christakos S. 2006 Novel mechanism of vitamin D receptor (VDR) activation: histone H3 lysine 9 methyltransferase is a transcriptional coactivator for VDR. J Bone Miner Res 2007;22(Suppl 1):S8.

34. Bai X, Miao D, Li J, et al. Transgenic mice overexpressing human fibroblast growth factor 23 (R176Q) delineate a putative role for parathyroid hormone in renal phosphate wasting disorders. Endocrinology 2004;145:5269–79.

35. Goetz R, Beenken A, Ibrahimi OA, et al. Molecular insights into the klotho-dependent, endocrine mode of action of fibroblast growth factor 19 subfamily members. Mol Cell Biol 2007;27:3417–28.

36. ADHR Consortium. Autosomal dominant hypophosphataemic rickets is associated with mutations in FGF23. Nat Genet 2000;26:345–8.

37. Shimada T, Mizutani S, Muto T, et al. Cloning and characterization of FGF23 as a causative factor of tumor-induced osteomalacia. Proc Natl Acad Sci U S A 2001;98:6500–5.

38. White KE, Carn G, Lorenz-Depiereux B, et al. Autosomal-dominant hypophosphatemic rickets (ADHR) mutations stabilize FGF-23. Kidney Int 2001;60:2079–86.

39. Weber TJ, Liu S, Indridason OS, et al. Serum FGF23 levels in normal and disordered phosphorus homeostasis. J Bone Miner Res 2003;18:1227–34.

40. Liu S, Tang W, Zhou J, et al. Fibroblast growth factor 23 is a counter-regulatory phosphaturic hormone for vitamin D. J Am Soc Nephrol 2006;17:1305–15.

41. Shimada T, Kakitani M, Yamazaki Y, et al. Targeted ablation of Fgf23 demonstrates an essential physiological role of FGF23 in phosphate and vitamin D metabolism. J Clin Invest 2004;113:561–8.

42. Kurosu H, Ogawa Y, Miyoshi M, et al. Regulation of fibroblast growth factor-23 signaling by klotho. J Biol Chem 2006;281:6120–3.

43. Imura A, Tsuji Y, Murata M, et al. Alpha-Klotho as a regulator of calcium homeostasis. Science 2007;316:1615–8.

44. Kuro-o M, Matsumura Y, Aizawa H, et al. Mutation of the mouse klotho gene leads to a syndrome resembling ageing. Nature 1997;390:45–51.

45. Tsujikawa H, Kurotaki Y, Fujimori T, et al. Klotho, a gene related to a syndrome resembling human premature aging, functions in a negative regulatory circuit of vitamin D endocrine system. Mol Endocrinol 2003;17:2393–403.

46. Urakawa I, Yamazaki Y, Shimada T, et al. Klotho converts canonical FGF receptor into a specific receptor for FGF23. Nature 2006;444:770–4.

47. Yoshida T, Fujimori T, Nabeshima Y. Mediation of unusually high concentrations of 1,25-dihydroxyvitamin D in homozygous klotho mutant mice by increased expression of renal 1alpha-hydroxylase gene. Endocrinology 2002;143:683.

48. Pike JW, Spanos E, Colston KW, et al. Influence of estrogen on renal vitamin D hydroxylases and serum 1alpha,25-(OH)2D3 in chicks. Am J Physiol 1978;235:E338–43.

49. Tanaka Y, Castillo L, Wineland MJ, et al. Synergistic effect of progesterone, testosterone, and estradiol in the stimulation of chick renal 25-hydroxyvitamin D3-1alpha-hydroxylase. Endocrinology 1978;103:2035–9.

50. Baksi SN, Kenny AD. Does estradiol stimulate in vivo production of 1,25-dihydroxyvitamin D3 in the rat? Life Sci 1978;22:787–92.

51. Shinki T, Ueno Y, DeLuca HF, et al. Calcitonin is a major regulator for the expression of renal 25-hydroxyvitamin D3-1alpha-hydroxylase gene in normocalcemic rats. Proc Natl Acad Sci U S A 1999;96:8253–8.

52. Kawashima H, Torikai S, Kurokawa K. Calcitonin selectively stimulates 25-hydroxyvitamin D3-1 alpha-hydroxylase in proximal straight tubule of rat kidney. Nature 1981;291:327–9.

53. Galante L, Colston KW, MacAuley SJ, et al. Effect of calcitonin on vitamin D metabolism. Nature 1972;238:271–3.

54. Stevenson JC, Hillyard CJ, MacIntyre I, et al. A physiological role for calcitonin: protection of the maternal skeleton. Lancet 1979;2:769–70.

55. Kumar R, Cohen WR, Silva P, et al. Elevated 1,25-dihydroxyvitamin D plasma levels in normal human pregnancy and lactation. J Clin Invest 1979;63:342–4.

56. Zhong Y, Armbrecht HJ, Christakos S. Calcitonin, a regulator of the 25-hydroxyvitamin D3 1alpha-hydroxylase gene. J Biol Chem 2009;284:11059–69.

57. Robinson CJ, Spanos E, James MF, et al. Role of prolactin in vitamin D metabolism and calcium absorption during lactation in the rat. J Endocrinol 1982;94:443–53.

58. Ajibade DV, Dhawan P, Christakos S. Prolactin: a regulator of the 25-hydroxyvitaminD3 1alpha hydroxylase gene. J Bone Miner Res 2009;24(Suppl 1). Available at: http://www.asbmr.org/Meetings/AnnualMeeting/AbstractDetail.aspx?aid=51d4e88b-f79d-47e2-a15b-134f0c57b52.e. Accessed September 17, 2009.

59. Cundy T, Haining SA, Guilland-Cumming DF, et al. Remission of hypoparathyroidism during lactation: evidence for a physiological role for prolactin in the regulation of vitamin D metabolism. Clin Endocrinol (Oxf) 1987;26:667–74.

60. Caplan RH, Beguin EA. Hypercalcemia in a calcitriol-treated hypoparathyroid woman during lactation. Obstet Gynecol 1990;76:485–9.

61. Zehnder D, Evans KN, Kilby MD, et al. The ontogeny of 25-hydroxyvitamin D(3) 1alpha-hydroxylase expression in human placenta and decidua. Am J Pathol 2002;161:105–14.

62. Evans KN, Nguyen L, Chan J, et al. Effects of 25-hydroxyvitamin D3 and 1,25-dihydroxyvitamin D3 on cytokine production by human decidual cells. Biol Reprod 2006;75:816–22.

63. Liu N, Kaplan AT, Low J, et al. Vitamin D induces innate antibacterial responses in human trophoblasts via an intracrine pathway. Biol Reprod 2009;80:398–406.

64. Novakovic B, Sibson M, Ng HK, et al. Placenta-specific methylation of the vitamin D 24-hydroxylase gene: implications for feedback autoregulation of active vitamin D levels at the fetomaternal interface. J Biol Chem 2009;284:14838–48.

65. Sharma OP. Hypercalcemia in granulomatous disorders: a clinical review. Curr Opin Pulm Med 2000;6:442–7.

66. Armbrecht HJ, Zenser TV, Davis BB. Effect of age on the conversion of 25-hydroxyvitamin D3 to 1,25-dihydroxyvitamin D3 by kidney of rat. J Clin Invest 1980;66:1118–23.

67. Matkovits T, Christakos S. Variable in vivo regulation of rat vitamin D-dependent genes (osteopontin, Ca, Mg-adenosine triphosphatase, and 25-hydroxyvitamin

D3 24-hydroxylase): implications for differing mechanisms of regulation and involvement of multiple factors. Endocrinology 1995;136:3971–82.

68. Tsai KS, Heath H 3rd, Kumar R, et al. Impaired vitamin D metabolism with aging in women. Possible role in pathogenesis of senile osteoporosis. J Clin Invest 1984; 73:1668–72.

69. Cheng S, Coyne D. Vitamin D and outcomes in chronic kidney disease. Curr Opin Nephrol Hypertens 2007;16:77–82.

70. Lee SW, Russell J, Avioli LV. 25-hydroxycholecalciferol to 1,25-dihydroxycholecal-ciferol: conversion impaired by systemic metabolic acidosis. Science 1977;195: 994–6.

71. Portale AA, Booth BE, Halloran BP, et al. Effect of dietary phosphorus on circu-lating concentrations of 1,25-dihydroxyvitamin D and immunoreactive parathyroid hormone in children with moderate renal insufficiency. J Clin Invest 1984;73: 1580–9.

72. Hsu CH, Vanholder R, Patel S, et al. Subfractions in uremic plasma ultrafiltrate inhibit calcitriol metabolism. Kidney Int 1991;40:868–73.

73. Gutierrez O, Isakova T, Rhee E, et al. Fibroblast growth factor-23 mitigates hyper-phosphatemia but accentuates calcitriol deficiency in chronic kidney disease. J Am Soc Nephrol 2005;16:2205–15.

The Vitamin D Receptor: New Paradigms for the Regulation of Gene Expression by 1,25-Dihydroxyvitamin D$_3$

J. Wesley Pike, PhD*, Mark B. Meyer, PhD

KEYWORDS

- Transcription • ChIP-chip analysis • Distal enhancers
- RNA polymerase II • Histone H4 acetylation • VDR gene

Research during the past 2 decades has established that the diverse biologic actions of 1,25-dihydroyxyvitamin D$_3$ (1,25(OH)$_2$D$_3$) are initiated through precise changes in gene expression that are mediated by an intracellular vitamin D receptor (VDR).[1] Activation of the VDR through direct interaction with 1,25(OH)$_2$D$_3$ prompts the receptor's rapid binding to regulatory regions of target genes, where it acts to nucleate the formation of large protein complexes whose functional activities are essential for directed changes in transcription.[2] In most target cells, these actions trigger the expression of networks of target genes whose functional activities combine to orchestrate specific biologic responses. These responses are tissue-specific and range from highly complex actions essential for homeostatic control of mineral metabolism to focal actions that control the growth, differentiation, and functional activity of numerous cell types including those of the immune system, skin, the pancreas and bone, as well as many other targets that are described in this issue devoted to vitamin D.[3] In these tissues, gene targets are numerous. New studies combined with new techniques are now revealing a surprising increase in mechanistic complexity wherein multiple regulatory regions, frequently located many kilobases upstream, within, or downstream of a target gene's transcription unit, seem to participate in transcriptional modulation.[4–7]

This work was supported by National Institutes of Health Grants DK-072281, DK-073995, DK-074993 and AR-045173.

Department of Biochemistry, University of Wisconsin-Madison, 433 Babcock Drive, Madison, WI 53706, USA

* Corresponding author.

E-mail address: pike@biochem.wisc.edu

Endocrinol Metab Clin N Am 39 (2010) 255–269

doi:10.1016/j.ecl.2010.02.007

0889-8529/10/$ – see front matter © 2010 Elsevier Inc. All rights reserved.

VDR STRUCTURE AND FUNCTION

The VDR is Structurally Organized to Mediate Changes in Transcription in Response to 1,25(OH)$_2$D$_3$

Despite nearly 2 decades of extensive biochemical characterization of the VDR after its discovery in 1974,[8,9] it was the cloning of this receptor's gene and the subsequent analysis of recombinant protein that led to key insights into its structure and its function.[10,11] As depicted in **Fig. 1A**, the VDR protein is comprised of 3 distinct regions, an N-terminal dual zinc finger DNA-binding domain, a C-terminal ligand-binding activity domain, and an extensive and unstructured region that links the 2 functional domains of this protein together. The C-terminal region of the molecule, whose three-dimensional structure has been solved by X-ray crystallography,[12,13] is the most complex and is comprised of 12 α-helices as illustrated in **Fig. 1B**. Amino acid contacts within a subset of these α-helices form a dynamic ligand-binding pocket, as shown in **Fig. 1C**. Selective occupancy by 1,25(OH)$_2$D$_3$ leads to the formation of 2 independent protein interaction surfaces on the VDR protein: 1 that facilitates interaction with a heterodimer partner required for specific DNA binding and 1 that is essential for the recruitment of large coregulatory complexes required for gene modulation.[14] Additional studies suggest that the VDR can also be posttranslationally modified through phosphorylation, an alteration in the protein that may be capable of modulating and fine-tuning its transcriptional activity.[15–17] Collectively, these domains within the VDR create a macromolecule receptive to physiologically relevant levels of circulating 1,25(OH)$_2$D$_3$ and capable of directing cellular regulatory machinery to specific subsets of genes whose protein products are key to 1,25(OH)$_2$D$_3$ response.

The VDR Specifies Target Genes Through its DNA-binding Properties

The zinc finger containing the DNA-binding domain of the VDR is typical of that found in all members of the steroid receptor gene family including those for estrogens, androgens, and glucocorticoids, as well as for thyroid hormone, retinoid acid, and other lipophilic regulators.[18,19] The VDR is now known to recognize a specific DNA sequence or vitamin D response element (VDRE) comprised of 2 hexameric nucleotide half-sites separated by 3 base pairs (bp).[1,20] Other response element structures also occur, although these appear much less frequently.[21] The 2 DNA half-sites accommodate the binding of a heterodimer comprised of a VDR molecule and a retinoid X receptor (RXR) molecule.[19] The latter forms a heterodimer with other members of the steroid receptor family as well, including receptors for retinoic acid and thyroid hormone, thus linking the activities of several different endocrine systems. Recent studies, described later, suggest that RXR is independently bound to many sites on the genome in the absence of an activating ligand, thereby marking potential regulatory sites for subsequent activation by 1,25(OH)$_2$D$_3$. 1,25(OH)$_2$D$_3$ via its receptor also suppresses the transcriptional expression of numerous genes.[1,22] The requirements for direct VDR DNA binding and for heterodimer formation with RXR in the suppression of gene activity are currently unclear.

The VDR Regulates Transcription Through its Ability to Recruit Coregulatory Complexes

Selective VDR DNA binding in a cell serves to highlight that subset of genes within a genome whose transcriptional activities are targeted under a specific set of conditions for modification by 1,25(OH)$_2$D$_3$. Changes in gene expression are not mediated directly via the VDR, however, but rather indirectly through the protein's ability to facilitate through its transactivation domain the recruitment of large and diverse coregulatory machines that directly mediate such changes.[2,23] This recruitment is often gene specific, suggesting a role for additional and as yet unidentified components. Coregulatory complexes generally contain 1 VDR-interacting component as well as many additional subunits, several of which can contain inherent enzymatic activity. These complexes include machines with ATPase-containing nucleosomal remodeling ability, enzymes such as acetyl- and deacetyltransferases and methyl- and demethyltransferases containing selective chromatin histone modifying capabilities, and complexes that play a role in RNA polymerase II (RNA pol II) recruitment and initiation such as Mediator, as documented in **Fig. 2**. Each of these groups of proteins identifies a key step in the process of transcription regulation and many more are likely to be identified in the future. The details of how these machines operate to enhance or suppress the expression of these gene targets are only now beginning to emerge.

VITAMIN D TARGET GENES
1,25(OH)$_2$D$_3$ Regulates Networks of Genes in a Tissue/Cell-specific Fashion

As described earlier, the role of ligand-activated VDR is to direct cellular transcription machinery to specific sites on the genome where these complexes can influence the production of RNA, which encodes proteins that are integral to specific biologic activities. It is in this manner that 1,25(OH)$_2$D$_3$ plays a central role in regulating mineral metabolism via its actions in intestinal and kidney epithelial cells and in specific bone cells. Although many target genes that play important roles in calcium and phosphorus homeostatic have been identified, additional targets important to these processes continue to be discovered. These include the calcium and phosphate transporters and their associated basolaterally located, energy-driven ion pumps in the intestine and kidney,[24–26] and the osteoblast-synthesized osteoclastogenic differentiation factor receptor activator of NF-κB ligand (RANKL),[27] which stimulates the activity of existing bone-resorbing osteoclasts, prolongs their lifespan, and induces the formation of new replacements.[28] Vitamin D also regulates gene networks involved in bile acid metabolism in the colon,[29] the degradation of xenobiotic compounds in several tissues,[24] the differentiation of keratinocytes in skin,[30] the development and cycling of dermal hair follicles,[31] and the functions of key cell types involved in innate and adaptive immunity.[32] The genes and gene networks that have been identified as responsible for these biologic actions of 1,25(OH)$_2$D$_3$ are extensive. Indeed, many have emerged as a consequence of contemporary genome-wide analyses that are almost routinely conducted by investigators currently, and which are capable of measuring the effects of the hormone on entire cellular or tissue transcriptomes. Many of these gene networks are regulated by the hormone in a tissue-specific fashion. Perhaps most interesting is the intricate regulatory controls exerted directly by 1,25(OH)$_2$D$_3$ and its receptor at genes involved in the vitamin D ligand's production and degradation, actions that contribute to the maintenance of biologically active levels of intracellular 1,25(OH)$_2$D$_3$. Thus, as outlined in **Fig. 3**, 1,25(OH)$_2$D$_3$ suppresses the renal expression of *Cyp27b1*,[33] whose protein product is responsible for its synthesis, and induces *Cyp24a1*,[33,34] whose product is responsible for its degradation to calcitroic acid. In addition to these activities, 1,25(OH)$_2$D$_3$ also autoregulates the expression of its own receptor gene (**Fig. 3**), thus modulating not only levels of the ligand but also of the VDR.[5,35] Some of the mechanistic details of this regulation are discussed later. Thus, 1,25(OH)$_2$D$_3$ also contributes directly to the maintenance of the key signaling components essential for generating and mediating hormonal response.

***Traditional Studies were Initiated by Identifying Target Genes and Defining Regions
that Mediate Regulation by the Vitamin D Hormone***

Identifying the site(s) of action of $1,25(OH)_2D_3$ at a target gene locus represents the first
step in defining the molecular processes that are essential for altering a gene's transcriptional output. This step is also important because it often leads to the identification of a region that is likely to provide important regulatory control after activation

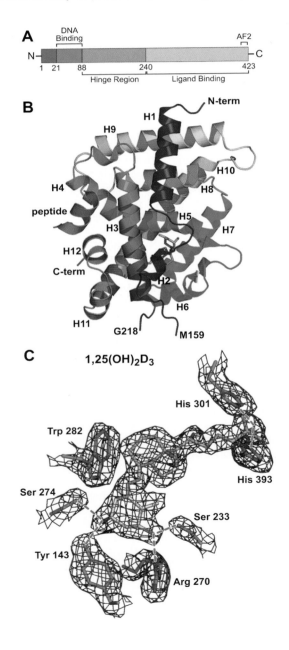

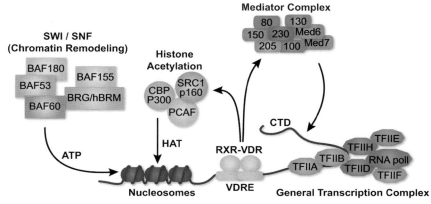

Fig. 2. Coregulatory complexes that are involved in mediating the actions of 1,25(OH)$_2$D$_3$ and the VDR. The general transcriptional apparatus is shown at the TSS and the VDR/RXR heterodimer is shown bound to its regulatory vitamin D response element or VDRE. Three regulatory complexes are shown that interact with the VDR: an ATPase-containing, chromatin remodeling complex termed SWI/SNF, a histone acetylation complex containing histone acetyltransferases (HAT) and Mediator complex. The latter facilitates the activation of RNA pol II through its C-terminal domain (CTD). Nucleosomes as well as individual proteins that comprise the individual coregulatory complexes are indicated.

through other signaling pathways as well. Early studies of the osteocalcin gene and its regulation by 1,25(OH)$_2$D$_3$ in bone cells provide an excellent example of this principle. Based on the ability of 1,25(OH)$_2$D$_3$ to induce osteocalcin in bone cells, our early molecular studies, using a traditional human osteocalcin promoter-reporter plasmid approach coupled to classic protein-DNA interaction analyses, revealed the first DNA-binding site for the VDR.[20,36] This site was located approximately 485 bp upstream of the human gene's transcriptional start site (TSS) and was comprised of 2 directly repeated 6-bp sequences separated by 3 bp. Follow-on studies confirmed the general location and highly conserved nature of this vitamin D responsive region in the rat[37] and mouse genes.[38] The latter was functionally suppressed by 1,25(OH)$_2$D$_3$

Fig. 1. Structure and key features of the VDR. (A) The VDR protein comprised of a DNA-binding domain, a large ligand-binding domain, and a hinge region that links the 2 functional domains of the protein together. N, amino terminal end; C, carboxy terminal end; AF2, activation function 2. Amino acid numbers are shown. (B) Crystal structure of the VDR ligand-binding domain comprised of 12 α-helices (H1–H12). The N-terminal and C-terminal portions of the molecule are shown. A deletion in the molecular from G218 to M159 was required to achieve the formation of crystals. The position of 1,25(OH)$_2$D$_3$ is shown in the ligand-binding pocket as a stick figure. The ligand-binding domain was crystallized in the presence of a short peptide (indicated) representing a key LxxLL motif located in all coregulatory proteins that interact directly with the VDR. The repositioning of H12 as a consequence of 1,25(OH)$_2$D$_3$ binding provides the structural change necessary for interaction of the VDR with the LxxLL motif. (C) An electron density map of 1,25(OH)$_2$D$_3$ and adjacent amino acids within the VDR protein that make direct contact with the ligand. (*Data from* Vanhooke JL, Benning MM, Bauer CB, et al. Molecular structure of the rat vitamin D receptor ligand-binding domain complexed with 2-carbon-substituted vitamin D$_3$ hormone analogues and a LXXLL-containing coactivator peptide. Biochemistry 2004;43(14):4101–10.)

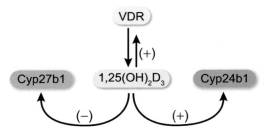

Fig. 3. Regulatory control of the synthesis (*Cyp27b1*), degradation (*Cyp24a1*), and mediation of activity (*Vdr*) of 1,25(OH)$_2$D$_3$ The concentration of 1,25(OH)$_2$D$_3$ in cells is determined through its synthesis and its degradation. Its functional activity is determined by the presence and intracellular concentration of the VDR.

as a result of a strategic change in the regulatory element's base structure thereby highlighting an important species-specific difference in vitamin D response. An extensive series of studies conducted more than a decade after these initial discoveries firmly established that this general region was a direct target for many different transcription factors some of which were activated by either separate or overlapping signal transduction pathways.[39] The ability of these proteins to influence response to 1,25(OH)$_2$D$_3$ and for the vitamin D hormone and its receptor to influence their actions was characterized. Perhaps the most important transcription factor to be discovered at the osteocalcin promoter was RUNX2, a regulatory protein now known to be essential to the formation and bone-forming activity of osteoblasts.[40,41] During the ensuing years, many genes have been explored for the location of regulatory sites that are capable of mediating 1,25(OH)$_2$D$_3$ action, binding the VDR and its heterodimer partner, and recruiting coregulatory complexes necessary for changes in transcriptional output. These include the genes for osteocalcin, osteopontin, bone sialoprotein, *TRPV6*, *PTH*, *PTHrp*, *Cyp24a1*, and *Cyp27b1* as well as many others. In the case of *Cyp24a1*, 2 sites located within 300 bp of the TSS were identified as significant mediators of the actions of 1,25(OH)$_2$D$_3$.[34]

NEW APPROACHES REVEAL NEW INSIGHTS INTO VITAMIN D$_3$–MEDIATED GENE REGULATION
Development of New Approaches to the Study of Transcription Research

The study of gene regulation in the past several decades has relied heavily on the analysis of transcriptional activity generated from gene promoter/reporter plasmids transfected into host cells to identify key components of regulatory processes. These analyses, together with biochemical assays that assess direct protein-protein and protein-DNA interactions have provided considerable insight into how genes are regulated. These approaches are inherently biased, however, because they rely on cellular transfection, involve the analysis of short segments of target genes that are not in context with the gene's normal chromatin environment, are often dependent on co-expression and/or over-expression of DNA-binding proteins and/or specific coregulators for measureable activity and, in many cases, use concentrations of reactants that are manyfold higher than that normally found in cells. These deficiencies as well as many others prompted the development and application of new techniques to assess the molecular details of transcriptional regulation. Perhaps the most important has been the development of chromatin immunoprecipitation (ChIP) analysis, a technique summarized in **Fig. 4** that permits the detection of regulatory proteins and/or the

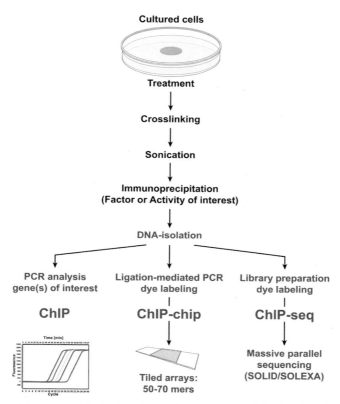

Fig. 4. Methodology associated with chromatin immunoprecipitation (ChIP) analysis and subsequent ChIP-DNA microarray (ChIP-chip) or massive parallel sequencing (ChIP-seq) analyses. Biologic samples are cross-linked, sonicated to prepare discrete size chromatin fragments, and then subjected to immunoprecipitation using selected antibodies. The precipitated DNA is then isolated and evaluated by polymerase chain reaction analysis or amplified and then subjected to either ChIP-chip or ChIP-seq analyses.

appearance of covalent activity at specific DNA targets in unmodified cells or tissues.[42,43] However, it has been the analysis of amplified ChIP products using tiled microarrays (ChIP-chip)[44] or massively parallel sequencing techniques (ChIP-seq),[45–47] as also shown in the figure, that has provided the most important new insights yet into how genes are regulated. These latter extensions to ChIP analysis impose no restrictions on the regions within the genome that can be evaluated. Thus, they can be used to examine at an equally high level of resolution a single gene locus of several hundreds of kilobases or an entire genome comprised of several billion bases. These techniques are currently being used to re-examine the mechanisms whereby $1,25(OH)_2D_3$ regulates known targets of vitamin D action, to explore regulated genes for which the underlying mechanisms have yet to be discovered, to identify and assess new gene targets, and to establish overarching principles of VDR gene regulation at the genome-wide level. One principle that seems to be emerging from these studies is that the regulation of most genes, including those that are targets of vitamin D action, is mediated by multiple regulatory regions often located many kilobases from their respective gene's start site. Specific examples of how ChIP-chip and

ChIP-seq analyses are being used to illuminate the transcriptional actions of $1,25(OH)_2D_3$ are provided in the following sections. As mentioned earlier, many of our preconceived notions of how this hormone regulates transcription were only partially correct.

Regulation of Cyp24a1 Expression by 1,25(OH)₂D₃ Before and After ChIP-Chip Analysis

As indicated earlier, $1,25(OH)_2D_3$ regulates the expression of *Cyp27b1* and *Cyp24a1*. Because the expression of these genes is central to the maintenance of an effective vitamin D endocrine system, the diverging mechanisms whereby $1,25(OH)_2D_3$ suppresses the expression of *Cyp27b1* while inducing the expression of *Cyp24a1* have receive considerable attention. Although many details remain to be worked out, it seems that $1,25(OH)_2D_3$ prompts the displacement of a key transcription factor at the *Cyp27b1* proximal promoter that is responsible for basal expression.[48] This displacement suppresses the expression of *Cyp27b1*. In the case of *Cyp24a1*, numerous studies have shown the presence of 2 regulatory elements (VDREs) located approximately 150 and 250 bp upstream of the TSS that mediate the inducing capability of $1,25(OH)_2D_3$ via the VDR and its partner RXR.[34,49] Several additional regulatory sites are also present in this proximal region that contribute to the up-regulation of *Cyp24a1*, including sites for the transcription factor C/EBPβ and for Ets-1.[50] Parathyroid hormone (PTH) also regulates *Cyp24a1*, although this action is indirect and mediated via either a modification of $1,25(OH)_2D_3$ response and/or through post-translational events.[51,52] Recent ChIP studies of $1,25(OH)_2D_3$-induced activation of *Cyp24a1* reveal that the hormone induces rapid binding of VDR and RXR to the proximal promoter elements and that this binding leads to the recruitment of coregulators such as the p160 family members, the integrators CBP and p300, the Med1 cofactor TRAP220, and RNA polymerase II (RNA pol II).[53] This region also undergoes rapid histone H4 acetylation, likely the result of the appearance of the p160 family members. The appearance of these factors at the *Cyp24a1* proximal promoter is cyclic within the first 3 hours, with a periodicity of approximately 45 minutes.[53] This periodicity has been observed for other nuclear receptors and its mechanism recently modeled for PPARγ in HEK293 cells.[54] These and other studies provide excellent overviews of *Cyp27b1* and *Cyp24a1* regulation by $1,25(OH)_2D_3$.

In recent studies, the authors used ChIP-chip and ChIP-seq analyses to examine the ability of $1,25(OH)_2D_3$ to induce not only VDR and RXR binding to the human *CYP24A1* promoter but also to stimulate the recruitment of RNA pol II to the gene's TSS and to promote changes in histone H4 acetylation.[55] These studies confirmed the earlier findings of a region located immediately proximal to the *CYP24A1* promoter to which the VDR/RXR heterodimer binds on induction by $1,25(OH)_2D_3$. The hormone also induced an increase in H4 acetylation and the recruitment of RNA pol II at this region, and at sites within the transcription unit. Surprisingly, ChIP-chip analysis also revealed that $1,25(OH)_2D_3$ induced VDR/RXR heterodimer binding to a robust cluster of intergenic sites located 50 to 70 kb downstream of the human *CYP24A1* gene. H4 acetylation and RNA pol II recruitment were increased across these sites in a fashion similar to that identified at the proximal promoter. This cluster of $1,25(OH)_2D_3$-regulated enhancers was also conserved, in position and function, in the mouse *Cyp24a1* gene locus. Functional analysis of these regions using large recombineered bacterial artificial chromosome (BAC) clones containing the entire mouse and human *CYP24A1* gene loci confirmed the contribution of these downstream clusters of enhancers. Thus, ChIP-chip analysis has revealed unexpectedly that *CYP24A1*, a quintessential target of $1,25(OH)_2D_3$ action, is regulated by multiple enhancers located not only proximal but also downstream of and distal to the promoter. This characteristic of the CYP24A1 gene is emerging as typical of most highly regulated genes, and highlights an important new feature of gene regulation, as revealed by ChIP-chip analysis.

$1,25(OH)_2D_3$ Autoregulates the Expression of the VDR Gene Through Intronic and Upstream Enhancers

The VDR is an absolute determinant of the biologic activity of $1,25(OH)_2D_3$.[1] Thus, the receptor's expression in cells is a requirement for response, and the receptor's concentration itself a key component of sensitivity to the hormone. Although little is known of the molecular determinants of basal expression of the VDR in cells, the VDR gene is known to be regulated by a variety of hormones including PTH, retinoic acid, and the glucocorticoids.[56] Perhaps most interesting is the ability of $1,25(OH)_2D_3$ to increase the level of VDR gene expression itself. Despite the discovery of this autoregulatory feature of the VDR gene several decades ago,[10,35,57] a general lack of a regulatory response to $1,25(OH)_2D_3$ at the promoter for the VDR gene left the mechanism unresolved. To elucidate this mechanism, however, the authors turned to ChIP-chip analysis and explored the entire mouse Vdr gene locus for the presence of regions that might mediate the inducing actions of $1,25(OH)_2D_3$. This analysis revealed the presence of several enhancers that bound the VDR and its heterodimer partner RXR that were located in 2 separate introns approximately 20 and 30 kb downstream of the gene's TSS.[5] No activity was observed at the Vdr gene's proximal promoter thus confirming the lack of activity observed in earlier studies. At least 1 of these regions contained a functional VDRE capable of mediating vitamin D hormone action when analyzed independently in host cells. More recent studies have now identified additional sites of regulation, at least 1 of which is located many kilobases upstream of the Vdr gene's TSS.[58] Subsets of these enhancers also mediate the actions of PTH, retinoic acid, and the glucocorticoids, through the binding of the transcription factors CREB, RAR, and GR, respectively, thus underscoring a previously known characteristic of enhancers, that of modularity. Further examination resulted in the identification of additional transcription factors such a C/EBPβ, which likely participate in the basal expression of the VDR in selected cell types. Subsequent BAC clone analysis, as described earlier, has confirmed the roles of these enhancers in the regulation of Vdr gene expression. Current studies are focused on the use of these large DNA constructs to recapitulate Vdr gene expression in vivo in transgenic mice.

$1,25(OH)_2D_3$ and PTH Regulates the Expression of the Mouse Rankl Gene Through Multiple Upstream Distal Enhancers

Rankl is a TNFα-like factor that is produced by stromal cells and osteoblasts and which regulates the differentiation, activation, and survival of osteoclasts, cells responsible for bone resorption.[28,59,60] The expression of this factor in osteoblast lineage cells is regulated by the 2 primary calciotropic hormones, $1,25(OH)_2D_3$ and PTH, as well as several of the inflammatory cytokines including IL-1, TNFα, and IL-6. These actions on Rankl expression facilitate the normal bone remodeling function of $1,25(OH)_2D_3$ and PTH in particular but also highlight the bone loss that is associated with increased levels of these hormones. As with the genes discussed earlier, early studies aimed at understanding the regulation of Rankl gene expression focused on the proximal promoter and regions immediately upstream. Although $1,25(OH)_2D_3$ was shown to manifest activity at the proximal promoter, this activity was modest and difficult to interpret.[61–63] Activity as a consequence of PTH treatment was not detected. These features of the mouse and human RANKL proximal promoters suggested the possibility that the genes might be regulated through additional unidentified control regions. To explore this possibility, the authors conducted a ChIP-chip analysis and explored the ability of 1,25(OH)$_2$D$_3$ to induce VDR binding across the mouse *Rankl* gene locus. This analysis revealed the presence of 5 regions capable of mediating the regulatory activity of the vitamin D hormone.[4] Surprisingly, these regions were located 16, 22, 60, 69, and 75 kilobases (kb) upstream of the *Rankl* TSS. The region at 75 kb was shown to contain several VDREs and was particularly active. Studies in parallel by Fu and colleagues[64] revealed that a region immediately upstream of the enhancer at −75 kb mediated the actions of PTH through CREB as well. This combined enhancer was thus termed the distal control region or DCR. Subsequent studies suggested that the actions of PTH were not limited to the DCR, but were also observed at several of the more proximal enhancers identified for the VDR.[65] Although basal levels of H4 acetylation were noted at many of these enhancers, 1,25(OH)$_2$D$_3$ and PTH induced a striking increase in this epigenetic activity. The vitamin D hormone also induced an increase in RNA pol II at these sites.[4,66] These studies suggested that the binding of VDR and CREB to these sites initiated changes in chromatin structure and function, thus supporting the hypothesis that they represent true regulatory enhancers. The central role of the enhancer located at −75/76 prompted Galli and colleagues[66] to delete this region in the mouse genome. Surprisingly, this deletion resulted in a significant suppression of the basal expression of *Rankl* in osteoblasts and limited responsiveness to exogenous 1,25(OH)$_2$D$_3$ and PTH. In addition, these mice displayed a modest increase in bone mineral density in adults that was similar to that observed in PTH-null mice. These studies support a distinct biologic role for a unique *Rankl* enhancer in basal and inducible Rankl gene expression and highlight the usefulness of ChIP-chip analysis in identifying this and additional regulatory regions. These results reinforce the emerging concept that many if not most genes are regulated through the actions of multiple enhancers that can be located in often remote regions surrounding a gene's transcription unit. More recent studies have now identified an even more distal region, located 88 kb upstream of the mouse *Rankl* TSS that mediates the actions of the gp130-activating cytokines such as IL-6 through the STAT3 transcription factor.[67]

GENOME-WIDE STUDIES REVEAL OVERARCHING PRINCIPLES OF GENE REGULATION BY STEROID HORMONES AND BY 1,25(OH)$_2$D$_3$

ChIP-chip analyses on a genome-wide scale have been conducted recently for several steroid hormones and their respective receptors.[42–44,46,47,68] These studies include an examination of binding sites for the estrogen, androgen, and peroxisome proliferator-activated receptors. These studies have revealed new insights into the sites of action of these transcription factors and are currently establishing not only new gene targets but new principles through which hormones activate genomic targets. In several cases, investigators have identified the effect of transcription factor binding on RNA pol II recruitment and changes in epigenetic marks. Genome-wide studies of VDR binding sites in tissues and cells are currently in progress and have yet to be published. However, an extensive analysis of subsets of known 1,25(OH)$_2$D$_3$ target genes has been examined, and these studies together with the earlier observations on *CYP24a1*, *Vdr*, *Rankl*, and *Lrp5* [6] indicate several common features. These features confirm those reported through the genome-wide studies conducted for other endocrine systems. First, it is now clear that the expression of target genes is commonly regulated by multiple control regions. Although many of these regulatory regions are located proximal to promoters, most are situated many kilobases from their respective promoters upstream and downstream, as well as at intronic and exonic sites within the transcription unit itself. Second, although the binding of the VDR to these regulatory regions is largely, although not exclusively, dependent on activation by 1,25(OH)$_2$D$_3$, RXR, the VDR's heterodimer partner, can be found frequently at these regulatory sites before activation. Thus, as indicated earlier in this article, RXR may mark certain regulatory sites for subsequent activation by 1,25(OH)$_2$D$_3$. RXR also forms homodimers with itself as well as heterodimers with other members of the steroid receptor family. Accordingly, the presence of RXR at a specific site could alternatively represent the means for gene activation by other endocrine factors. Third, bioinformatic analysis of these regulatory sites of VDR/RXR activity has revealed that they are almost always associated with a recognizable regulatory element (VDREs) to which the heterodimer complex can bind directly. Functional studies of these elements have generally confirmed the validity of these projected binding sites. Fourth, the binding of the VDR/RXR heterodimer to regulatory sites within genes can be demonstrated by ChIP-chip analysis to be associated with subsequent genetic activity and frequently with a change in gene expression. Thus, VDR/RXR binding at enhancers correlates with the recruitment of many of the coregulators described earlier, including acetyltransferases, cointegrators such as CBP, corepressor such as SMRT or NCoR, and members of the Mediator complex. The appearance of regulatory complexes at these sites of VDR action are likely responsible for striking increases in histone H4 acetylation or methylation that are observed at these sites and for the increase in RNA pol II that is recruited to these sites and to transcriptional start sites. Thus, the binding of the VDR facilitates downstream molecular activities that are integral to changes in the transcriptional output of target genes. An investigation of the regulation of these same genes by other hormones and signaling pathways demonstrates that these regulatory regions also bind other transcription factors, thereby supporting the idea that regulatory regions are modular in nature and mediate the activity of multiple signaling inputs at target genes. These and additional features of gene regulation that have emerged as a result of ChIP-chip analyses provide new perspectives on the underlying mechanisms through which the expression of target genes is controlled.

SUMMARY

This article represents a summary of what is known of the VDR protein and its molecular mechanism of action at target genes. New methodologies now used, such as ChIP-chip and ChIP-seq, as well as novel reporter studies using large BAC clones stably transfected into culture cells or introduced as transgenes in mice, are providing new insights into how 1,25(OH)$_2$D$_3$-activated VDR modulates the expression of genes at single gene loci and at the level of gene networks. Many of these insights are unexpected and suggest that gene regulation is even more complex than previously appreciated. These studies also highlight new technologies and their central role in establishing fundamental biologic principles.

ACKNOWLEDGMENTS

The author thanks the members of the Pike laboratory for helpful discussions related to the work described and Laura Vanderploeg for preparing the figures.

REFERENCES

1. Haussler MR, Whitfield GK, Haussler CA, et al. The nuclear vitamin D receptor: biological and molecular regulatory properties revealed. J Bone Miner Res 1998;13(3):325–49.
2. Sutton AL, MacDonald PN. Vitamin D: more than a "bone-a-fide" hormone. Mol Endocrinol 2003;17(5):777–91.
3. Bouillon R, Carmeliet G, Verlinden L, et al. Vitamin D and human health: lessons from vitamin D receptor null mice. Endocr Rev 2008;29(6):726–76.
4. Kim S, Yamazaki M, Zella LA, et al. Activation of receptor activator of NF-kappaB ligand gene expression by 1,25-dihydroxyvitamin D_3 is mediated through multiple long-range enhancers. Mol Cell Biol 2006;26(17):6469–86.
5. Zella LA, Kim S, Shevde NK, et al. Enhancers located within two introns of the vitamin D receptor gene mediate transcriptional autoregulation by 1,25-dihydroxyvitamin D_3. Mol Endocrinol 2006;20(6):1231–47.
6. Fretz J, Zella L, Kim S, et al. 1,25-Dihydroxyvitamin D_3 regulates the expression of low-density lipoprotein receptor-related protein 5 via deoxyribonucleic acid sequence elements located downstream of the start site of transcription. Mol Endocrinol 2006;20(9):2215–30.
7. Meyer M, Watanuki M, Kim S, et al. The human transient receptor potential vanilloid type 6 distal promoter contains multiple vitamin D receptor binding sites that mediate activation by 1,25-dihydroxyvitamin D_3 in intestinal cells. Mol Endocrinol 2006;20(6):1447–61.
8. Brumbaugh PF, Haussler MR. 1α,25-Dihydroxycholecalciferol receptors in intestine. I. Association of 1α,25-dihydroxycholecalciferol with intestinal mucosa chromatin. J Biol Chem 1974;249(4):1251–7.
9. Brumbaugh PF, Haussler MR. 1α,25-Dihydroxycholecalciferol receptors in intestine. II. Temperature-dependent transfer of the hormone to chromatin via a specific cytosol receptor. J Biol Chem 1974;249(4):1258–62.
10. McDonnell DP, Mangelsdorf DJ, Pike JW, et al. Molecular cloning of complementary DNA encoding the avian receptor for vitamin D. Science 1987;235(4793):1214–7.
11. Baker AR, McDonnell DP, Hughes M, et al. Cloning and expression of full-length cDNA encoding human vitamin D receptor. Proc Natl Acad Sci U S A 1988; 85(10):3294–8.
12. Rochel N, Wurtz JM, Mitschler A, et al. The crystal structure of the nuclear receptor for vitamin D bound to its natural ligand. Mol Cell 2000;5(1):173–9.
13. Vanhooke JL, Benning MM, Bauer CB, et al. Molecular structure of the rat vitamin D receptor ligand binding domain complexed with 2-carbon-substituted vitamin D_3 hormone analogues and a LXXLL-containing coactivator peptide. Biochemistry 2004;43(14):4101–10.
14. Smith CL, O'Malley BW. Coregulator function: a key to understanding tissue specificity of selective receptor modulators. Endocr Rev 2004;25(1):45–71.
15. Jurutka P, Hsieh J, Nakajima S, et al. Human vitamin D receptor phosphorylation by casein kinase II at Ser-208 potentiates transcriptional activation. Proc Natl Acad Sci U S A 1996;93(8):3519–24.
16. Hilliard GT, Cook R, Weigel N, et al. 1,25-Dihydroxyvitamin D_3 modulates phosphorylation of serine 205 in the human vitamin D receptor: site-directed mutagenesis of this residue promotes alternative phosphorylation. Biochemistry 1994; 33(14):4300–11.
17. Jurutka P, Hsieh J, MacDonald P, et al. Phosphorylation of serine 208 in the human vitamin D receptor. The predominant amino acid phosphorylated by

casein kinase II, in vitro, and identification as a significant phosphorylation site in intact cells. J Biol Chem 1993;268(9):6791–9.

18. Mangelsdorf DJ, Thummel C, Beato M, et al. The nuclear receptor superfamily: the second decade. Cell 1995;83(6):835–9.

19. Mangelsdorf DJ, Evans RM. The RXR heterodimers and orphan receptors. Cell 1995;83(6):841–50.

20. Ozono K, Liao J, Kerner SA, et al. The vitamin D-responsive element in the human osteocalcin gene. Association with a nuclear proto-oncogene enhancer. J Biol Chem 1990;265(35):21881–8.

21. Carlberg C. Molecular basis of the selective activity of vitamin D analogues. J Cell Biochem 2003;88(2):274–81.

22. Demay MB, Kiernan MS, DeLuca HF, et al. Sequences in the human parathyroid hormone gene that bind the 1,25-dihydroxyvitamin D_3 receptor and mediate transcriptional repression in response to 1,25-dihydroxyvitamin D_3. Proc Natl Acad Sci U S A 1992;89(17):8097–101.

23. Dowd DR, Sutton AL, Zhang C, et al. Comodulators of vitamin D receptor-mediated gene expression. In: Feldman D, Pike JW, Glorieux FH, editors. Vitamin D. 2nd edition. New York: Elsevier/Academic Press; 2005. p. 291–304.

24. Bouillon R, Bischoff-Ferrari H, Willett W. Vitamin D and health: perspectives from mice and man. J Bone Miner Res 2008;23(7):974–9.

25. Bouillon R, Carmeliet G, Boonen S. Ageing and calcium metabolism. Baillieres Clin Endocrinol Metab 1997;11(2):341–65.

26. Benn BS, Ajibade D, Porta A, et al. Active intestinal calcium transport in the absence of transient receptor potential vanilloid type 6 and calbindin-D9k. Endocrinology 2008;149(6):3196–205.

27. Jimi E, Akiyama S, Tsurukai T, et al. Osteoclast differentiation factor acts as a multifunctional regulator in murine osteoclast differentiation and function. J Immunol 1999;163(1):434–42.

28. Leibbrandt A, Penninger J. RANK/RANKL: regulators of immune responses and bone physiology. Ann N Y Acad Sci 2008;1143:123–50.

29. Makishima M, Lu TT, Xie W, et al. Vitamin D receptor as an intestinal bile acid sensor. Science 2002;296(5571):1313–6.

30. Bikle DD. Vitamin D regulated keratinocyte differentiation. J Cell Biochem 2004; 92(3):436–44.

31. Demay M, MacDonald P, Skorija K, et al. Role of the vitamin D receptor in hair follicle biology. J Steroid Biochem Mol Biol 2007;103(3-5):344–6.

32. Adorini L. Regulation of immune responses by vitamin D receptor ligands. In: Feldman D, Pike JW, Glorieux FH, editors. Vitamin D. 2nd edition. New York: Elsevier/Academic Press; 2005. p. 631–48.

33. Prosser DE, Jones G. Enzymes involved in the activation and inactivation of vitamin D. Trends Biochem Sci 2004;29(12):664–73.

34. Zierold C, Darwish HM, DeLuca HF. Two vitamin D response elements function in the rat 1,25-dihydroxyvitamin D 24-hydroxylase promoter. J Biol Chem 1995; 270(4):1675–8.

35. Costa EM, Hirst MA, Feldman D. Regulation of 1,25-dihydroxyvitamin D_3 receptors by vitamin D analogs in cultured mammalian cells. Endocrinology 1985;117(5):2203–10.

36. Kerner SA, Scott RA, Pike JW. Sequence elements in the human osteocalcin gene confer basal activation and inducible response to hormonal vitamin D_3. Proc Natl Acad Sci U S A 1989;86(12):4455–9.

37. Terpening C, Haussler C, Jurutka P, et al. The vitamin D-responsive element in the rat bone Gla protein gene is an imperfect direct repeat that cooperates with other

cis-elements in 1,25-dihydroxyvitamin D₃- mediated transcriptional activation. Mol Endocrinol 1991;5(3):373–85.

38. Clemens T, Tang H, Maeda S, et al. Analysis of osteocalcin expression in transgenic mice reveals a species difference in vitamin D regulation of mouse and human osteocalcin genes. J Bone Miner Res 1997;12(10):1570–6.

39. Lian JB, Stein GS, Javed A, et al. Networks and hubs for the transcriptional control of osteoblastogenesis. Rev Endocr Metab Disord 2006;7(1–2):1–16.

40. Stein GS, Lian JB, Stein JL, et al. Combinatorial organization of the transcriptional regulatory machinery in biological control and cancer. Adv Enzyme Regul 2005; 45:136–54.

41. Ducy P, Zhang R, Geoffroy V, et al. Osf2/Cbfa1: a transcriptional activator of osteoblast differentiation. Cell 1997;89(5):747–54.

42. Shang Y, Hu X, DiRenzo J, et al. Cofactor dynamics and sufficiency in estrogen receptor-regulated transcription. Cell 2000;103(6):843–52.

43. Shang Y, Myers M, Brown M. Formation of the androgen receptor transcription complex. Mol Cell 2002;9(3):601–10.

44. Carroll J, Meyer C, Song J, et al. Genome-wide analysis of estrogen receptor binding sites. Nat Genet 2006;38(11):1289–97.

45. Lin C, Vega V, Thomsen J, et al. Whole-genome cartography of estrogen receptor alpha binding sites. PLoS Genet 2007;3(6):e87.

46. Welboren W, van Driel M, Janssen-Megens E, et al. ChIP-Seq of ERalpha and RNA polymerase II defines genes differentially responding to ligands. EMBO J 2009;28(10):1418–28.

47. Lefterova M, Zhang Y, Steger D, et al. PPARgamma and C/EBP factors orchestrate adipocyte biology via adjacent binding on a genome-wide scale. Genes Dev 2008;22(21):2941–52.

48. Murayama A, Takeyama K, Kitanaka S, et al. Positive and negative regulations of the renal 25-hydroxyvitamin D₃ 1α-hydroxylase gene by parathyroid hormone, calcitonin, and 1α,25(OH)₂D₃ in intact animals. Endocrinology 1999;140(5):2224–31.

49. Ohyama Y, Ozono K, Uchida M, et al. Functional assessment of two vitamin D-responsive elements in the rat 25-hydroxyvitamin D₃ 24-hydroxylase gene. J Biol Chem 1996;271(48):30381–5.

50. Dwivedi P, Omdahl J, Kola I, et al. Regulation of rat cytochrome P450C24 (CYP24) gene expression. Evidence for functional cooperation of Ras-activated Ets transcription factors with the vitamin D receptor in 1,25-dihydroxyvitamin D(3)-mediated induction. J Biol Chem 2000;275(1):47–55.

51. Yang W, Friedman P, Kumar R, et al. Expression of 25(OH)D₃ 24-hydroxylase in distal nephron: coordinate regulation by 1,25(OH)₂D₃ and cAMP or PTH. Am J Physiol 1999;276(4 Pt 1):E793–805.

52. Zierold C, Mings J, DeLuca H. Regulation of 25-hydroxyvitamin D₃-24-hydroxylase mRNA by 1,25-dihydroxyvitamin D₃ and parathyroid hormone. J Cell Biochem 2003;88(2):234–7.

53. Kim S, Shevde NK, Pike JW. 1,25-Dihydroxyvitamin D₃ stimulates cyclic vitamin D receptor/retinoid X receptor DNA-binding, co-activator recruitment, and histone acetylation in intact osteoblasts. J Bone Miner Res 2005;20(2):305–17.

54. Degenhardt T, Rybakova K, Tomaszewska A, et al. Population-level transcription cycles derive from stochastic timing of single-cell transcription. Cell 2009;138(3): 489–501.

55. Meyer MB, Goetsch PD, Pike JW. A downstream intergenic cluster of regulatory enhancers contributes to the induction of *CYP24A1* expression by 1α,25-dihydroxyvitamin D₃. J Biol Chem 2010, in press. DOI:10.1074/jbc.M110.119958.

56. Esteban L, Eisman J, Gardiner E. Vitamin D receptor promoter and regulation of receptor expression. In: Feldman D, Pike JW, Glorieux FH, editors. Vitamin D. 2nd edition. New York: Elsevier/Academic Press; 2005. p. 193–217.

57. Santiso-Mere D, Sone T, Hilliard GM 4th, et al. Positive regulation of the vitamin D receptor by its cognate ligand in heterologous expression systems. Mol Endocrinol 1993;7(7):833–9.

58. Zella LA, Meyer MB, Nerenz RD, et al. Multifunctional enhancers regulate mouse and human vitamin D receptor gene transcription. Mol Endocrinol 2010;24(1): 128–47.

59. Kong YY, Feige U, Sarosi I, et al. Activated T cells regulate bone loss and joint destruction in adjuvant arthritis through osteoprotegerin ligand. Nature 1999; 402(6759):304–9.

60. Kong YY, Yoshida H, Sarosi I, et al. OPGL is a key regulator of osteoclastogenesis, lymphocyte development and lymph-node organogenesis. Nature 1999; 397(6717):315–23.

61. Kitazawa S, Kajimoto K, Kondo T, et al. Vitamin D_3 supports osteoclastogenesis via functional vitamin D response element of human RANKL gene promoter. J Cell Biochem 2003;89(4):771–7.

62. Kitazawa R, Mori K, Yamaguchi A, et al. Modulation of mouse RANKL gene expression by Runx2 and vitamin D_3. J Cell Biochem 2008;105(5):1289–97.

63. Mori K, Kitazawa R, Kondo T, et al. Modulation of mouse RANKL gene expression by Runx2 and PKA pathway. J Cell Biochem 2006;98(6):1629–44.

64. Fu Q, Manolagas SC, O'Brien CA. Parathyroid hormone controls receptor activator of NF-kappaB ligand gene expression via a distant transcriptional enhancer. Mol Cell Biol 2006;26(17):6453–68.

65. Kim S, Yamazaki M, Shevde NK, et al. Transcriptional control of receptor activator of nuclear factor-kappaB ligand by the protein kinase A activator forskolin and the transmembrane glycoprotein 130-activating cytokine, oncostatin M, is exerted through multiple distal enhancers. Mol Endocrinol 2007;21(1):197–214.

66. Galli C, Zella LA, Fretz JA, et al. Targeted deletion of a distant transcriptional enhancer of the receptor activator of nuclear factor-kappaB ligand gene reduces bone remodeling and increases bone mass. Endocrinology 2008; 149(1):146–53.

67. Bishop KA, Meyer MB, Pike JW. A novel distal enhancer mediates cytokine induction of mouse RANKL gene expression. Mol Endocrinol 2009;23(12):2095–110.

68. Welboren W, Stunnenberg H, Sweep F, et al. Identifying estrogen receptor target genes. Mol Oncol 2007;1(2):138–43.

Assessment and Interpretation of Circulating 25-Hydroxyvitamin D and 1,25-Dihydroxyvitamin D in the Clinical Environment

Bruce W. Hollis, PhD[a,b,*]

KEYWORDS

- Vitamin D • 25-Hydroxyvitamin D
- 1,25-Dihydroxyvitamin D • Calcidiol • Calcitriol

Vitamin D is a 9,10-seco steroid, as shown by the numbering of its carbon skeleton. Vitamin D has 2 distinct forms: vitamin D_2 and vitamin D_3. Vitamin D_2 is a 28-carbon molecule derived from the plant sterol ergosterol, whereas vitamin D_3 is a 27-carbon derivative of cholesterol. Vitamin D_2 differs from vitamin D_3 in that it contains an extra methyl group and a double bond between carbons 22 and 23.

The most important aspects of vitamin D chemistry center on its *cis*-triene structure. This unique structure makes vitamin D and related metabolites susceptible to oxidation, ultraviolet (UV) light-induced conformational changes, heat-induced conformational changes, and attacks by free radicals. Most of these transformation products have less biologic activity than does vitamin D. Research has now shown that vitamin D_2 is much less bioactive than vitamin D_3 in humans.[1] The parent compounds vitamin D_2 and vitamin D_3 are sometimes referred to as calciferol.

Hydroxylation reactions at both carbon 25 of the side chain and, subsequently, carbon 1 of the A ring result in the metabolic activation of vitamin D. Metabolic inactivation of vitamin D takes place primarily through a series of oxidative reactions at carbons 23, 24, and 26 of the molecule's side chain. Metabolic activation and inactivation are well characterized and result in a plethora of vitamin D metabolites.[2] Of

[a] Department of Biochemistry and Molecular Biology, Children's Research Institute, Medical University of South Carolina, 173 Ashley Avenue, Charleston, SC 29425, USA
[b] Department of Pediatrics, Children's Research Institute, Medical University of South Carolina, 173 Ashley Avenue, Charleston, SC 29425, USA
* Corresponding author. Department of Pediatrics, Children's Research Institute, Medical University of South Carolina, 173 Ashley Avenue, Charleston, SC 29425.
E-mail address: hollisb@musc.edu

Endocrinol Metab Clin N Am 39 (2010) 271–286
doi:10.1016/j.ecl.2010.02.012
0889-8529/10/$ – see front matter © 2010 Elsevier Inc. All rights reserved.

these metabolites, only 25-hydroxyvitamin D (25(OH)D) and 1,25-dihydroxyvitamin D (1,25(OH)$_2$D) provide any clinically relevant information. 25(OH)D$_2$ and 25(OH)D$_3$ are commonly known as calcifediol and the 1,25(OH)$_2$D metabolites as calcitriol.

In this review the current state of the science on the clinical assessment of circulating 25(OH)D and 1,25(OH)$_2$D is described.

METHODS OF 25(OH)D QUANTITATION

The assessment of circulating 25(OH)D started its journey approximately 4 decades ago with the advent of the competitive protein-binding assay (CPBA).[3] From that early time to the present we have progressed to radioimmunoassay (RIA), high-performance liquid chromatography (HPLC), and liquid chromatography coupled with mass spectrometry (LC/MS). A brief description of each technique is given here.

Competitive Protein-Binding Assay

A major factor responsible for the explosion of information on vitamin D metabolism and its relation to clinical disease was the introduction of a CPBA for 25(OH)D. Haddad and Chyu[3] introduced this CPBA almost 4 decades ago. The assay assessed circulating 25(OH)D concentrations using the vitamin D–binding protein (DBP) as a primary binding agent and [3]H-25(OH)D$_3$ as a reporter. Although this CPBA was valid, it was also relatively cumbersome. Technicians had to extract the sample with organic solvent, dry it under nitrogen, and purify it using column chromatography. This assay was suitable for the research laboratory but did not meet the requirements of a high-throughput clinical laboratory.

The major difficulty in measuring 25(OH)D is attributable to the molecule itself. 25(OH)D is probably the most hydrophobic compound measured by protein-binding assay (PBA), which constitutes either CPBA or radioimmunoassay (RIA). The fact that the molecule exists in 2 forms, 25(OH)D$_2$ and 25(OH)D$_3$, compounds the difficulties with its quantitation by PBA. 25(OH)D's lipophilic nature renders it especially vulnerable to the matrix effects of any PBA. Anything present in the sample assay vessel that is not present in the calibrator assay vessel can cause matrix effects. These matrix effect substances are usually lipid but in the newer direct assays, they could be anything contained in the serum or plasma sample. These matrix factors change the ability of the binding agent, antibody, or binding protein to associate with 25(OH)D in the sample or standard in an equal fashion. When this occurs, it markedly diminishes the assay's validity. Experience has demonstrated that the DBP is more susceptible to these matrix effects than antibodies.[4] The original Haddad procedure overcame the matrix problem by using chromatographic sample purification before CPBA.[3]

Researchers had a strong desire to simplify this cumbersome CPBA for 25(OH)D, so Belsey and colleagues[5] developed a streamlined CPBA in 1974. The goal of this second-generation CPBA was to eliminate chromatographic sample purification as well as individual sample recovery using [3]H-25(OH)D$_3$. However, after several years of trying, researchers were unable to validate the Belsey assay due to matrix problems originating from ethanolic sample extraction.[6]

The 25(OH)D CPBAs did have the advantage of being cospecific for 25(OH)D$_2$ and 25(OH)D$_3$ and thus provided a "total" 25(OH)D value if the assay was valid. The DBP's binding cospecificity for 25(OH)D$_2$ and 25(OH)D$_3$ as well as its stability made it an attractive candidate for incorporation into automated direct chemiluminescent assays. In fact, Nichols Institute Diagnostics used this approach when its researchers developed the Advantage 25(OH)D Assay. The US Food and Drug Administration (FDA) approved this assay for clinical use, but Nichols ultimately withdrew it from the market place due to its propensity to overestimate total circulating 25(OH)D concentrations and its surprising inability to detect circulating 25(OH)D$_2$.[7,8] Although never described, these problems were probably linked to the DBP's inability to resolve the matrix problems associated with direct sample assay. At present, the CPBA for 25(OH)D is rarely used. Also, one cannot accurately compare most CPBA results for circulating 25(OH)D concentrations from the past with values from current methods because many of the matrix interferences were not linear in the old CPBAs.

Radioimmunoassay

In the early 1980s, the author's group decided that a nonchromatographic RIA for circulating 25(OH)D would be the best approach to measuring the substance. This group therefore designed an antigen that would generate an antibody that was cospecific for 25(OH)D$_2$ and 25(OH)D$_3$.[9] In addition, a simple extraction method was designed that allowed simple nonchromatographic quantification of circulating 25(OH)D.[9] In 1985 Immunonuclear Corp., now known as DiaSorin, introduced this ^{3}H-based RIA as a kit on a commercial basis. This RIA was further modified in 1993 to incorporate a ^{125}I-labeled reporter and calibrators (standards) in a serum matrix.[10] This modification finally made mass assessment of circulating 25(OH)D possible. In that same year this assay became the first FDA-approved device for the clinical diagnosis of nutritional vitamin D deficiency. Further, during the past 23 years these DiaSorin tests have been used in the vast majority of large clinical studies worldwide to define "normal" circulating 25(OH)D levels in a variety of disease states. This test still remains today the only RIA-based assay that provides a "total" 25(OH)D value.

Random-Access Automated Instrumentation

DiaSorin Corporation, Roche Diagnostics, and the now defunct Nichols Institute Diagnostics all introduced methods for the direct (no extraction) quantitative determination of 25(OH)D in serum or plasma using completive protein assay chemiluminescence technology.[11] These assays appear quite similar on the surface but they are not.

In 2001, Nichols Diagnostics introduced the fully automated chemiluminescence Advantage 25(OH)D assay system. In this assay system, nonextracted serum or plasma was added directly into a mixture containing human DBP, acridinium-ester labeled anti-DBP, and 25(OH)D$_3$-coated magnetic particles. Note that the primary binding agent was human DBP. Thus, this assay was a CPBA, much like the manual procedure introduced in 1974 by Belsey and colleagues.[5] The major difference between these procedures was that Belsey depotenized the sample with ethanol before assaying it. The calibrators for the Belsey assay were in ethanol. In the Advantage assay, the calibrators were in a serum-based matrix, and its developers assumed that this matrix would replicate the serum or plasma sample introduced directly into the assay system. In the end, the 1974 Belsey assay never worked and neither did the Advantage 25(OH)D Assay. The company removed the assay from the market in 2006.

In 2004, the DiaSorin Corporation introduced the fully automated chemiluminescence Liaison 25(OH)D Assay System.[11] This assay is very similar to the late Advantage assay, with one major difference: the Liaison assay uses an antibody as a primary binding agent as opposed to the human DBP in the Advantage system. Thus, the Liaison is a true RIA method. Details on this procedure are available elsewhere.[11] The Liaison 25(OH)D assay is cospecific for 25(OH)D$_2$ and 25(OH)D$_3$, so it reports a "total" 25(OH)D concentration. DiaSorin recently introduced a second-generation Liaison 25(OH)D assay. This new version has increased functional sensitivity and much improved assay precision. The Liaison 25(OH)D assay is the single most widely used 25(OH)D assay in the world for clinical diagnosis.

The most recent addition to the automated 25(OH)D assay platforms is from Roche Diagnostics. Their test is an RIA called vitamin D_3(25-OH), which can be performed on their Elecsys and Cobas systems. Roche only released this assay in 2007, so very little information on it is available. However, the assay can only detect 25(OH)D_3, so it will not be a viable product in countries in which vitamin D_2 is used clinically, including the United States.[12]

Direct Physical Detection Methods

Direct detection methodologies for determining circulating 25(OH)D include both HPLC and LC/MS procedures.[13–17] The HPLC methods separate and quantitate circulating 25(OH)D_2 and 25(OH)D_3 individually. HPLC followed by UV detection is highly repeatable and, in general, most people consider it the gold standard method. However, these methods are cumbersome and require a relatively large sample as well as an internal standard. Sample throughout is slow and is not suited to a high-demand clinical laboratory processing up to 10,000 25(OH)D assays per day.

Researchers have recently revitalized LC/MS as a viable method to assess circulating 25(OH)D.[14–17] As with HPLC, LC/MS quantitates 25(OH)D_2 and 25(OH)D_3 separately. When performed properly, LC/MS is a very accurate testing method. However, the equipment is very expensive and its overall sample throughput cannot, when performed properly, match that of the automated instrumentation format. As a methodology, LC/MS can compare favorably with RIA techniques.[15,16] One unique problem with LC/MS is its relative inability to discriminate between 25(OH)D_3 and its inactive isomer 3-epi-25(OH)D_3. This problem has been especially noticeable in the circulation of newborn infants.[14] Next to the DiaSorin assays, LC/MS is the next most used procedure for the clinical assessment of circulating 25(OH)D.

DETERMINING ANALYTICAL RECOVERY OF 25(OH)D_2 AND 25(OH)D_3 IN HUMAN SERUM OR PLASMA

Questions constantly arise regarding the various 25(OH)D assay procedures' ability to accurately measure total 25(OH)D (25(OH)D_2 + 25 (OH)D_3) levels in human samples.[8] A brief study recently has described the ability of the DiaSorin Liaison Total-D 25(OH)D Assay System to perform this task as compared with the gold standard HPLC/UV quantitation of 25(OH)D_2 and 25(OH)D_3.[18] Baseline serum samples that contained only 25(OH)D_3 were obtained from 9 volunteers. All subjects then consumed 50,000 IU/d vitamin D_2 for a period of 14 days. Seven days following the final dose serum samples were again obtained. For exogenous in vitro recovery experiments 32 ng/mL of either 25(OH)D_2 or 25(OH)D_3 were added, in a small volume of ethanol, to each baseline serum sample. All samples were then subjected to direct HPLC/UV quantitation to determine individual levels of 25(OH)D_2 and 25(OH)D_3[9] or the DiaSorin Liaison Total-D Assay.

25(OH)D calibrators from The National Institute of Standards and Technology (NIST) were also tested. NIST describes the samples as Level 1, "normal" human serum; Level 2, "normal" human serum diluted 1:1 with horse serum; and Level 3, "normal" human serum "spiked" with 25(OH)D_2 attempting to equal the amount of endogenous 25(OH)D_3 contained in the sample. Horse serum from Sigma Chemical Company was also accessed.

In the group of volunteers the baseline total 25(OH)D was 48.3 ± 19.0 and 43.7 ± 16.8 ng/mL ($\bar{x}$ ± SD) by HPLC-UV and Liaison, respectively. In these baseline samples HPLC-UV analysis demonstrated 99% of the circulating 25(OH)D to be of the D_3 form, and only 2 of 9 subjects had detectable (>1.0 ng/mL) 25(OH)D_2. Following 14 days of oral vitamin D_2 supplementation, total 25(OH)D levels were determined to be 81.1 ± 21.9 and 80.0 ± 25.5 ng/mL by HPLC-UV and Liaison, respectively. By HPLC analysis the elevations in 25(OH)D_2 ranged from 25 to 88 ng/mL. In these postsupplementation samples, HPLC-UV analysis also revealed 25(OH)D_3 to be 43.5% of the total while the remaining 56.5% was 25(OH)D_2. The regression relationship of pre and post samples between HPLC-UV and Liaison was Liaison Total-D = 1.04 (HPLC-UV) − 5.27, r^2 = 0.95 (**Fig. 1**). The recovery of exogenously added 25(OH)D_2 or 25(OH)D_3 to baseline samples was 98.3% ± 5.7% and 99.0% ± 6.7%, respectively by HPLC-UV analysis, and 22.8% ± 19.7% and 62.7% ± 24.8%, respectively by Liaison analysis.[18]

NIST Level 1 concentrations measured by the Liaison compared favorably with HPLC results. However, NIST Level 2 was higher (Liaison vs HPLC) and Level 3 was lower (Liaison vs HPLC). The higher concentration in the NIST Level 2 can be attributed to the impact of the horse serum matrix, and lower levels in NIST Level 3 can be attributed to the lack of recovery of exogenous material by the Liaison system.

The data reveal an important artifact that could lead to false conclusions about the ability of direct competitive antibody-based chemiluminescence assays to quantitatively detect 25(OH)D_2 and/or 25(OH)D_3 in patient samples. It has proven difficult to produce an antibody that is cospecific for the detection of 25(OH)D_2 and 25(OH)D_3 in human serum. In fact, only one such antibody has been reported, being the antibody used in the DiaSorin 25(OH)D assays.[9]

In the United States it is imperative that any 25(OH)D assay used for clinical diagnosis has the ability to detect total 25(OH)D, a sum of 25(OH)D_2 and 25(OH)D_3. With a single exception, all competitive protein-binding assays introduced commercially have discriminated against 25(OH)D_2 including the now defunct Nichols Advantage 25(OH)D assay system . It is also a fact that approximately 99% of the United States population has undetectable 25(OH)D_2 in their circulation, because vitamin D_2 is rarely

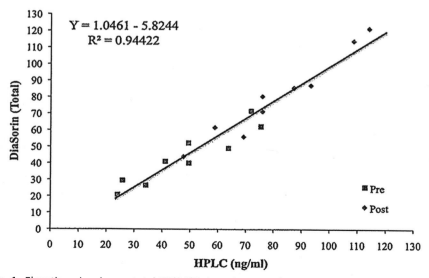

Fig. 1. Elevations in plasma total 25(OH)D in volunteers following supplementation with vitamin D_2 as measure by the DiaSorin Liaison Total method versus HPLC. Volunteers were given vitamin D_2. Presupplementation concentrations are represented by the closed boxes and postsupplementation by the closed diamonds.

used as a supplement nowadays and patients only receive it when being treated for vitamin D deficiency by a physician. Because blood samples in the general population rarely contain significant amounts of 25(OH)D$_2$, and because the compound is usually discriminated against by most antibody-based assays, it is the compound most often added exogenously to human serum to assess cross-reactivity and determine analytical recovery.

We have assumed since the early 1970s that when one adds exogenous 25(OH)D to a blood sample it rapidly binds to its carrier protein, the DBP, with little interaction to other blood components.[19] Up to this point in vitamin D assay technology, exogenous addition of 25(OH)D$_2$ or 25(OH)D$_3$ has served clinicians well in the testing of quantitative analytical recoveries of these compounds.[9] Problems were never encountered because extraction procedures were based on organic solvents of one kind or another, and they all destroyed the DBP and liberated the 25(OH)D into solution. The direct serum or plasma assays emerging today do not destroy the carrier proteins. Instead they rely on pH changes and/or blocking agents that liberate the 25(OH)D from its carrier protein but do not affect the ability of the steroid to bind to a specific antibody. This later disruption method is the one employed in the Liaison assay.[11]

The results clearly demonstrate that exogenously added 25(OH)D$_2$ or 25(OH)D$_3$ do not distribute themselves on the DBP as occurs when assembled in vivo. The other possibility is that exogenously added 25(OH)D distribute to moieties other than the DBP, suggested by the clear linear relationship observed from in vivo human samples containing elevated amounts of 25(OH)D$_2$ when assayed by the Liaison method versus HPLC-UV. On the other hand, the failure of quantitative recovery is apparent from exogenously added 25(OH)D$_2$ or 25(OH)D$_3$ to the same samples when the assay methods are compared (**Table 1**). This study describes an in vitro anomaly that really has no physiologic relevance, but could result in erroneous conclusions about 25(OH)D assay performance when comparing sample destruction methods such as HPLC-UV versus the newer sample disruption method such as the Liaison assay.[18] Extreme caution is warranted when preparing samples for such comparisons, as is being done by the Vitamin D External Quality Assessment Scheme (DEQAS) and NIST.

Table 1
Comparison of 25(OH)D concentrations measured by the DiaSorin Liaison and HPLC as a result of various exogenous and endogenous treatments.

Sample ID	DiaSorin Liaison	HPLC
	Total 25(OH)D (ng/mL)	
Baseline	43.7 ± 16.8	48.3 ± 19.0
Vitamin D$_2$	81.1 ± 21.9	80.0 ± 23.5
Baseline+25(OH)D$_2$[a]	51.0 ± 16.8 (22.8%)	79.7 ± 19.0 (98.3%)
Baseline+25(OH)D$_3$[a]	63.7 ± 20.4 (62.7%)	80.0 ± 18.5 (99.0%)
Horse serum	12.7 ± 1.0	4.7 ± 0.2
NIST Level 1 [22–24][b]	24.4 ± 0.8 (106%)	26.0 ± 1.1 (113%)
NIST Level 2 [12–14][b]	19.8 ± 0.5 (152%)	15.9 ± 0.7 (122%)
NIST Level 3 [42–46][b]	27.2 ± 1.0 (61.8%)	48.1 ± 3.0 (109%)

[a] 32 ng/mL was added to each of 9 samples. Values in parentheses represent amount of 25(OH)D recovered as a percentage of mean values.
[b] Values in brackets are expected values provided by NIST. Values in parentheses represent amount of 25(OH)D recovered as a percentage of mean values.

DETERMINING AND DEFINING A "NORMAL" CIRCULATING 25(OH)D LEVEL

To define a "normal" circulating level of a given substance or nutrient, one usually obtains blood samples from a diverse population, measures the substance in question, plots the data by Gaussian distribution, and determines normality. This method works well for nutrients such as folate or vitamin E, and was precisely how normative circulating levels of 25(OH)D were defined in humans beginning about 40 years ago by Haddad and Chyu,[3] who sampled a population of "normal" individuals whom were asymptomatic for disease, assessed circulating 25(OH)D, and determined a mean value. In their study Haddad and Chyu also assessed 25(OH)D in a group of lifeguards and demonstrated their levels to be 2.5 times those of the "normals". Countless similar studies performed over the ensuing decades reiterated the same conclusion. The author, however, interpreted the original Haddad data differently, suggesting that the 25(OH)D levels in the lifeguards were normal and the "normals" were actually vitamin D deficient.[20] This interpretation has largely been validated by the current research.

For all practical purposes, vitamin D does not naturally occur in foodstuffs that humans eat. There are exceptions such as oily fish and fish liver oil. In fact, from an evolutionary standpoint, humans did not require vitamin D in their food supply because over millions of years humans evolved a photosynthetic mechanism in their skin to produce large amounts of vitamin D_3. Thus, our skin is part of the vitamin D endocrine system, and vitamin D_3 is really a preprohormone. The problem now is that humans avoid the sun, wear sunscreen, and reside in latitudes for which they are not programmed to live. To make matters worse, the dietary requirement for vitamin D in adults is 200 IU/d, as defined by the Adequate Intake (AI) by the Food and Nutrition Board, and is essentially meaningless.[21] As a result of these factors, a "normal" circulating 25(OH)D range is now defined using various biomarkers of physiology or disease as opposed to a random population Gaussian distribution.

The first use of biomarkers to define "normal" 25(OH)D levels, of course, started with parameters that affected skeletal integrity such as parathyroid hormone, bone mineral density, and intestinal calcium absorption.[20] These parameters demonstrated that a minimum circulating level of 25(OH)D should be at least 32 ng/mL (80 nmol).[20,22] At present, the "normal" circulating 25(OH)D level also relies on data based on the other diverse physiologic functions of 25(OH)D including cancer prevention,[23–31] infectious disease,[32–37] cardiovascular health,[38–45] diabetes,[45–48] and autoimmune control.[49–51] Because of the diverse interaction of vitamin D with our genome, this list is certain to grow.[52] For the present it is generally agreed that a normal level of circulating 25(OH)D is 32 to 100 ng/mL (80–250 nmol). It must be noted that 32 ng/mL is not an "optimum" level but a minimum "normal" level. What constitutes an "optimum" level remains to be determined, and may well be different for varied physiologic processes.

CLINICAL REPORTING OF CIRCULATING 25(OH)D CONCENTRATIONS

As highlighted earlier, all DiaSorin 25(OH)D assays are approved by the FDA for clinical utility. Thus, the diagnostic 25(OH)D tests sold by DiaSorin and IDS Diagnostics (Fountain Hills, AZ, USA) are under strict FDA control and monitoring for assay performance and reliability. In what is considered a distributing trend, many clinical reference laboratories are replacing these FDA-approved tests with "home-brew" LC/MS methods that are diverse and not under FDA scrutiny. The reasons for this switch in use are the "perceived" advantages of LC/MS technology being more accurate, precise, specific, cost effective, and providing the separate determination of 25(OH)D_2 and 25(OH)D_3. First, with respect to accuracy and precision, the DiaSorin and IDS RIA methods perform at least as well as LC/MS methods according to the DEQAS operated out of London, United Kingdom. As far as specificity goes, the DiaSorin tests appear more specific than LC/MS methodology in that the DiaSorin assays do not detect the inactive 3-epimer of 25(OH)D$_3$.[14] Finally, LC/MS assays are marketed on their ability to separately measure 25(OH)D$_2$ and 25(OH)D$_3$ in a blood sample. However, clinically there is no advantage to this separate measurement claim. Not a single scientific publication exists that demonstrates separate 25(OH)D$_2$ and 25(OH)D$_3$ whose measurements are superior to a "total" 25(OH)D value as supplied by the DiaSorin tests. In fact, this separate reporting has been shown to confuse clinicians.[53] The truth is that LC/MS laboratories report separate values because that is how LC/MS technology has to report the data,[14–17] and is not a reason to "spin" it to a clinical advantage. Also, the FDA has made its opinion on the separate reporting of 25(OH)D$_2$ and 25(OH)D$_3$ clear. In 2007, ESA Biosciences Inc (Chelmsford, MA, USA) submitted a 510K application to the FDA seeking approval of an HPLC procedure to determine 25(OH)D$_2$ and 25(OH)D$_3$ separately in blood. The FDA responded "Assays intended for clinical use must have a clinical indication as well as an analytical claim. Please provide additional information to establish the clinical validity of separate 25(OH)D$_2$ and 25(OH)D$_3$ in diagnosis." Of course, no such data exist so ESA's test was only approved after they agreed to report only "total" 25(OH)D. Thus, separate reporting of 25(OH)D$_2$ and 25(OH)D$_3$ in the eyes of the FDA is of no medical advantage or use. Some LC/MS laboratories have actually billed inappropriate Current Procedural Terminology codes to enhance return for these separate reported values. The author considers this practice to be abusive and fraudulent, and believe it must end. Further, 99% of all patient samples assayed will not contain any 25(OH)D$_2$.

Replacement of FDA-controlled devices such as the DiaSorin and IDS assays with "home-brew" LC/MS assays from a clinical diagnostic standpoint is, again, disturbing, because the DiaSorin assays have and continue to be the standard of clinical 25(OH)D assessment. One can say this because the "normal" range of circulating 25(OH)D is almost entirely based on clinical studies using the DiaSorin tests. In fact, Labcorp (Burlington, NC, USA) uses a publication by Hollis[20] on which to base its clinical range of 25(OH)D levels. In turn, this publication is based on DiaSorin assay–based clinical studies, so unless a given LC/MS method is calibrated against the DiaSorin methods, this reference range should not be reported against.

Many years and clinical studies have gone into establishing the DiaSorin reference range and, as stated earlier, this consists of thousands of scientific publications. To prove the point the author has selected some large significant clinical studies on which the "normal" circulating level of 25(OH)D is based, most of which used DiaSorin and some IDS assays as their method of analysis. No LC/MS clinical studies are included because basically none exist, which is the author's point exactly.

The DiaSorin RIA has been used to generate all of the 25(OH)D data from the third National Health and Nutrition Examination Survey (NHANES III). Selected references on this topic are included to validate this claim.[38,48,53–56] Many more studies from NHANES exist with respect to vitamin D and all use the DiaSorin RIA. Studies from the huge National Institutes of Health (NIH)-sponsored Women's Health Initiative (WHI) used the DiaSorin LIAISON assay for the first 2 major publications,[31,57] with others to follow.

The Harvard-based studies, the Health Professionals' Follow-up Study (HPFAS), and the Nurses' Health Study (NHS) have been used to establish much of the information in the last decade regarding the relationship of circulating 25(OH)D levels and various disease states such as cancer, autoimmune, cardiovascular, and renal. All of these studies again used DiaSorin-based assays.[24–30,34,35,45–49] Of course, one cannot forget the relationship of vitamin D status, parathyroid hormone, and skeletal integrity. Hundreds of articles have been published on this topic; most using DiaSorin assays and none using LC/MS testing.

What then should LC/MS laboratories do? If they are going to use the current DiaSorin-based reference range[20] they had better target their values to that of the DiaSorin test. In fact, this is basically how the FDA has been approving new devices for 25(OH)D assessment through the 510K process since the DiaSorin RIA was the first device approved in 1993. The alternative is that each LC/MS site establish their own reference range, which will take years of clinical study because a normal Gaussian distribution is useless in establishing a normative 25(OH)D range. In fact, this "normalization" of values is common between other 25(OH)D assays and DiaSorin testing, as recent articles demonstrate.[58]

Finally, clinical reference laboratories should simply use a single reference range to report circulating 25(OH)D levels, as does Labcorp, 32 to 100 ng/mL. Compare this to the Mayo Clinic, which reports 4 different "classes" of 25(OH)D status. This type of reporting is confusing and should be discontinued.

METHODS OF 1,25(OH)$_2$D QUANTITATION

Of all the steroid hormones, 1,25(OH)$_2$D represented the most difficult challenge to the analytical biochemist with respect to quantitation. 1,25(OH)$_2$D circulates at picomolar concentrations (too low for direct UV or MS quantitation), is highly lipophilic, and its precursor, 25(OH)D, circulates at nanomolar levels. The development of simple, rapid assay for this compound has proven to be a daunting task.

Radioreceptor Assays

The first radioreceptor assay (RRA) for 1,25(OH)$_2$D was introduced in 1974.[59] Although this initial assay was extremely cumbersome, it did provide invaluable information with respect to vitamin D homeostasis. This initial RRA required a 20-mL serum sample, which was extracted using Bligh-Dyer organics. The extract had to be purified by 3 successive chromatographic systems, and chickens had to be euthanized and the vitamin D receptor (VDR) harvested from their intestines. By 1976, the volume requirement for this RRA had been reduced to a 5-mL sample, and sample prepurification had been modified to include HPLC.[60] However, the sample still had to be extracted using a modified Bligh-Dyer procedure and then prepurified on Sephadex LH-20. Chicken intestinal VDR was still used as a binding agent.

A major advancement occurred in 1984 with the introduction of a radically new concept for the RRA determination of circulating 1,25(OH)$_2$D.[61] This new RRA used solid-phase extraction of 1,25(OH)$_2$D from serum along with silica cartridge purification of 1,25(OH)$_2$D. As a result, the need for HPLC sample prepurification was eliminated. Also, this assay used VDR isolated from calf thymus, which proved to be quite stable and thus had to be prepared only periodically. Further, the volume requirement was reduced to 1 mL of serum or plasma. This assay opened the way for any laboratory to measure circulating 1,25(OH)$_2$D. This procedure also resulted in the production of the first commercial kit for 1,25(OH)$_2$D measurement. This RRA was further simplified in 1986 by decreasing the required chromatographic purification steps.[62] This method has become a citation classic.[63]

As good as the calf thymus RRA for 1,25(OH)$_2$D was, it still possessed 2 serious shortcomings. First, VDR had to be isolated from thymus glands. Second, because the VDR is so specific for its ligand, only ^{3}H-1,25(OH)$_2$D$_3$ could be used as a reporter, eliminating the use of ^{125}I or chemiluminescent reporter; this was a major handicap, especially for the commercial laboratory.

Radioimmunoassay

In 1978, the first RIA for 1,25(OH)$_2$D was introduced.[64] Although it was an advantage not to have to isolate the VDR as a binding agent, this RIA was relatively nonspecific, so the cumbersome sample preparative steps were still required. Over the next 18 years all RIAs developed for 1,25(OH)$_2$D suffered from the same shortcomings. In 1996, the author's group developed the first significant advance in 1,25(OH)$_2$D quantification in a decade.[65] This RIA incorporated a ^{125}I reporter, as well as standards in an equivalent serum matrix, so individual sample recoveries were no longer required. The sample purification procedure is the same one previously used for the rapid RRA procedure.[62] This assay has 100% cross-reactivity between 1,25(OH)$_2$D$_2$ and 1,25(OH)$_2$D$_3$ and is FDA-approved for clinical diagnosis in humans.

Another ^{125}I-based RIA for 1,25(OH)$_2$D is also commercially available from IDS Ltd. The basis of this kit is a selective immunoextraction of 1,25(OH)$_2$D from serum or plasma with a specific monoclonal antibody bound to a solid support. This antibody is directed toward the H-hydroxylated A ring of 1,25(OH)$_2$D.[66] This assay procedure has never been published in detail, so critical evaluation is difficult. The author concluded that this immunoextraction procedure was highly specific for the 1-hydroxylated forms of vitamin D. However, he also believes that this procedure overestimated circulating 1,25(OH)$_2$D levels. Evidence of this overestimation is evident in a recent publication that shows a correlation of circulating 25(OH)D and 1,25(OH)$_2$D at physiologic levels,[67] indicating that 25(OH)D may be interfering with the assay.

Enzyme-linked immunosorbent assays for circulating 1,25(OH)$_2$D determinations do exist commercially from Immunodiagnostik and IDS. However, their performance has never been published in detail.

Direct Physical Detection Methods

Direct detection methodology for determining circulating 1,25(OH)$_2$D is very problematic because of the low concentration (pmol) in the blood. Because of this fact, direct UV detection is not possible. Recently 2 commercial laboratories, Mayo Clinic and Quest Diagnostics, have begun to offer LC/MS detection of circulating 1,25(OH)$_2$D. However, details of these analyses are not in the public domain.

DETERMINING AND DEFINING A "NORMAL" CIRCULATING 1,25(OH)$_2$D LEVEL

Unlike 25(OH)D, a normal circulating level of 1,25(OH)$_2$D can be determined from a Gaussian distribution of subjects. Over the last 3 decades this has been accomplished, and a normal adult level has been defined as 16 to 56 pg/mL with a mean of 37.6 pg/mL.[68] Circulating 1,25(OH)$_2$D is diagnostic for several clinical conditions, including vitamin D–dependent rickets types I and II, hypercalcemia associated with sarcoidosis, and other hypercalcemic disorders causing increased 1,25(OH)$_2$D levels. These other disorders include tuberculosis, fungal infections, Hodgkin disease, lymphoma, and Wegener granulomatosis. In all other clinical conditions involving the vitamin D endocrine system, including hypoparathyroidism, hyperparathyroidism, and chronic renal failure, the assay of 1,25(OH)$_2$D is a confirmatory test. It is also important to remember that circulating 1,25(OH)$_2$D provides essentially no information with respect to the patient's nutritional vitamin D status. Thus, circulating 1,25(OH)$_2$D should not be used as an indicator for hypo- or hypervitaminosis D when nutritional factors are suspected.

A very interesting condition that has a profound effect on circulating 1,25(OH)D levels is pregnancy.[69] During pregnancy, circulating 1,25(OH)$_2$D increases dramatically. In the author's recently completed NIH-funded pregnancy and vitamin D trial, circulating $1,25(OH)_2D$ levels averaged 130 pg/mL with levels of 300 to 400 pg/mL observed in some patients. These levels are so dramatic they could almost be used as a pregnancy test. The physiologic purpose of this dramatic elevation remains to be determined.

STABILITY OF 25(OH)D AND 1,25(OH)₂D IN SERUM OR PLASMA

Researchers have known for nearly 30 years that endogenous 25(OH)D and $1,25(OH)_2D$ are extremely stable in serum or plasma.[70] Lissner and colleagues[70] showed that vitamin D metabolites in blood stored at 24°C for up to 72 hours remain intact. Recent studies on the stability of 25(OH)D in plasma or serum that has undergone many freeze-thaw cycles have reported the same stability.[71] The author has used the same pooled human 25(OH)D and $1,25(OH)_2D$ internal controls stored at −20°C for more than 10 years with no detectable degradation of either compound. The DEQAS, a major vitamin D quality assessment organization, ships its serum samples used by laboratories for quality assessment by ground post worldwide without affecting 25(OH)D and $1,25(OH)_2D$ values.

The author has performed experiments with the aim of destroying endogenous 25(OH)D and $1,25(OH)_2D$ in plasma to obtain a vitamin D–free human plasma to prepare various immunoassay procedure calibrators. When crystalline $25(OH)D_3$ or $1,25(OH)_2D_3$ was placed in ethanol in an open glass Petri dish and the dish exposed to intense UV light, the UV light destroyed the compounds within a few minutes. When the same experiment was conducted using serum or plasma, however, the $25(OH)D_3$ and $1,25(OH)_2D_3$ levels did not change after 2 days of UV light exposure. The author therefore stopped trying to use this procedure to produce vitamin D–free plasma.

Why are vitamin D and its metabolites so stable in serum or plasma when they are insulted with UV light, temperature shifts, or oxidation? One reason is that UV light penetrates aqueous media very poorly. However, the main reason is probably that in serum or plasma, vitamin D and its metabolites are essentially bound completely to the serum DBP, and this complex resists potential insults to the vitamin D molecule very effectively. In conclusion, 25(OH)D and $1,25(OH)_2D$ are very stable in serum or plasma, so they require only minimal attention to storage conditions.

STANDARDIZATION OF 25(OH)D AND 1,25(OH)₂D ANALYSIS

DEQAS (Internet: www.deqas.org) was founded in 1989 to compare the performance of then-available 25(OH)D tests. DEQAS has since become the largest vitamin D quality assessment program in the world, with approximately 600 participating laboratories worldwide. The organization's major aim today is to assess the analytical reliability of 25(OH)D and $1,25(OH)_2D$ assays. The organization achieves this goal by:

- Distributing serum pools at regular intervals
- Conducting statistical analyses of submitted results
- Appropriately manipulating pools to provide information on assay specificity and recovery
- Assigning gas chromatography-MS target values to selected 25(OH)D pools
- Helping participants and manufacturers evaluate methods by providing samples, technical support, and impartial advice
- Offering advice and support to participants having difficulty achieving an acceptable level of assay performance
- Providing a forum for exchanging information on all aspects of vitamin D assay methodology.

The author's laboratory has participated in both the DEQAS 25(OH)D and DEQAS 1,25(OH)$_2$D survey since 1997, and the survey has been invaluable in maintaining the integrity of his assay procedure. When DEQAS leaders question manufacturers about inconsistencies in their methods, most manufacturers attempt to address the issue identified.

One example of the value DEQAS offers occurred when DEQAS informed Nichols Institute Diagnostics that its Advantage 25(OH)D automated assay was overestimating total 25(OH)D concentrations and that, contrary to the manufacturer's claims, the method could not detect circulating 25(OH)D$_2$ concentrations.[8] Nichols Institute Diagnostics chose not to respond to the concerns that DEQAS identified. The company subsequently went out of business and its Advantage 25(OH)D assay is no longer on the market. As this example shows, DEQAS provides an invaluable service to the vitamin D assay community. In the future, it is hoped that DEQAS can incorporate the new NIST 25(OH)D calibrators into its survey in some fashion.

The DEQAS survey has shown that most current 25(OH)D assay protocols perform in a comparable fashion with respect to absolute values, assay linearity, and assay precision. However, the survey results also show that the only assays that quantitatively detect total 25(OH)D are HPLC methods, LC/MS methods, and the DiaSorin assays.

SUMMARY

The assessment of circulating 25(OH)D and, to a lesser degree, 1,25(OH)$_2$D is rapidly becoming an important clinical tool in the diagnosis and management of many diverse pathologies. At present, the reference ranges for circulating 25(OH)D and 1,25(OH)$_2$D are 32 to 100 ng/mL and 16 to 56 ng/mL, respectively, and are largely based on clinical data derived from the FDA-cleared DiaSorin assay procedures.

REFERENCES

1. Armas LAG, Hollis BW, Heaney RP. Vitamin D$_2$ is much less effective than vitamin D$_3$ in humans. J Clin Endocrinol Metab 2004;89:5387–91.
2. Bouillon R, Okamura WH, Norman AW. Structure-function relationships in the vitamin endocrine system. Endocr Rev 1995;16:200–57.
3. Haddad JG, Chyu KJ. Competitive protein-binding radioassay for 25-hyroxycholecalciferol. J Clin Endocrinol Metab 1971;33:992–5.
4. Bouillon R, Van Herck E, Jans I, et al. Two direct nonchromatographic assays for 25-hydroxyvitamin D. Clin Chem 1984;30:1731–6.
5. Belsey RE, DeLuca HF, Potts JT. A rapid assay for 25-OH-vitamin D$_3$ without preparative chromatography. J Clin Endocrinol Metab 1974;38:1046–51.
6. Dorantes LM, Amaud SB, Arnaud CD, et al. Importance of the isolation of 25 hydroxyvitamin D before assay. J Lab Clin Med 1978;91:791–6.
7. Leventis HC, Garrison L, Sibley M, et al. Underestimation of serum 25-hydroxyvitamin D by the Nichols Advantage Assay in patients receiving vitamin D$_2$ replacement therapy. Clin Chem 2005;51:1072–4.
8. Carter GD, Jones JC, Berry JL. The anomalous behavior of exogenous 25-hydroxyvitamin D in competitive binding assays. J Steroid Biochem Mol Biol 2007;103:480–2.
9. Hollis BW, Napoli JL. Improved radioimmunoassay for vitamin D and its use in assessing vitamin D status. Clin Chem 1985;31:1815–9.
10. Hollis BW, Kamerud JO, Selvaag SR, et al. Determination of vitamin D status by radioimmunoassay with a ^{125}I-labeled tracer. Clin Chem 1993;39:529–33.

11. Ersfeld DL, Rao DS, Body JJ, et al. Analytical and clinical; validation of the 25 OH vitamin D assay for the LIAISON automated analyzer. Clin Biochem 2004;37: 867–74.

12. Cavalier E, Wallac AM, Knox S, et al. Vitamin D measurement may not reflect what you give to our patients. J Bone Miner Res 2008;23:1864–5.

13. Lensmeyer GL, Wiege DA, Binkley N, et al. HPLC measurement for 25-hydroxy-vitamin D measurement: comparison with contemporary assays. Clin Chem 2006; 52:1120–6.

14. Singh RJ, Taylor RL, Reddy GS, et al. C-3 epimers can account for a significant proportion of total circulating 25(OH)D in infants, complicating accurate measurement and interpretation of vitamin D status. J Clin Endocrinol Metab 2006;91:3055–61.

15. Mansell Z, Wright DJ, Rainbow SJ. Routine isotope-dilution liquid chromatography-tandem mass spectrometry assay for simultaneous measurement of the 25-hydroxy metabolites of vitamins D_2 and D_3. Clin Chem 2005;51: 1683–90.

16. Chen H, McCoy LF, Schleicher RL, et al. Measurement of $25(OH)D_2$ and $25(OH)D_3$ in human serum using liquid chromatography-tandem mass spectrometry and its comparison to a radioimmunoassay method. Clin Chim Acta 2008; 391:6–12.

17. Saenger AK, Laha TJ, Bremner DE, et al. Quantification o f serum 25-hydroxyvitamin D2 and D3 using HPLC-tandem mass spectrometry and examination if reference intervals for diagnosis of vitamin D deficiency. Am J Clin Pathol 2006; 125:914–20.

18. Horst RL. In vivo versus in vitro recovery of $25(OH)D_2$ and D_3 in human samples using high-performance liquid chromatography and the DiaSorin Liaison Total-D assay: Limitations of the NIST controls. J Steroid Biochem Molec Biol 2010, in press.

19. Belsey R, Clark MB, Bernat M, et al. The physiologic significance of plasma transport of vitamin D and metabolites. Am J Med 1973;57:50–6.

20. Hollis BW. Circulating 25-hydroxyvitamin D levels indicative of vitamin D sufficiency: implications for establishing a new effective dietary intake recommendation for vitamin D. J Nutr 2005;135:317–22.

21. Institute of Medicine. Dietary reference intakes: calcium, phosphorus, magnesium, vitamin D, fluoride. Washington, DC: National Academy Press; 1997. p. 250–516.

22. Hollis BW, Wagner CL. Normal serum vitamin D levels. N Engl J Med 2005;352: 515–6.

23. Abbas S, Linseisen J, Slanger T, et al. Serum 25-hydroxyvitamin D and risk of postmenopausal breast cancer—results of a large case-control study. Carcinogenesis 2008;29:93–9.

24. Betone-Johnson ER, Chen WY, Holick MF, et al. Plasma 25-hydroxyvitamin D and 1,25-dihydroxyvitamin D and risk of breast cancer. Cancer Epidemiol Biomarkers Prev 2005;14:1991–7.

25. Feskanich D, Ma J, Fuchs CS, et al. Plasma vitamin D metabolites and risk of colorectal cancer in women. Cancer Epidemiol Biomarkers Prev 2004;13:1502–8.

26. Giovannucci E, Liu Y, Rimm EB, et al. Prospective study of predictors of vitamin D status and cancer incidence and mortality in men. J Natl Cancer Inst 2006;98: 451–9.

27. Zhou W, Heist RS, Liu G, et al. Circulating 25-hydroxyvitamin D levels predict survival in early-state nonsmall-cell lung cancer patients. J Clin Oncol 2007;25: 474–85.

28. Tworoger SS, Lee IM, Buring JE, et al. Plasma 25-hydroxyvitamin D and 1,25-dihydroxyvitamin D and risk of incident ovarian cancer. Cancer Epidemiol Biomarkers Prev 2007;16:783–8.
29. Mikhak B, Hunter DJ, Speigelman D, et al. Vitamin D receptor (VDR) gene polymorphisms and haplotypes, interactions with plasma 25-hydroxyvitamin D and 1,25-dihydroxyvitamin D, and prostate cancer risk. Prostate 2007;67:911–23.
30. Wu K, Feskanich D, Fuchs CS, et al. A nested case control study of plasma 25-hydroxyvitamin D concentrations and risk of colorectal cancer. J Natl Cancer Inst 2007;99:1120–9.
31. Wactawski-Wende J, Kotchen JM, Anderson GL, et al. Calcium plus vitamin D supplementation and the risk of colorectal cancer. N Engl J Med 2006;354:684–96.
32. Liu PT, Sterdger S, Li H, et al. Toll-like receptor triggering of a vitamin D-mediated human antimicrobial response. Science 2006;311:1770–3.
33. Zasloff M. Fighting infections with vitamin D. Nat Med 2006;12:388–90.
34. Dietrich T, Nunn M, Dawson-Hughes B, et al. Association between serum concentrations of 25-hydroxyvitamin D and gingival inflammation. Am J Clin Nutr 2005;82:575–80.
35. Dietrich T, Joshipura KJ, Dawson-Hughes B, et al. Association between serum concentrations of 25-hydroxyvitamin D and periodontal disease in the US population. Am Clin Nutr 2004;80:108–13.
36. Bodnar LM, Krohn MA, Simhan HN. Maternal vitamin D deficiency is associated with bacterial vaginosis in the first trimester of pregnancy. J Nutr 2009;139:1157–61.
37. Cannell JJ, Zasloff M, Garland CF, et al. On the epidemiology of influenza. Virol J 2008;5:1–12.
38. Scragg R, Sowers MF, Bell C. Serum 25-hydroxyvitamin D, ethnicity and blood pressure in the third National Health and Nutrition Examination Survey. Am J Hypertens 2007;7:713–9.
39. Forman JP, Giovannucci E, Holmes MD, et al. Plasma 25-hydroxyvitamin D levels and risk of incident hypertension. Hypertension 2007;49:1063–9.
40. Martins D, Wolf M, Pan D, et al. Prevalence of cardiovascular risk factors and the serum levels of 25-hydroxyvitamin D in the United States. Arch Intern Med 2007;167:1159–65.
41. Wang TJ, Pencina MJ, Booth SL, et al. Vitamin D deficiency and risk of cardiovascular disease. Circulation 2008;117:503–11.
42. Giovannucci E, Liu Y, Hollis BW, et al. A prospective study of 25-hydroxyvitamin D and risk of myocardial infarction in men. Arch Intern Med 2008;168:1174–80.
43. Pilz JS, Marz W, Wellnitz B, et al. Association of vitamin D deficiency with heart failure and sudden cardiac death in a large cross-sectional study of patients referred for coronary angiography. J Clin Endocrinol Metab 2008;93:3927–35.
44. Pilz S, Dobnig H, Fischer JE, et al. Low vitamin D levels predict stroke in patients referred to coronary angiography. Stroke 2008;39:2611–3.
45. Dobnig H, Pilz S, Scharnagl H, et al. Independent association of low 25(OH)D and 1,25(OH)$_2$D levels will all-cause and cardiovascular mortality. Arch Intern Med 2008;168:1340–9.
46. Chiu KC, Chu A, Go V, et al. Hypovitamninosis D is associated with insulin resistance and beta cell dysfunction. Am J Clin Nutr 2004;79:820–5.
47. Zipitis CS, Abodeng AK. Vitamin D supplementation in early childhood and risk of type 1 diabetes: a systematic review and meta-analysis. Arch Dis Child 2008;93:512–7.

48. Chonchol M, Scragg R. 25-hydroxyvitamin D, insulin resistance and kidney function in the third national health and nutrition examination survey. Kidney Int 2007; 71:134–9.
49. Munger KL, LI Levin, Hollis BW, et al. Serum 25-hydroxyvitamin D levels and risk of multiple sclerosis. JAMA 2006;20:2832–8.
50. Ramagopalan SV, Maugeri NJ, Handunnetthi L, et al. Expression of multiple sclerosis-associated MHC class II allele HLA-DRB1*1501 is regulated by vitamin D. PLoS Genet 2009;5:e1000369.
51. Cantorna MT, Yu S, Bruce D. The paradoxical effects of vitamin D on type 1 mediated immunity. Mol Aspects Med 2008;29:369–75.
52. Tavera-Mendoza LE, White JH. Cell defenses and sunshine vitamin. Sci Am 2007; 297:62–72.
53. Binkley N, Drezner MK, Hollis BW. Laboratory reporting of 25-hydroxyvitamin D results: potential for clinical misinterpretation. Clin Chem 2006;52:2124–5.
54. Nesby-O'Dell S, Scanion KS, Cogswell ME, et al. Hypovitaminosis D prevalence and determinants among African American and white women of reproductive age: third national health and nutrition examination survey, 1988-1994. Am J Clin Nutr 2002;76:187–92.
55. Looker JAC, Mussolino Me. Serum 25-hydroxyvitamin D and hip fracture risk in older white adults. J Bone Miner Res 2008;23:143–50.
56. Dawson-Hughes B. Calcium plus vitamin D and the risk of fractures. N Engl J Med 2006;354:2285–7.
57. Jackson RD, LaCroix AZ, Gass M, et al. Calcium plus vitamin D supplementation and the risk of fractures. N Engl J Med 2006;354:669–83.
58. Rovner AJ, Stallings VA, Schall JL, et al. Vitamin D insufficiency in children, adolescents, and young adults with cystic fibrosis despite routine oral supplementation. Am J Clin Nutr 2007;86:1694–9.
59. Brumbaugh PF, Haussler DH, Bressler R, et al. Radioreceptor assay for $1\alpha,25$-dihydroxyvitamin D3. Science 1974;183:1089–91.
60. Eisman JA, Hamstra AJ, Kream BE, et al. A sensitive, precise, and convenient method for determination of 1,25-dihydroxyvitamin D in human plasma. Arch Biochem Biophys 1976;176(1):235–43.
61. Reinhardt TA, Horst RL, Orf JW, et al. A microassay for 1,25-dihydroxyvitamin D not requiring high performance liquid chromatography: application to clinical studies. J Clin Endocrinol Metab 1984;58:91–8.
62. Hollis BW. Assay of circulating 1,25-dihydroxyvitamin D involving a novel single-cartridge extraction and purification. Clin Chem 1986;32(11):2060–3.
63. Hollis BW. Phase switching SPE for faster $1,25(OH)_2D$ analysis 1986. Clin Chem 2008;54:446–7.
64. Clemens TL, Hendy GN, Graham RF, et al. A radioimmunoassay for 1,25-dihydroxycholecalciferol. Clin Sci Mol Med 1978;54:329–32.
65. Hollis BW, Kamerud JQ, Kurkowski A, et al. Quantification of circulating 1,25-dihydroxyvitamin D by radioimmunoassay with ^{125}I-labeled tracer. Clin Chem 1996;42(4):586–92.
66. Fraser WD, Durham BH, Berry JL, et al. Measurement of plasma 1,25 dihydroxyvitamin D using a novel immunoextraction technique and immunoassay with iodine labeled vitamin D tracer. Ann Clin Biochem 1997;34(Pt 6): 632–7.
67. El-Hajj Feleihan G, Nabulsi M, Tamim H, et al. Effect of vitamin D replacement on musculoskeletal parameters in school children: a randomized controlled trial. J Clin Endocrinol Metab 2006;91(2):405–12.

68. Favus MJ, editor. Primer on the metabolic bone diseases and disorders of mineral metabolism. 6th edition. Washington, DC: The American Society for Bone and Mineral Research; 2006. p. 492.

69. Kumar R, Cohen WR, Silva P, et al. Elevated 1,25(OH)$_2$D plasma levels in normal human pregnancy and lactation. J Clin Invest 1979;63:342–4.

70. Lissner D, Mason RS, Posen S. Stability of vitamin D metabolites in human blood serum and plasma. Clin Chem 1981;27:773–4.

71. Antoniucci DM, Black DM, Sellmeyer DE. Serum 25-hydroxyvitamin D is unaffected by multiple freeze-thaw cycles. Clin Chem 2004;51:258–60.

Low Vitamin D Status: Definition, Prevalence, Consequences, and Correction

Neil Binkley, MD*, Rekha Ramamurthy, MD, Diane Krueger, BS

KEYWORDS

- Vitamin D • 25-Hydroxyvitamin D • Supplementation
- Deficiency • Insufficiency

Vitamin D is obtained either by ingestion or cutaneous production. When skin is exposed to ultraviolet B radiation, 7-dehydrocholesterol is converted to vitamin D_3 (cholecalciferol). Dietary sources may provide either vitamin D_3 or vitamin D_2 (ergocalciferol).[1,2] However, few foods contain appreciable amounts of vitamin D, as such dietary intake is often low. Combining low intake with indoor lifestyle and sun-avoiding behaviors including sunscreen use, it is not surprising that low vitamin D status is endemic.[3–6] The skeletal health consequences of vitamin D deficiency (calcium malabsorption and skeletal fragility) have long been recognized. More recently it has become appreciated that low vitamin D status leads to muscle weakness, falls, and potentially a multitude of nonskeletal morbidities.[7,8] This review considers the definition and prevalence, potential health consequences, and approaches to correcting low vitamin D status.

VITAMIN D BACKGROUND AND ASSESSMENT

Vitamin D must be metabolized to become physiologically active. Specifically, vitamin D (either D_2 or D_3) is converted to 25-hydroxyvitamin D (25(OH)D) in the liver and subsequently to the active or "hormonal" form, 1,25-dihydroxyvitamin D (1,25(OH)$_2$D) in the kidneys.[9] Measurement of 25(OH)D is the accepted indicator of an individual's vitamin D status.[10] This evaluation is not intuitive, as it would seem logical that measurement of the active form, 1,25(OH)$_2$D, would be the appropriate measure of an individual's vitamin D status. It is not rare anecdotally to see health

University of Wisconsin-Madison Osteoporosis Clinical Center and Research Program, 2870 University Avenue, Suite 100, Madison, WI 53705, USA
* Corresponding author.
E-mail address: nbinkley@wisc.edu

Endocrinol Metab Clin N Am 39 (2010) 287–301
doi:10.1016/j.ecl.2010.02.008
0889-8529/10/$ – see front matter © 2010 Elsevier Inc. All rights reserved.

endo.theclinics.com

care providers obtain measurement of 1,25(OH)$_2$D purportedly to evaluate an individual patient's vitamin D status. However, measurement of circulating 1,25(OH)$_2$D does not provide a useful assessment of an individual's vitamin D status, as vitamin D deficiency leads to parathyroid hormone (PTH) elevation, which enhances renal 1α-hydroxylase activity thereby promoting conversion of available 25(OH)D to 1,25(OH)$_2$D. As 25(OH)D is present in much higher concentration than 1,25(OH)$_2$D (ng/mL vs pg/mL) given the enhanced conversion induced by PTH elevation, 1,25(OH)$_2$D may be normal even in the setting of low vitamin D status.

The clinical measurement of 25(OH)D has been problematic, with substantial variability present between laboratories.[11,12] It is not the purpose of this review to detail approaches to and challenges with vitamin D measurement; this topic is reviewed elsewhere in this issue. Suffice it to say that current evaluations find that clinical 25(OH)D measurement has improved,[13] allowing health care providers to have reasonable confidence in clinical 25(OH)D measurements. Moreover, the recent availability of standard reference materials from the National Institute of Standards and Technology seems destined to further improve between-laboratory agreement. However, despite 25(OH)D assay improvements, health care providers must appreciate that assay variability is present for all laboratory results. The analytical imprecision and inaccuracy present in all quantitative medical procedures is due to method, human, and instrument limitations that confound application of rigid diagnostic cutpoint approaches. For example, if one were using a 25(OH)D value of 30 ng/mL to differentiate "low" from "optimal" vitamin D status, it must be recognized that a laboratory result of 29 ng/mL does not differ from 31 ng/mL.[14]

LOW VITAMIN D STATUS: DEFINITION AND PREVALENCE

A spectrum of vitamin D status has been proposed wherein individuals whose serum 25(OH)D value is less than approximately 10 ng/mL are classified as deficient and may sustain impaired bone mineralization (rickets/osteomalacia), while those with a value less than approximately 30 ng/mL are identified as insufficient (**Fig. 1**) and may sustain long-term adverse health consequences.[15] However, the cutpoint values selected, and even the verbiage to describe low vitamin D status, remain controversial. For example, terminology including deficiency, insufficiency, inadequacy, and hypovitaminosis has been variously, and interchangeably, applied to describe low vitamin D status. To avoid what seems to be a nonproductive debate, the terminology "low vitamin D status" is used here. Moreover, as noted above, 25(OH)D assay variability and absence of accepted standards has confounded agreement on a single definition of "low."

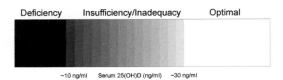

Deficiency   Insufficiency/Inadequacy   Optimal

~10 ng/ml   Serum 25(OH)D (ng/ml)   ~30 ng/ml

Fig. 1. Spectrum of vitamin D status. The spectrum of low vitamin D status is depicted. At very low vitamin D levels, (25(OH)D of approximately 10 ng/mL or less) calcium malabsorption, osteomalacia/rickets and myopathy occur. Less marked vitamin D deficiency (often referred to as inadequacy or insufficiency) has been associated with a variety of adverse health consequences. Consensus regarding an "optimal" 25(OH)D concentration continues to evolve; however, there seems to be increasing agreement that values greater than approximately 30 to 32 ng/mL are associated with optimal physiologic function.

Recognizing that controversy exists, there seems to be increasing consensus that circulating 25(OH)D values less than approximately 30 to 32 ng/mL indicate less than ideal vitamin D status.[16] These cutpoint values were suggested based on the long-established role of vitamin D to facilitate calcium and phosphorus absorption with deficiency leading to rickets/osteomalacia.[17–19] Thus, less severe vitamin D "deficiency" appears to cause calcium malabsorption, leading to secondary hyperparathyroidism with resulting elevated bone turnover and ultimately, bone loss.[20] The 25(OH)D to PTH relationship has been extensively reported, with various studies finding an apparent inflection point at around 20 to 30 ng/mL.[16,21] Moreover, some work demonstrates improved calcium absorption at 25(OH)D levels within what had previously been accepted as the "normal" range.[22] However, others have challenged this seemingly cardinal tenant of low vitamin D status by reporting that calcium malabsorption does not occur until severe vitamin D deficiency is present, due to PTH-mediated maintenance of 1,25-dihydroxyvitamin D levels.[23,24] Finally, it has recently been suggested by Heaney and colleagues[25] that the point at which hepatic 25(OH)D production becomes zero order could be used to define the lower end of normal vitamin D status. In this work, the investigators found serum 25(OH)D to rapidly increase as circulating vitamin D_3 (cholecalciferol) increased. When circulating vitamin D_3 exceeds approximately 5.8 ng/mL, the hepatic 25-hydroxylase appears to become saturated and this reaction switches from first order to zero order. Taking this approach would define the lower limit of normal at approximately 35 ng/mL,[25] obviously quite close to the 30 to 32 ng/mL suggested by other end points such as the relationship with PTH.

It is plausible that some of the debate surrounding what value defines "optimal" 25(OH)D status is being confounded by different levels for various tissues and end points; that is, the cutpoint for various nonclassic targets of vitamin D might vary from that for bone.[26] Furthermore, it is possible that the 25(OH)D value for "optimal" physiologic functioning might differ between individuals. Having a range of "normal" for virtually all clinically measured biologic parameters is well known by clinicians. As vitamin D is, in essence, an endogenously produced hormone, it is not surprising that between-individual variability and regulation would exist. In this regard, the skin of humans,[27] and other animals,[28] possesses the ability to regulate cholecalciferol production. Moreover, limited data suggest that variation in vitamin D degradation may exist, in that differences in 24-hydroxylase capacity between individuals may be based on race.[29] Data from a study of adults in Hawaii supports between-individual differences despite abundant sun exposure.[30] In fact, inspection of serum 25(OH)D concentration in that cohort reveals a virtually normal or Gaussian distribution (**Fig. 2**). Indeed, other studies of highly UV-exposed adults[31,32] find some individuals with "low" 25(OH)D despite high UV exposure and a fairly broad range of what it would seem logical to define as "normal," as noted in **Fig. 2**. Thus, it seems likely that some of these people with "low" 25(OH)D levels could in fact be "optimal" for them. It is clearly accepted that a range exists for multiple physiologic functions that is considered "normal" for healthy adults; it is not known whether the same should apply to 25(OH)D.

Given these data, it is not surprising that an exact 25(OH)D cutpoint to define suboptimal vitamin D status remains somewhat controversial.[33] Despite this, there is increasing agreement that values less than approximately 30 to 32 ng/mL be identified as "low."[34,35] When this cutpoint is applied, low vitamin D status is extremely common worldwide. For example, recent reports classify 52% to 77% of the studied cohorts as "low" using 30 ng/mL as a cutpoint.[21,36–38] Even the more restrictive cutpoint of less than 20 ng/mL identifies 18% to 36% as "low" (**Fig. 3**). It is not surprising that studies report a variable prevalence of low vitamin D status as the studied cohorts differ in

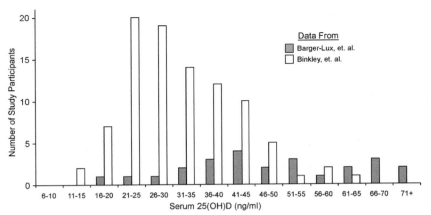

Fig. 2. Distribution of serum 25(OH)D in highly sun-exposed adults. In these 2 studies in which the average total body sun exposure was approximately 11 hours per week, a broad, and somewhat Gaussian, distribution of circulating 25(OH)D is apparent. Note that the study by Barger-Lux and colleagues used a 25(OH)D assay that measures approximately 10% higher than the HPLC assay used in the report by Binkley and colleagues. (*Data from* Binkley N, Novotny R, Krueger D, et al. Low vitamin D status despite abundant sun exposure. J Clin Endocrinol Metab 2007;92:2130–5; and Barger-Lux MJ, Heaney RP. Effects of above average summer sun exposure on serum 25-hydroxyvitamin D and calcium absorption. J Clin Endocrinol Metab 2002;87:4952–6.)

age, sex, race, body mass index, and dietary vitamin D intake. Although it is often assumed that some of the variable prevalence of low vitamin D reflects limited availability of sun exposure due to living at higher latitudes, it is of interest that a recent meta-analysis involving 394 studies comprising more than 32,000 subjects found no

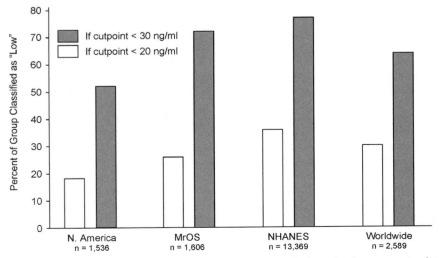

Fig. 3. Prevalence of low vitamin D status in various populations. In these recent cohort studies, low vitamin D status, whether defined as a 25(OH)D level below 20 ng/mL or below 30 ng/mL, is extremely common. (*Data from* Refs.[21,36–38].)

influence of latitude on 25(OH)D concentration.[39] It seems likely that the absence of an effect based on latitude reflects current human indoor lifestyles, clothing, and sun-avoidance behavior. Moreover, it is probable that these factors are contributing to worsening population vitamin D status. Although measurement issues confound data interpretation, recent National Health and Nutrition Examination Survey data report a decline in mean 25(OH)D concentration from the 1988 to 1994 data collection to that of 2000 to 2004.[36,40] In summary, despite variation in 25(OH)D methodology, cutpoint selected, and cohort studied, it is clear that low vitamin D status is common worldwide.

LOW VITAMIN D STATUS: CONSEQUENCES
Bone

Low vitamin D status has long been associated with osteomalacia/rickets, and a role in osteoporosis pathogenesis via calcium malabsorption and secondary hyperparathy-roidism has more recently been suggested. Consistent with an important role of low vitamin D status in osteoporosis, recent meta-analyses find low 25(OH)D to be asso-ciated with higher fracture risk.[41–43] In addition, a dose effect was reported, with greater vitamin D intakes and higher achieved 25(OH)D concentrations providing superior fracture reduction benefit.[43] In summary, while one can debate the cutpoint, low vitamin D status leads to adverse bone consequences.

Muscle Function and Falls

Both genomic and nongenomic effects of vitamin D on muscle have been proposed.[44,45] Regardless of the mechanism, patients with osteomalacia due to vitamin D deficiency develop muscle pain and weakness that is improved with vitamin D therapy.[46–48] Muscle biopsy in such people reveals atrophy of the fast twitch (type II) fibers. As type II fibers are first to be recruited to avoid falling, this observation may explain the increased falls risk in vitamin D deficient individuals.[49] Of note, randomized prospective studies find vitamin D to reduce risk of falls by more than 20%.[50] It seems likely that reducing falls contributes in a major way to the fracture reduction efficacy observed with vitamin D.[51] Moreover, similar to the relationship observed with frac-ture, a higher vitamin D dose provides greater reduction in the risk of falls.[52] The 25(OH)D concentration needed to optimize leg function has been explored, with various cutpoints (eg, 16–24 ng/mL) suggested.[35,53] A recent review finds 25(OH)D concentrations less than approximately 16 ng/mL to be associated with substantially poorer leg function, but additionally finds values greater than approximately 36 to 40 ng/mL to be optimal.[26]

Cancer

Vitamin D has antiproliferative and prodifferentiating effects on many cell types.[54] It has been proposed that these effects are related to local production of 1,25-dihydrox-yvitamin D, thus favorably impacting genes affecting cellular proliferation/differentia-tion and thereby reducing cancer risk.[7] Consistent with this, an extensive, albeit largely associational, literature exists relating higher latitude, low vitamin D intake, and/or less sunlight exposure to increased risk of, or mortality from, multiple types of cancer.[55–59] Prospective trials of vitamin D supplementation with cancer as an end point are very limited; the Women's Health Initiative did not demonstrate a reduc-tion in colon cancer risk, perhaps related to the low daily dose (400 IU) of vitamin D used.[60] However, a smaller prospective study of postmenopausal women found calcium plus vitamin D_3 (1100 IU daily) to reduce overall cancer risk by approximately

60%.[61] To summarize, physiologically logical hypotheses, observational data, and one small randomized trial find low vitamin D status to be associated with higher cancer risk. Additional prospective studies are needed.

Other Conditions

It is likely that vitamin D has immune modulating effects. It has long been recognized that vitamin D deficiency is associated with respiratory infections, which perhaps contributed to the use of cod liver oil in antituberculous therapy.[62,63] More recently, it has become appreciated that calcitriol enhances monocyte mycobacterial killing, likely by facilitating production of the antimicrobial protein, cathelicidin.[64] Moreover, helper type 1 and 2 cells are vitamin D targets, with vitamin D causing a shift toward an anti-inflammatory profile.[65–68] Thus, it is not surprising that low vitamin D status is associated with an increased risk of autoimmune and potentially infectious diseases.[69–71] In addition, inflammation is increasingly being recognized as a contributor to the pathogenesis of various diseases, and vitamin D modulates inflammatory cytokine production.[72–74]

It has been suggested that endemic low vitamin D status is contributing to the increased prevalence of diabetes mellitus. Multiple potential mechanisms have been proposed, including vitamin D increasing insulin production/secretion.[75–77] In addition, observational studies associate low vitamin D status with diabetes type 1 and type 2.[78–80] Prospective studies of vitamin D supplementation are clearly indicated; however, on the whole it appears that low vitamin D status impairs glucose metabolism.[78]

Observational studies report an association between low vitamin D status and cardiovascular disease.[81–85] Potential mechanisms include a vitamin D effect on the endothelium,[86] vascular smooth muscle,[87,88] and/or cardiomyocytes,[89] all of which possess the vitamin D receptor. Prospective studies to further evaluate this reported association are needed.

In summary, low vitamin D status has been associated with a variety of diseases, and biologically plausible hypotheses exist to suggest a possible causal role. However, until confirmed by randomized studies, it is wise to be cautious and recognize that association does not prove causation.

WHEN SHOULD VITAMIN D STATUS BE ASSESSED?

Given the multitude of potential adverse health consequences ascribed to low vitamin D status, it is not surprising that screening 25(OH)D measurement has been advocated.[90,91] Such screening may in fact be appropriate, if it becomes established that low vitamin D status contributes in a causal manner to multiple adverse health outcomes, for example, cardiovascular disease, diabetes, hypertension, and so forth, with which it is currently associated. However, in the absence of randomized trials documenting benefit for these varied outcomes, population-based screening seems premature.

At this time, rather than advocating a population screening approach, it seems reasonable to measure 25(OH)D in those identified as being at high risk of vitamin D deficiency and those for whom a prompt musculoskeletal response to optimization of vitamin D status could be expected. Such groups include those with osteoporosis, a history of falls or with high risk of falls, malabsorption (eg, celiac disease, radiation enteritis, bariatric surgery, and so forth), individuals with liver disease, and those requiring medications known to alter vitamin D status, for example, certain anticonvulsants. Given the relationship of low vitamin D status with cancer, it also seems rational to measure 25(OH)D in those with malignancy.[92]

Alternatively, it could be argued that simple treatment of all individuals with vitamin D should be advocated, thereby making 25(OH)D measurement unnecessary. Although this approach is attractive, it is unfortunately problematic in that no expert consensus exists regarding a recommended dose. For example, the National Osteoporosis Foundation recommends 800 to 1000 IU daily,[93] whereas some vitamin D experts suggest values over 2000 IU.[94] Moreover, as discussed later, vitamins D_2 and D_3 appear to not be equally potent in maintaining 25(OH)D.[95,96] As such, daily intake of 1000 IU of vitamin D_2 may well not be equal to 1000 IU of vitamin D_3. In addition, vitamin D dosing may differ by age in that older adults likely require higher vitamin D intakes because of to the lower capability of skin to produce vitamin D with advancing age.[97] Similarly, clear differences exist between races, with African Americans requiring higher intakes than Caucasian Americans; Hispanic individuals may have intermediate requirements.[98] Some of these differences in required intake may reflect differences in cutaneous melanin content[99]; however, other less well understood between-individual differences in vitamin D absorption and subsequent metabolism may well play a role. In this regard, even among individuals of similar age and race/ethnicity, substantial between-individual variability in response to equal vitamin D intake is noted (**Fig. 4**). Thus, if a health care provider wishes to assure optimal vitamin D status in an individual patient, it is necessary to obtain a 25(OH)D measurement.

APPROACHES TO VITAMIN D REPLETION/SUPPLEMENTATION

Increasing exposure to sunlight would be an effective and free approach to improving vitamin D status. However, this does not seem to be a viable approach, given

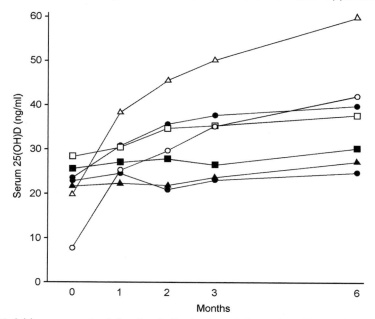

Fig. 4. Variable response to daily vitamin D_3. In these 7 Caucasian older adults (age 66–88 years), all of whom started the study with a 25(OH)D level less than 30 ng/mL, the variable response to daily administration of 1600 IU vitamin D_3 is apparent. (*From* Binkley N, Gemar D, Woods A, et al. Effect of vitamin D_2 or vitamin D_3 supplementation on serum 25OHD. J Bone Miner Res 2008;23(Suppl 1):S350; with permission.)

widespread sun-avoidance campaigns[100–103] based on the association of UV exposure with skin cancer.[104] Sun avoidance and sunscreen use [55,100,105,106] reduce skin exposure to UV radiation and thereby reduce skin vitamin D production.[2,107] In the face of such pervasive and powerful efforts, advocating sun exposure as a population-based measure to improve vitamin D status faces grave obstacles. Despite this, exposure to sunlight in moderation, perhaps for 15 minutes prior to sunscreen application, seems reasonable and is free. It should be noted that due to differences in skin pigmentation, season, latitude, time of day of sun exposure, and amount of body surface exposed, simple recommendations such as "15 minutes of sun on the hands and face" are overly simplistic and will not assure optimal vitamin D status in all people.

Higher dose vitamin D treatment approaches to the clinical correction of vitamin D deficiency, and when to monitor 25(OH)D status during and following vitamin D treatment/supplementation, have received surprisingly little attention. Various "high-dose" repletion approaches, for example, 50,000 IU 3 times weekly, weekly or monthly, have been evaluated.[108–111] A recent evaluation of clinical approaches found vitamin D_2 regimens using more than 600,000 IU administered over an average time of 2 months achieved 25(OH)D values greater than 30 ng/mL in 64% of patients, with the highest value being 100 ng/mL.[108] An additional clinical report of "high-dose" vitamin D_2 (50,000 IU once weekly for up to 3 years) achieved a 25(OH)D level above 30 ng/mL in 23 of 24 patients, with the highest reported value being 100 ng/mL.[112]

Maintenance of vitamin D status with daily doses from 1000 to 4000 IU have been studied.[96,113,114] As noted above, between-individual variability exists. However, a reasonable clinical "rule of thumb" is that the addition of 1000 IU of vitamin D_3 daily can be expected to increase circulating 25(OH)D by approximately 10 ng/mL.

Although daily vitamin D supplementation is very inexpensive (approximately $1 per month), available data find daily vitamin D supplementation to be less effective than expected at increasing serum 25(OH)D status, simply due to failure to reliably take the supplements.[115,116] This finding is hardly surprising in that suboptimal adherence to prescribed therapies for a variety of conditions is well known to clinicians.[117] However, based on the increasing calcium intake of the United States population over time[118] (perhaps related to widespread educational programs), it seems feasible that similar approaches to informing the public about health benefits of vitamin D supplementation could improve endemic low vitamin D status. An alternative, and highly viable, approach is increased availability of vitamin D fortified foods coupled with higher amounts of vitamin D per serving in such food.

How best to monitor 25(OH)D status in individuals receiving vitamin D therapy has not been systematically evaluated. However, as compliance/adherence with many daily therapies (including vitamins) is often poor, monitoring 25(OH)D status 4 to 6 months after initiating treatment in those at high risk (eg, patients with osteomalacia, fragility fractures, or high risk of falls) seems reasonable. Repeat evaluation at earlier time points seems inappropriate, as it takes 3 to 6 months for serum 25(OH)D to plateau following initiation of supplementation.

WHAT IS VITAMIN D TOXICITY?

Both clinicians and patients may express concern that the "high" amounts of vitamin D noted here will lead to toxicity. It is clear that huge doses of vitamin D do lead to hypercalcemia and hypercalciuria. However, there is no clear-cut definition of which level of serum 25(OH)D should be considered "toxic." This doubt has led to variability in the clinical reporting of 25(OH)D results, with some laboratories reporting possibly toxic levels as being above 80 ng/mL while others include up to 100 ng/mL as being within the reference range. Such variability is not surprising, as recent expert opinion suggests "the serum 25(OH)D concentration that is the threshold for vitamin D toxicity has not been established."[119] However, a review of the published vitamin D toxicity cases finds all reports of hypercalcemia due to vitamin D intoxication to be associated with 25(OH)D concentrations greater than 88 ng/mL.[120]

Regarding what constitutes "high" 25(OH)D values, it seems reasonable that highly sun-exposed individuals could be used to assist in the determination of "normal" vitamin D status.[33] When such individuals are evaluated, it appears that the highest attainable 25(OH)D values from cutaneous production are in the 70 to 80 ng/mL range.[30,31] Thus, the current approach of reporting 80 to 100 ng/mL as the upper limit of normal seems appropriate.

DOES THE EFFECT OF VITAMIN D$_2$ DIFFER FROM THAT OF VITAMIN D$_3$?

Two chemically distinct forms of vitamin D exist: vitamin D$_3$ (cholecalciferol) is a 27-carbon molecule, whereas vitamin D$_2$ (ergocalciferol) contains 28 carbons and differs from vitamin D$_3$ by the presence of an additional methyl group and a double bond between carbons 22 and 23. Although clear chemical differences exist, whether vitamin D$_2$ and vitamin D$_3$ are equally effective at increasing 25(OH)D and have equivalent physiologic effects remains unclear. At present, these 2 forms are regarded as equal and interchangeable. However, some data suggest that vitamin D$_2$ is less "potent" at maintaining serum 25(OH)D than is vitamin D$_3$.[95,96,121] Although a recent report challenges this[113] and found D$_2$ and D$_3$ to be equally effective, the vast majority of studies find vitamin D$_3$ to be somewhat more potent. It seems possible that this reflects lower affinity of vitamin D$_2$ for vitamin D binding protein in the circulation, leading to more rapid clearance. As such, use of supplements containing vitamin D$_3$, rather than vitamin D$_2$, seems appropriate.[122] It is unfortunate that vitamin D$_2$ is the only high-dose prescription vitamin D preparation in the United States and some other countries. Despite its lower potency, use of high-dose vitamin D$_2$ does increase circulating 25(OH)D concentration.

SUMMARY

Low vitamin D status is extremely common worldwide due to low dietary intake and low skin production. Suboptimal vitamin D status contributes to many conditions, including osteomalacia/rickets, osteoporosis, falls, and fractures. It is possible or even likely that low vitamin D status increases risk for a multitude of other conditions. Although consensus does not exist, it appears that circulating 25(OH)D concentrations greater than 30 to 32 ng/mL are needed for optimal health. To achieve this, daily intakes of at least 1000 IU of D$_3$ daily are required, and it is probable that substantially higher amounts are required to achieve such values on a population basis. It seems premature to recommend widespread screening for 25(OH)D measurement. Targeted measurement in those at increased risk for vitamin D deficiency and those most likely to have a prompt positive response to supplementation is appropriate. Widespread optimization of vitamin D status likely will lead to prevention of many diseases with attendant reduction of morbidity, mortality, and expense.

REFERENCES

1. Holick MF. Environmental factors that influence the cutaneous production of vitamin D. Am J Clin Nutr 1995;61:638S–45S.

2. Holick MF. The photobiology of vitamin D and its consequences for humans. Ann N Y Acad Sci 1985;453:1–13.

3. Looker AC, Dawson-Hughes B, Calvo MS, et al. Serum 25-hydroxyvitamin D status of adolescents and adults in two seasonal subpopulations from NHANES III. Bone 2002;30:771–7.

4. Rucker D, Allan JA, Fick GH, et al. Vitamin D insufficiency in a population of healthy western Canadians. Can Med Assoc J 2002;166:1517–24.

5. Nesby-O'Dell S, Scanlon KS, Cogswell ME, et al. Hypovitaminosis D prevalence and determinants among African American and white women of reproductive age: Third National Health and Nutrition Examination Survey, 1988-1994. Am J Clin Nutr 2002;76:187–92.

6. Calvo MS, Whiting SJ. Prevalence of vitamin D insufficiency in Canada and the United States: importance to health status and efficacy of current food fortification and dietary supplement use. Nutr Rev 2003;61:107–13.

7. Holick MF. Vitamin D deficiency. N Engl J Med 2007;357:266–81.

8. Binkley N. Does low vitamin D status contribute to "age-related" morbidity? J Bone Miner Res 2007;22:V55–8.

9. DeLuca HF. The vitamin D story: a collaborative effort of basic science and clinical medicine. FASEB J 1988;2:224–36.

10. Standing Committee on the Scientific Evaluation of Dietary Reference Intakes Food and Nutrition Board, Institute of Medicine. Dietary reference intakes for calcium phosphorus, magnesium, vitamin D and fluoride. Washington, DC: National Academy Press; 1997.

11. Lips P, Chapuy MC, Dawson-Hughes B, et al. An international comparison of serum 25-hydroxyvitamin D measurements. Osteoporos Int 1999;9: 394–7.

12. Binkley N, Krueger D, Cowgill C, et al. Assay variation confounds hypovitaminosis D diagnosis: a call for standardization. J Clin Endocrinol Metab 2003;89: 3152–7.

13. Binkley N. Vitamin D: clinical measurement and use. J Musculoskelet Neuronal Interact 2006;6:338–40.

14. Binkley N, Krueger D, Engelke JA, et al. What is your patient's vitamin D status? Clinical consideration of variability in a 25(OH)D measurement. J Bone Miner Res 2008;23(Suppl 1):S351.

15. Heaney RP. Functional indices of vitamin D status and ramifications of vitamin D deficiency. Am J Clin Nutr 2004;80(Suppl):1706S–9S.

16. Dawson-Hughes B, Heaney RP, Holick MF, et al. Estimates of optimal vitamin D status. Osteoporos Int 2005;16:713–6.

17. McCollum EV, Simmonds N, Becker JE, et al. An experimental demonstration of the existence of a vitamin which promotes calcium deposition. J Biol Chem 1922;53:293–312.

18. Steenbock H. The induction of growth promoting and calcifying properties in a ration by exposure to light. Science 1924;60:224–5.

19. DeLuca HF. Overview of general physiologic features and functions of vitamin D. Am J Clin Nutr 2004;80(Suppl):1689S–96S.

20. Lips P. Vitamin D deficiency and secondary hyperparathyroidism in the elderly: Consequences for bone loss and fractures and therapeutic implications. Endocr Rev 2001;22:477–501.

21. Holick MF, Siris ES, Binkley N, et al. Prevalence of vitamin D inadequacy among postmenopausal North American women receiving osteoporosis therapy. J Clin Endocrinol Metab 2005;90:3215–24.

22. Heaney RP, Dowell MS, Hale CA, et al. Calcium absorption varies within the reference range for serum 25-hydroxyvitamin D. J Am Coll Nutr 2003;22:142–6.

23. Need AG, Nordin BEC. Misconceptions—vitamin D insufficiency causes malabsorption of calcium. Bone 2008;42:1021–4.

24. Need AG, O'Loughlin PD, Morris HA, et al. Vitamin D metabolites and calcium absorption in severe vitamin D deficiency. J Bone Miner Res 2008; 23:1859–63.

25. Heaney RP, Armas LAG, Shary JR, et al. 25-hydroxylation of vitamin D_3: relation to circulating vitamin D_3 under various input conditions. Am J Clin Nutr 2008;87: 1738–42.

26. Bischoff-Ferrari HA, Giovannucci E, Willett WC, et al. Estimation of optimal serum concentrations of 25-hydroxyvitamin D for multiple health outcomes. Am J Clin Nutr 2006;84:18–28.

27. Holick MF, MacLaughlin JA, Doppelt SH. Regulation of cutaneous previtamin D_3 photosynthesis in man: skin pigment is not an essential regulator. Science 1981; 211:590–3.

28. Ferguson GW, Gehrmann WH, Karsten KB, et al. Ultraviolet exposure and vitamin D synthesis in a sun-dwelling and a shade-dwelling species of Anolis: are there adaptations for lower ultraviolet B and dietary vitamin D_3 availability in the shade? Physiol Biochem Zool 2005;78:193–200.

29. Awumey EMK, Mitra DA, Hollis BW, et al. Vitamin D metabolism is altered in Asian Indians in the Southern United States: a clinical research center study. J Clin Endocrinol Metab 1998;83:169–73.

30. Binkley N, Novotny R, Krueger D, et al. Low vitamin D status despite abundant sun exposure. J Clin Endocrinol Metab 2007;92:2130–5.

31. Barger-Lux MJ, Heaney RP. Effects of above average summer sun exposure on serum 25-hydroxyvitamin D and calcium absorption. J Clin Endocrinol Metab 2002;87:4952–6.

32. Tangpricha V, Turner A, Spina C, et al. Tanning is associated with optimal vitamin D status (serum 25-hydroxyvitamin D concentration) and higher bone mineral density. Am J Clin Nutr 2004;80:1645–9.

33. Hollis BW. Circulating 25-hydroxyvitamin D levels indicative of vitamin D sufficiency: Implications for establishing a new effective dietary intake recommendation for vitamin D. J Nutr 2005;135:317–22.

34. Hollis BW. Assessment of vitamin D status and definition of a normal circulating range of 25-hydroxyvitamin D. Curr Opin Endocrinol Diabetes Obes 2008;15: 489–94.

35. Kuchuk NO, Pluijm SMF, van Schoor NM, et al. Relationships of serum 25-hydroxyvitamin D to bone mineral density and serum parathyroid hormone and markers of bone turnover in older adults. J Clin Endocrinol Metab 2009;94:1244–50.

36. Ginde AA, Liu MC, Camargo CA. Demographic differences and trends of vitamin D insufficiency in the US population, 1988-2004. Arch Intern Med 2009;169:626–32.

37. Lips P, Hosking D, Lippuner K, et al. The prevalence of vitamin D inadequacy amongst women with osteoporosis: an international epidemiological investigation. J Intern Med 2006;260:245–54.

38. Orwoll E, Nielson CM, Marshall LM, et al. Vitamin D deficiency in older men. J Clin Endocrinol Metab 2009;94:1214–22.

39. Hagenau T, Vest R, Gissel TN, et al. Global vitamin D levels in relation to age, gender, skin pigmentation and latitude: an ecologic meta-regression analysis. Osteoporos Int 2009;20:133–40.

40. Looker AC, Pfeiffer CM, Lacher DA, et al. Serum 25-hydroxyvitamin D status of the US population: 1988-1994 compared with 2000-2004. Am J Clin Nutr 2008; 88:1519–27.

41. Cauley JA, La Croix A, Wu L, et al. Serum 25-hydroxyvitamin D concentrations and risk for hip fractures. Ann Intern Med 2008;149:242–50.

42. Bischoff-Ferrari HA, Willett WC, Wong JB, et al. Fracture prevention with vitamin D supplementation: a meta-analysis of randomized controlled trials. JAMA 2005; 293:2257–64.

43. Bischoff-Ferrari HA, Willett WC, Wong JB, et al. Prevention of nonvertebral fractures with oral vitamin D and dose dependency. Arch Intern Med 2009;169:551–61.

44. Pfeifer M, Begerow B, Minne HW. Vitamin D and muscle function. Osteoporos Int 2002;13:187–94.

45. Janssen HCJP, Samson MM, Verhaar HJJ. Vitamin D deficiency, muscle function, and falls in elderly people. Am J Clin Nutr 2002;75:611–5.

46. Mingrone D, Greco AV, Castagneto M, et al. A woman who left her wheelchair. Lancet 1999;353:806.

47. Skaria J, Katiyar BC, Srivastava TP, et al. Myopathy and neuropathy associated with osteomalacia. Acta Neurol Scand 1975;51:37–58.

48. Glerup H, Mikkelsen K, Poulsen L, et al. Hypovitaminosis D myopathy without biochemical signs of osteomalacic bone involvement. Calcif Tissue Int 2000; 66:419–24.

49. Flicker L, Mead K, MacInnis RJ, et al. Serum vitamin D and falls in older women in residential care in Australia. J Am Geriatr Soc 2003;51:1533–8.

50. Bischoff-Ferrari HA, Dawson-Hughes B, Willett WC, et al. Effect of vitamin D on falls: a meta-analysis. JAMA 2004;291:1999–2006.

51. Dawson-Hughes B, Harris SS, Krall EA, et al. Effect of calcium and vitamin D supplementation on bone density in men and women 65 years of age or older. N Engl J Med 1997;337:670–6.

52. Broe KE, Chen TC, Weinberg J, et al. A higher dose of vitamin D reduces the risk of falls in nursing home residents: a randomized, multiple-dose study. J Am Geriatr Soc 2007;55:234–9.

53. Wicherts IS, van Schoor NM, Boeke AJP, et al. Vitamin D status predicts physical performance and its decline in older persons. J Clin Endocrinol Metab 2007;92: 2058–65.

54. Bikle D. Nonclassic actions of vitamin D. J Clin Endocrinol Metab 2009;94: 26–34.

55. Garland CF, Garland FC, Gorham ED, et al. The role of vitamin D in cancer prevention. Am J Public Health 2006;96:252–61.

56. Gorham ED, Garland CF, Garland FC, et al. Optimal vitamin D status for colorectal cancer prevention A quantitative meta analysis. Am J Prev Med 2007; 32:210–6.

57. Giovannucci E, Liu Y, Rimm EB, et al. Prospective study of predictors of vitamin D status and cancer incidence and mortality in men. J Natl Cancer Inst 2006;98:451–9.

58. Feskanich D, Ma J, Fuchs CS, et al. Plasma vitamin D metabolites and risk of colorectal cancer in women. Cancer Epidemiol Biomarkers Prev 2004;13: 1502–8.

59. Garland CF, Gorham ED, Mohr SB, et al. Vitamin D and prevention of breast cancer: pooled analysis. J Steroid Biochem 2007;103:708–11.

60. Wactawski-Wende J, Kotchen JM, Anderson GL, et al. Calcium plus vitamin D supplementation and the risk of colorectal cancer. N Engl J Med 2006;354: 684–96.

61. Lappe JM, Travers-Gustafson D, Davies KM, et al. Vitamin D and calcium supplementation reduces cancer risk: results of a randomized trial. Am J Clin Nutr 2007;85:1586–91.
62. Martineau AR, Honecker FU, Wilkinson RJ, et al. Vitamin D in the treatment of pulmonary tuberculosis. J Steroid Biochem Mol Biol 2007;103:793–8.
63. Russell B. The history of lupus vulgaris: its recognition, nature, treatment and prevention. Proc R Soc Med 1954;48:127–32.
64. Liu PT, Stenger S, Li H, et al. Toll-like receptor triggering of a vitamin D-mediated human antimicrobial response. Science 2006;311:170–3.
65. van Etten E, Mathieu C. Immunoregulation by 1,25-dihydroxyvitamin D_3: Basic concepts. J Steroid Biochem Mol Biol 2005;97:93–101.
66. Bemiss CJ, Mahon BD, Henry A, et al. Interleukin-2 is one of the targets of 1,25-dihydroxyvitamin D_3 in the immune system. Arch Biochem Biophys 2002;402:249–54.
67. Mahon BD, Wittke A, Weaver V, et al. The targets of vitamin D depend on the differentiation and activation status of CD4 positive T cells. J Cell Biochem 2003;402:922–33.
68. Cantorna MT, Humpal-Winter J, DeLuca HF. In vivo upregulation on interleukin-4 is one mechanism underlying the immunoregulatory effects of 1,25-dihydroxyvitamin D_3. Arch Biochem Biophys 2000;377:135–8.
69. Peterlik M, Cross HS. Vitamin D and calcium deficits predispose for multiple chronic diseases. Eur J Clin Invest 2005;35:290–304.
70. Froicu M, Weaver V, Wynn TA, et al. A crucial role for the vitamin D receptor in experimental inflammatory bowel diseases. Mol Endocrinol 2003;17:2386–92.
71. Cantorna MT, Hayes CE, DeLuca HF. 1,25-dihydroxyvitamin D_3 reversibly blocks the progression of relapsing encephalomyelitis, a model of multiple sclerosis. Proc Natl Acad Sci U S A 1996;93:7861–4.
72. Boonstra A, Barrat FJ, Craine C, et al. 1 alpha 25-dihydroxyvitamin D_3 has a direct effect on naive CD4+ T cells to enhance the development of TH2 cells. J Immunol 2001;167:4974–80.
73. Willheim M, Thien R, Schrattbauer K, et al. Regulatory effects of 1 alpha 25 dihydroxyvitamin D_3 on cytokine production of human peripheral blood lymphocytes. J Clin Endocrinol Metab 1999;84:3739–44.
74. Rigby WF, Denome S, Fanger MW. Regulation of lymphokine production and human T-lymphocyte activation by 1,25 dihydroxyvitamin D_3: Specific inhibition at the level of messenger RNA. J Clin Invest 1987;79:1659–64.
75. Kadowaki S, Norman AW. Demonstration that the vitamin D metabolite $1,25(OH)_2$-vitamin D_3 and not $24R,25(OH)_2$-vitamin D_3 is essential for normal insulin secretion in the perfused rat pancreas. Diabetes 1985;34:315–20.
76. Norman AW, Frankel JB, Heldt AM, et al. Vitamin D deficiency inhibits pancreatic secretion of insulin. Science 1980;209:823–5.
77. Rabinovitch A, Suarez-Pinzon WL, Sooy K, et al. Expression of calbindin-D28K in a pancreatic islet b-cell line protects against cytokine-induced apoptosis and necrosis. Endocrinology 2001;142:3649–55.
78. Mathieu C, Gysemans C, Guilietti A, et al. Vitamin D and diabetes. Diabetologia 2005;48:1247–57.
79. Zipitis CS, Akobeng AK. Vitamin D supplementation in early childhood and risk of type 1 diabetes: a systematic review and meta-analysis. Arch Dis Child 2008;93:512–7.

80. Pittas AG, Lau J, Hu FB, et al. The role of vitamin D and calcium in type 2 diabetes. A systematic review and meta-analysis. J Clin Endocrinol Metab 2007;92:2017–29.
81. Grimes DS, Hindle E, Dyer T. Sunlight, cholesterol and coronary heart disease. QJM 1996;89:579–89.
82. Voors AW, Johnson WD. Altitude and arteriosclerotic heart disease mortality in white residents of 99 of the 100 largest cities in the United States. J Chronic Dis 1979;32:157–62.
83. Rostand SG. Ultraviolet light may contribute to geographic and racial blood pressure differences. Hypertension 1997;30:150–6.
84. Scragg R, Jackson RD, Holdaway IM, et al. Myocardial infarction is inversely associated with plasma 25-hydroxyvitamin D_3 levels: A community based study. Int J Epidemiol 1990;19:559–63.
85. Poole KE, Loveridge N, Barker PJ, et al. Reduced vitamin D in acute stroke. Stroke 2006;37:243–5.
86. Merke J, Milde P, Lewicka S, et al. Identification and regulation of 1,25-dihydroxyvitamin D_3 receptor activity and biosynthesis of 1,25-dihydroxyvitamin D_3: studies in cultured bovine aortic endothelial cells and human dermal capillaries. J Clin Invest 1989;83:1903–15.
87. Somjen D, Weisman Y, Kohen F, et al. 25-hydroxyvitamin D_3-1 alpha hydroxylase is expressed in human vascular smooth muscle cells and is upregulated by parathyroid hormone and estrogenic compounds. Circulation 2005;111:1666–71.
88. Merke J, Hofmann W, Goldschmidt D, et al. Demonstration of 1,25 $(OH)_2$ vitamin D_3 receptors and actions in vascular smooth muscle cells in vitro. Calcif Tissue Int 1987;41:112–4.
89. Holick MF. High prevalence of vitamin D inadequacy and implications for health. Mayo Clin Proc 2006;81:353–73.
90. Holick MF. Too little vitamin D in premenopausal women: why should we care? Am J Clin Nutr 2002;76:3–4.
91. Giovannucci E. Can vitamin D reduce total mortality? Arch Intern Med 2007;167:1709–10.
92. Anonymous. Vitamin D deficiency: information for cancer patients. New York: The Bone and Cancer Foundation; 2008.
93. Anonymous. Clinician's guide to prevention and treatment of osteoporosis. Washington, DC: National Osteoporosis Foundation; 2008.
94. Heaney RP. Barriers to optimizing vitamin D_3 intake for the elderly. J Nutr 2006;136:1123–5.
95. Armas LAG, Hollis BW, Heaney RP. Vitamin D_2 is much less effective than vitamin D_3 in humans. J Clin Endocrinol Metab 2004;89:5387–91.
96. Binkley N, Gemar D, Woods A, et al. Effect of vitamin D_2 or vitamin D_3 supplementation on serum 25OHD. J Bone Miner Res 2008;23(Suppl 1):S350.
97. MacLaughlin JA, Holick MF. Aging decreases the capacity of human skin to produce vitamin D_3. J Clin Invest 1985;76:1536–8.
98. Weaver CM, Fleet JC. Vitamin D requirements: current and future. Am J Clin Nutr 2004;80:1735S–9S.
99. Matsuoka LY, Wortsman J, Haddad JG, et al. Racial pigmentation and the cutaneous synthesis of vitamin D. Arch Dermatol 1991;127:536–8.
100. Anonymous. National coalition for sun safety. Available at: http://www.aad.org/public/sunsafetydb.htm. Accessed February 10, 2010.
101. Task Force on Community Preventive Services. Recommendations to prevent skin cancer by reducing exposure to ultraviolet radiation. Am J Prev Med 2004;27:467–70.

102. Kirsner RS, Parker DF, Brathwaite N, et al. Sun protection policies in Miami-Dade county public schools: opportunities for skin cancer prevention. Pediatr Dermatol 2005;22:513–9.

103. Anonymous. Saving your skin from sun damage. Am Fam Physician 2006;74: 815–6.

104. Randle HW. Suntanning: differences in perceptions throughout history. Mayo Clin Proc 1997;72:461–6.

105. Skin cancer primary prevention and education initiative 2006 Sun safety at school: What you can do. Center for Disease Control; Guidelines for School. Available at: www.cdc.gov/cancer/skin/pdf/sunsafety_v0908.pdf. Accessed February 10, 2010.

106. US Environmental Protection Agency. SunWise Program. Available at: www.epa. gov/sunwise. Accessed February 10, 2010.

107. Matsuoka LY, Wortsman J, Hanafin N, et al. Chronic sunscreen use decreases circulating concentrations of 25-hydroxyvitamin D. Arch Dermatol 1988;124: 1802–4.

108. Pepper KJ, Judd SE, Nanes MS, et al. Evaluation of vitamin D repletion regimens to correct vitamin D status in adults. Endocr Pract 2009;15:95–103.

109. Przybelski R, Agrawal S, Krueger D, et al. Rapid correction of low vitamin D status in nursing home residents. Osteoporos Int 2008;19:1621–8.

110. Malabanan A, Veronikis IE, Holick MF. Redefining vitamin D insufficiency. Lancet 1998;351:805–6.

111. Geller JL, Adams JS. Vitamin D therapy. Current Osteoporos Rep 2008;6:5–11.

112. Ramamurthy R, Przybelski R, Gemar D, et al. Long-term high-dose vitamin D supplementation in the elderly is both safe and efficacious. J Clin Densitom 2009;12:375–6.

113. Holick MF, Biancuzzo RM, Chen TC, et al. Vitamin D_2 is as effective as vitamin D_3 in maintaining circulating concentrations of 25-hydroxyvitamin D. J Clin Endocrinol Metab 2008;93:677–81.

114. Heaney RP, Davies KM, Chen TC, et al. Human serum 25-hydroxycholecalciferol response to extended oral dosing with cholecalciferol. Am J Clin Nutr 2003;77: 204–10.

115. The Record Trial Reporting Group. Oral vitamin D_3 and calcium for secondary prevention of low-trauma fractures in elderly people (Randomized Evaluation of Calcium or vitamin D, RECORD): a randomized-placebo-controlled trial. Lancet 2005;365:1621–8.

116. Wactawski-Wende J, Jackson RD, LaCroix AZ, et al. Calcium plus vitamin D supplementation and the risk of fractures. N Engl J Med 2006;354:669–83.

117. Chesnut CHI. Treating osteoporosis with bisphosphonates and addressing adherence. Drugs 2006;66:1351–9.

118. Briefel RR, Johnson CL. Secular trends in dietary intake in the United States. Annu Rev Nutr 2004;24:401–31.

119. Vieth R. Vitamin D toxicity, policy and science. J Bone Miner Res 2007;22(Suppl 2):V64–8.

120. Vieth R. Vitamin D supplementation, 25-hydroxyvitamin D concentrations and safety. Am J Clin Nutr 1999;69:842–56.

121. Trang HM, Cole DEC, Rubin LA, et al. Evidence that vitamin D_3 increases serum 25-hydroxyvitamin D more efficiently than does vitamin D_2. Am J Clin Nutr 1998; 68:854–8.

122. Houghton LA, Vieth R. The case against ergocalciferol (vitamin D2) as a vitamin supplement. Am J Clin Nutr 2006;84:694–7.

Maternal Vitamin D Status: Implications for the Development of Infantile Nutritional Rickets

Kebashni Thandrayen, MBBCh, FCPaed(SA), MMed(Paeds)*,
John M. Pettifor, MBBCh, FCPaed(SA), PhD(Med)

KEYWORDS

- Vitamin D • Calcium • Infantile rickets • Pregnancy • Lactation
- Vitamin D requirements • Vitamin D deficiency

Infantile nutritional rickets is re-emerging as a worldwide health problem despite having been nearly eradicated in many countries, including the United States, in the 1930s and 1940s with the introduction of foods fortified with vitamin D, such as milk.[1] The resurgence of vitamin D deficiency and rickets in developed countries and its continued presence in many developing countries have raised considerable concern and questions about the epidemiology and prevention of vitamin D deficiency rickets during infancy.

Vitamin D fortification of food and/or milk (including infant milk formulas) and the provision of vitamin D supplements had eradicated the problem in North America and many parts of Europe[2] but the immigration of large numbers of dark-skinned families, and the emphasis on exclusive breastfeeding and "breast is best", have led to a rising incidence of vitamin D deficiency in most developed countries. Other reasons for the resurgence of rickets include the use of sunscreens[3] to reduce the risk of developing skin malignancies from ultraviolet (UV) radiation and religious/social practices that limit adequate sun exposure in pregnant and lactating mothers and their young children.[4]

Developing countries have also not been spared. Rapid urbanization and the movement of rural families into overcrowded shanty towns associated with increased atmospheric pollution[5] are some of the factors that have seen a continuation of or increase in the prevalence of rickets in young children.

MRC Mineral Metabolism Research Unit, Department of Pediatrics, Faculty of Health Sciences, University of Witwatersrand, Johannesburg, South Africa
* Corresponding author.
E-mail address: kebashni.thandrayen@wits.ac.za

Endocrinol Metab Clin N Am 39 (2010) 303–320
doi:10.1016/j.ecl.2010.02.006
0889-8529/10/$ – see front matter © 2010 Elsevier Inc. All rights reserved.

endo.theclinics.com

Over the last 20 years, there has been an increasing realization of the role played by maternal vitamin D status during pregnancy and lactation in influencing the vitamin D status of the newborn and young infant.

This article briefly describes the pathophysiology of vitamin D homeostasis in the mother-infant pair and the interrelationship between maternal vitamin D status and infantile nutritional rickets, and discusses ways of improving maternal vitamin D status and thus reducing the prevalence of vitamin D deficiency in the young infant.

CAUSE AND EPIDEMIOLOGY OF INFANTILE NUTRITIONAL RICKETS

The clinical picture of nutritional rickets was first described by Whistler (1645) and Glisson (1650), who reported that the disease rarely occurred before 6 months of age and was most prevalent between 6 months and 2.5 years of age.[6] Although the classic features of vitamin D deficiency rickets are most commonly seen during this period, studies have shown that symptomatic vitamin D deficiency can develop early in infancy.[7–12] In Turkey, for example, in a 2-year period, 42 infants less than 3 months of age were diagnosed with vitamin D deficiency and/or nutritional rickets,[8] and isolated cases of congenital rickets have been described from countries such as Greece and India.

As the clinical features of vitamin D deficiency may be absent or not pathognomonic of rickets in early infancy,[8,13] there may be an underestimation of the real prevalence of vitamin D deficiency in many studies.

Symptoms of hypocalcemia itself are frequently the presenting features of symptomatic vitamin D deficiency in infants less than 6 months of age, and asymptomatic hypocalcemia may be missed. At this early stage, radiographs generally do not show the typical features of rickets, although there may be some bone demineralization.[14] The development of symptomatic hypocalcemia, which occurs before any radiological changes, has been attributed to the high demand for calcium during the rapid growth characteristic of early infancy. Ladhani and colleagues[14] have reported that the ages of infants/children presenting with symptomatic hypocalcemia correlate with periods of rapid growth (**Fig. 1**). During childhood before the pubertal growth spurt, the slower bone growth and thus lower calcium demands allow the body to avoid symptomatic hypocalcemia by drawing on bone stores of calcium through secondary hyperparathyroidism in situations of vitamin D deficiency.[13] Symptomatic hypocalcemia in young infants caused by vitamin D deficiency has been reported from several countries, including the United Kingdom,[14,15] Turkey, where the infants were exclusively breastfed,[8] and Australia, where hypocalcemia was the mode of presentation in 50% of patients presenting at less than 6 months of age.[12] In the last study, hypocalcemic seizures were more common in the winter and spring months than in summer and autumn months.[12] In an Indian study of 13 exclusively breastfed infants presenting with hypocalcemic seizures secondary to proven vitamin D deficiency, the youngest was 2 months old and the oldest 6 months old.[7] As is typical of this group of infants, none had received vitamin D supplements and all the mothers had low circulating 25-hydroxyvitamin D (25-OHD) concentrations. It is clear from the literature that there is an increasing awareness among health practitioners of vitamin D deficiency presenting as hypocalcemic seizures during the first 6 months of life.[7,12] Whether or not the incidence is increasing is unclear as most studies are case reports.

Adequate endogenous synthesis of vitamin D is essential to establish and maintain vitamin D sufficiency and to prevent rickets in most children, as few foods, unless fortified, contain adequate amounts of vitamin D to maintain vitamin D sufficiency. The cutaneous production of vitamin D (cholecalciferol or vitamin D_3) depends on the

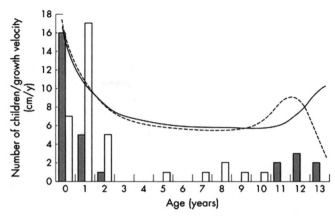

Fig. 1. Ages of children with vitamin D deficiency presenting with (*dark bars*) and without (*light bars*) hypocalcaemic symptoms. Growth velocity lines for boys (*solid*) and girls (*dotted lines*) have been superimposed onto the graph. (*Adapted from* Ladhani S, Srinivasan L, Buchanan C, et al. Presentation of vitamin D deficiency. Arch Dis Child 2004;89(8):782; with permission.)

amount of skin exposed and the dose of UV radiation with a wavelength of between 290 and 315 nm. Thus time of day, season, latitude, length of sunlight exposure, percentage of body surface exposed to sunlight (clothing), and skin pigmentation are all important factors influencing vitamin D formation.[16] The amount of UV-B radiation available for vitamin D synthesis is reduced in early morning, late evening, in the winter, and at latitudes greater than 37° N or S.[17,18] Evidence shows that 1 erythemal dose of sunlight, which is equivalent to a healthy young or middle-aged adult being on a sunny beach and obtaining enough sun to cause a slight pinkness to the skin, synthesizes approximately 20,000 IU D_3.[19] It has been suggested that for white infants to maintain vitamin D sufficiency, 2 hours of sunlight exposure per week are the minimum required if only the face is exposed, or 30 min/wk if the upper and lower extremities are exposed.[20] Dark-skinned persons are more at risk of vitamin D deficiency than light-skinned persons because increased melanin content of the skin absorbs more UV radiation.[21] Dark-skinned persons require 5 to 10 times the exposure of sunlight to produce the same amount of vitamin D_3 in their skin as does a white person with light skin.[21,22] Preventable factors and practices that are perceived to be health beneficial but detrimental to cutaneous vitamin D synthesis include limiting skin exposure to sunshine by avoiding direct sunlight, ensuring good skin coverage by clothing, and the use of sunscreens to prevent UV radiation penetrating the skin. Religious and cultural practices may also limit vitamin D synthesis, for example, purdah (seclusion of women from public observation) and veiling are primarily responsible for vitamin D deficiency in Muslim women and their infants,[4] and the practice of zuo yuezi or "doing the month" (confinement of new mothers and their babies to their beds) in China predisposes children to developing rickets.[23]

The burden and prevalence of infantile nutritional rickets have been reported in studies in the past few decades from developing regions such as the Middle East[24] and Asia[25,26], and from developed countries such as the United States,[1,25] United Kingdom,[14,15] Canada,[26] Australia,[27] and Greece.[28] Common factors that seem to be important in most of the studies include maternal vitamin D deficiency, being breastfed, birth during winter and spring, and increased skin pigmentation. In Canada, the overall confirmed cases of vitamin D deficiency were 2.9 cases per 100,000 children less than 7 years of age in a 2-year period[26] and in the United Kingdom the annual incidence rate was 7.5 per 100,000 children less than 5 years of age.[29] Both studies observed higher rates of vitamin D deficiency among darker-skinned and black African or African Caribbean individuals.[26,29] Furthermore, pregnant South Asian women residing in the United Kingdom have a high incidence of hypovitaminosis D, which is exacerbated by the low availability of overhead sun together with the risk factors of darker skin pigmentation, low amounts of outdoor activity, and excessive skin coverage by clothing.[30,31] A high prevalence of hypovitaminosis D has also been observed in Northern India, a tropical country with abundant sunshine, among pregnant Asian women and their newborns not observing purdah.[32] Despite the sunshine in Greece, mothers and their exclusively breastfed infants were found to be vitamin D deficient, especially during the winter and spring months.[28] Other risk factors in Greece included a lack of vitamin D enriched foods and use of sun-block creams, as well as women in urban areas spending little time outdoors because of indoor jobs.[28] Studies performed in the United States suggest that hypovitaminosis D affects healthy children of all ages and all races/ethnicities even although it is more common in dark-skinned infants and their mothers and those living in the northern states.[7,33–35] A study of 200 black and 200 white newborns in Pittsburgh, Pennsylvania found that 9.7% of white compared with 45.6% of black neonates had vitamin D deficiency (25-OHD <15 ng/mL), whereas approximately half of black and white neonates were vitamin D insufficient (25-OHD 15–32 ng/ml). There was no seasonal effect on vitamin D status in black neonates, which probably reflects the low vitamin D status of their mothers throughout the year.[36] Maternal vitamin D deficiency during pregnancy has been documented in many recent reports (**Table 1**); these studies raise the concern that most infants are being born with limited vitamin D reserves and in many, circulating 25-OHD concentrations indicate vitamin D deficiency.[37]

The pathogenesis of rickets in the Middle East is multifactorial, but maternal vitamin D deficiency plays a major role.[24] In Turkey, rickets is a disease of the underprivileged,[24,38] strongly correlated with poor social background and insufficient exposure to sunlight, and a lack of vitamin D supplementation seems to be decisive for the development of the disease.[24] Recent findings by Ozkan and colleagues[39] confirmed that 89% of patients with rickets had veiled mothers whose bodies were not directly exposed to sunlight. Overcrowding, smaller houses, lower family incomes, and lower parental education levels were all correlated with the prevalence of nutritional rickets.[38,39] Andiran and colleagues[38] have also emphasized that in Turkey the

Table 1
The prevalence of vitamin D deficiency (defined as 25-OHD<25 nmol/L) in pregnant women

Country	Percentage
United Kingdom	18
United Arab Emirates	25
Iran	80
North India	42
New Zealand	61
Netherlands	60–84 of non-Western women

Data from Dawodu A, Wagner CL. Mother-child vitamin D deficiency: an international perspective. Arch Dis Child 2007;92(9):737–40.

2 most important risk factors for a low serum 25-OHD level in a newborn are maternal 25-OHD concentrations less than 25 nmol/L (odds ratio [OR]=15.2, $P = .002$), and a covered mother (OR= 6.8, $P = .011$). Among maternal factors, interlude to the next pregnancy, prenatal care, physician visits, nutrition during nursing, and exposed body surface were lower in mothers of infants with rickets.[24] Sociocultural practices of mothers seem to be more important than nutritional factors in the pathogenesis of infantile nutritional rickets.

Robinson and colleagues[12] reported on the re-emerging burden of rickets in Sydney, Australia, which is a modern city with good nutritional health standards and high sunlight hours. These investigators implicated the immigration trends from North African, Middle Eastern, and Asian countries as the cause for the increasing prevalence of vitamin D deficiency. In their study, immigrant infants or first-generation offspring of immigrant parents with maternal vitamin D deficiency and exclusive or prolonged breastfeeding were prominent factors.[12] It is likely that the vitamin D status of immigrant women deteriorated after arriving in Australia, as less time was probably spent outdoors.[36]

In developing and developed countries, vitamin D deficiency has resurfaced. Despite adequate sunshine in certain regions, the fortification of food and dairy products in many countries and preventive strategies, the prevalence and burden of vitamin D deficiency are probably not diminishing and may be increasing. The major worldwide problems are lack of sun exposure, breastfeeding without vitamin D supplementation, and maternal vitamin D deficiency.

VITAMIN D AND CALCIUM HOMEOSTASIS IN THE MOTHER-INFANT PAIR DURING PREGNANCY AND LACTATION

Major changes in maternal calcium homeostasis take place during pregnancy and lactation, as the mother must provide enough calcium for fetal development during pregnancy and to meet breast milk calcium concentrations during lactation. In the nonpregnant and nonlactating woman, vitamin D sufficiency is essential to maintain normal calcium and bone homeostasis. However, during pregnancy and lactation, the vitamin D endocrine system probably plays little role in the physiologic alterations in maternal calcium homeostasis. In utero, the fetus too probably does not require the transplacental transfer of vitamin D to maintain normal calcium homeostasis as the placental transfer of calcium between mother and fetus is independent of vitamin D.[40] It is only after birth that the infant's dependency on vitamin D becomes evident, at least with respect to calcium metabolism and skeletal health in the infant.[41]

The placenta actively transports calcium (25–250 mg/d)[40] (**Fig. 2**) to the fetus, whose total and ionized serum calcium concentrations are maintained at about 1 mg/dL more than maternal levels.[42,43] To meet the needs for fetal bone development and growth, maternal intestinal calcium absorption increases by approximately 33%, with the maximum rate occurring in the last trimester.[43] These processes are mediated during pregnancy in part by increased 1,25-$(OH)_2$D concentrations but also through the actions of other regulating factors such as parathyroid hormone-related protein (PTHrP), estradiol, placental lactogen, and prolactin.[41,44]

Approximately 80% of fetal skeletal mineral is deposited between 25 weeks of gestation and term. At birth, neonatal total body calcium is approximately 30 g, of which 99% is in the skeleton.[45]

Fetal plasma calcium and phosphorus concentrations are higher than those of the neonate after delivery, which are higher than those of adults. The fetus has increased circulating levels of calcitonin and low levels of parathyroid hormone and the active

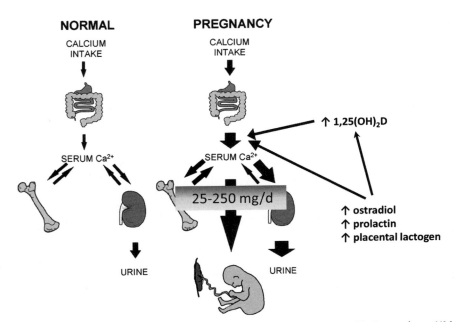

Fig. 2. Calcium homeostasis during pregnancy. (*Adapted from* Kovacs CS, Kronenburg HM. Maternal-fetal calcium and bone metabolism during pregnancy, puerperium, and lactation. Endocr Rev 1997;18(6):859; with permission.)

metabolite of vitamin D, 1,25-dihydroxyvitamin D (1,25-(OH)$_2$D).[46,47] At birth, maternal transfer of calcium and phosphorus ceases when the umbilical cord is cut, with the result that parathyroid hormone levels increase during the first 24 to 48 hours of extra-uterine life.[48] By 24 to 36 hours serum total calcium concentrations reach their nadir of about 9.0 mg/dL (2.25 mmol/L), whereas ionized calcium levels reach a nadir of 4.9 mg/dL (1.2 mmol/L) by approximately 16 hours of life.[33,49] The rapid decline in circulating calcium is believed to reflect continued incorporation of mineral substrate into bone in the face of a reduced influx caused by low dietary intakes and the absence of placental transfer in association with initially low levels of parathyroid hormone (PTH) and 1,25-(OH)$_2$D.[33] In the immediate postnatal period, the neonate becomes dependent on PTH and 1,25-(OH)$_2$D to maintain calcium homeostasis; thus vitamin D deficiency in the neonate may cause a prolongation of the neonatal hypocalcemia and a more severe decrease in serum calcium concentrations postnatally.[41]

During pregnancy 25-OHD readily crosses the placenta[50–52] (**Fig. 3**) such that cord blood 25-OHD levels are between 80% and 100% of maternal concentrations.[53–55] Vitamin D and 1,25-(OH)$_2$D do not cross the placenta into the fetus in appreciable amounts. Thus, the newborn is dependent on the maternal supply of 25-OHD to ensure an adequate vitamin D status at birth. As 25-OHD has a short half-life (2–3 weeks), newborn concentrations decrease rapidly during the neonatal period unless an exogenous source of vitamin D is provided.[34] Thus if maternal vitamin D status is poor, the low 25-OHD concentrations in the neonate decrease rapidly into the deficient range.

The mechanism by which the increased demands for calcium during lactation are met by the mother is different from that which occurs during pregnancy. Maternal losses of calcium and phosphorus through breast milk are more than 4 times greater than

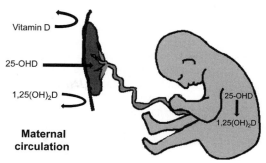

Fig. 3. Fetal vitamin D homeostasis during pregnancy. 25-OHD crosses the placenta; vitamin D and 1.25-(OH)₂ D do not.

those that are required by the fetus during pregnancy[40,44] (**Fig. 4**). During lactation the major source of calcium is the maternal skeleton, with 5% to 10% of bone mass being lost over the course of 6 months of lactation.[41] As mentioned earlier, during pregnancy the increased calcium demands are met by an increase in intestinal calcium absorption, and bone mass changes little during pregnancy. The probable mechanism by which bone mineral is mobilized during lactation is through the production of PTHrP in breast tissue and its secretion into the maternal circulation, mobilizing bone mineral and suppressing maternal PTH secretion. Further, the low estrogen levels characteristic of lactation enhance skeletal mobilization. Although serum calcitonin levels are

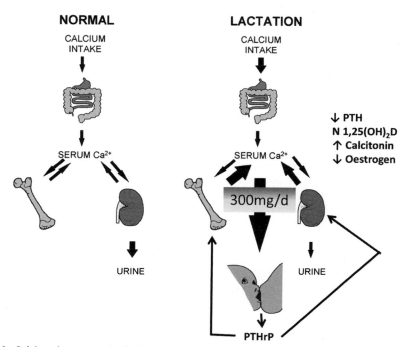

Fig. 4. Calcium homeostasis during lactation. (*Adapted from* Kovacs CS, Kronenburg HM. Maternal-fetal calcium and bone metabolism during pregnancy, puerperium, and lactation. Endocr Rev 1997;18(6):859; with permission.)

increased and may help to protect the calcium stores, these are insufficient to prevent rapid bone loss. Intestinal calcium absorption during lactation returns to normal from the increased rate that occurs during pregnancy. Neither habitual calcium intake nor calcium supplementation influences the rate or extent of maternal bone loss during lactation.[35] In general, maternal bone mass recovers to prepregnancy values within 3 to 6 months following the cessation of lactation by mechanisms that are unclear at present.[41]

Unlike the pattern of vitamin D and its metabolite transfer across the placenta during pregnancy, when the major transferred metabolite is 25-OHD, during lactation it seems that the parent vitamin D crosses readily into breast milk, whereas only about 1% of maternal circulating 25-OHD and no 1,25-(OH)$_2$D crosses. Thus breast milk contains the parent vitamins (D$_2$ and D$_3$) and small amounts of their 25-hydroxylation products (25-OHD$_2$ and 25-OHD$_3$) as well as other metabolites that are present in plasma.[56] The small amount of maternal circulating 25-OHD that crosses into breast milk provides a steady supply of antirachitic activity that is resistant to daily fluctuations in vitamin D supply,[57] although in most women the amount in breast milk is too small to prevent vitamin D deficiency in the breastfed infant. In contrast, 20% to 30% of maternal circulating vitamin D is expressed in breast milk.[57] However, maternal circulating vitamin D concentrations are low unless the mother has recently been exposed to sunlight or vitamin D supplements [58]; thus in the normal urban situation the parent vitamin D content of breast milk is low, resulting in the characteristically low antirachitic activity of breast milk.[57,59,60] It has been estimated that breast milk from an unsupplemented vitamin D replete mother contains the equivalent of 20 and 60 IU/L of antirachitic activity in the form of various metabolites,[61] which is insufficient to meet the vitamin D requirements of the exclusively breastfed infant[56] and contributes little to the infant's vitamin D status[38,56,61,62] (**Fig. 5**). Using the Heaney regression model[63] the currently recommended supplement of 400 IU/d vitamin D$_3$ during lactation would increase the maternal circulating 25-OHD concentration by 2.8 ng/mL following 5 months of supplementation, thus doing little to sustain the vitamin D status of the mother or her nursing infant.[57] However, this calculation does not take into account the possible increase in circulating maternal vitamin D levels and thus the possible resultant increase in parent vitamin D transfer into breast milk.

The lower vitamin D activity in breast milk of African American women is well documented,[59] and reflects the generally poorer vitamin D status of black women compared with white women in the United States. The cutaneous synthesis of vitamin D in individuals with darker skin pigmentation requires longer sun exposure or higher doses of UV-B radiation to produce comparable serum 25-OHD to that produced in

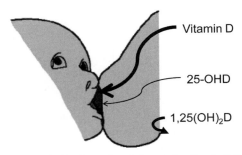

Fig. 5. Vitamin D homeostasis during lactation. It is mainly vitamin D (the parent compound) that crosses in breast milk.

individuals with lighter skin pigmentation.[64] The high incidence of obesity in African American women may also play a role in reducing 25-OHD concentrations, as has been reported by Parikh and colleagues,[65] who found a significant negative correlation between body mass index (calculated as weight in kilograms divided by the square of height in meters) or obesity and serum 25-OHD in African Americans.

The association between low maternal 25-OHD concentrations and poor vitamin D status in their breastfed infants has been noted in studies conducted in many different countries. This association probably reflects a combination of 2 major factors: first, the lack of adequate vitamin D activity in the breast milk of the vitamin D insufficient or deplete mother, and second, the exposure of the infant to similar social and environmental factors to those that induced vitamin D insufficiency in the mother (mainly a lack of sunlight exposure). This combination is highlighted in studies conducted in the Middle East, where there are large amounts of sunshine for most of the year. Despite the abundance of sunshine in the United Arab Emirates, exclusively breastfed, healthy, term infants and their mothers have a high prevalence of hypovitaminosis D without supplemental vitamin D.[66] In this study, rachitic infants were almost all breastfed (92% compared with 58% in age-matched controls), were not on vitamin D supplements (92% vs 62%), had limited sunlight exposure (0 min/d vs 45 min/d), and their mothers had lower 25-OHD concentrations (5.3 ng/mL vs 9.6 ng/mL) than mothers of nonrachitic children. In a study from Johannesburg, South Africa, which has an average of more than 8 hours of sunshine per day throughout the year, low maternal 25-OHD concentrations (10.6 ng/mL) during the winter months were believed to be responsible for the low 25-OHD concentrations in exclusively breastfed young infants.[34] Similarly in Pakistan, a high prevalence of vitamin D deficiency in breastfed infants (55%) and nursing mothers (45%) was observed.[67] In Sydney, Australia, 91% of a pediatric cohort with rickets had a 25-OHD level of less than 20 ng/mL if they were breastfed by a vitamin D deficient mother (<20 ng/mL).[12] All these studies highlight the importance of maternal vitamin D deficiency during lactation in the pathogenesis of rickets in breastfed infants. It is also important to ensure that the maternal vitamin D status during pregnancy is optimized so that the neonate starts life with a good 25-OHD concentration, as vitamin D stores in the neonate are limited because of the lack of passage of the parent vitamin D across the placenta.[68] Thus, in early infancy, the vitamin D status of breastfed infants depends on the 25-OHD transferred across the placenta during intrauterine life.[34,54] Thereafter, because of the short 3-week half-life of 25-OHD, either an exogenous supply of vitamin D through breast milk or infant supplementation or the endogenous production through sunlight exposure is necessary to maintain vitamin D sufficiency.

CONSEQUENCES OF VITAMIN D DEFICIENCY IN MOTHER-INFANT PAIRS

Besides the increased incidence of infantile rickets, neonatal hypocalcaemia, and the rare entity of congenital rickets, there is new evidence to suggest that there may be other consequences of maternal and infant vitamin D deficiency on the growing infant, child, and adolescent.

Intrauterine programming is important for neonatal and adult health, including bone health, and is determined by among other factors, adequate maternal nutritional and mineral homeostasis and the fetal hormonal milieu.[69] An adequate vitamin D status and normal calcium homeostasis during pregnancy may be essential components of intrauterine programming.

Furthermore, the vitamin D receptor is present in most tissues of the body, including osteoblasts, small intestine, colon, activated T and B lymphocytes, β islet cells, brain, heart, skin, gonads, prostate, breast, and mononuclear cells; thus a deficiency in vitamin D may affect not only the skeletal system.[70] It is possible that the maternal and infant vitamin D status might influence many tissue functions. These nonskeletal actions of vitamin D are discussed, see the articles by Hewison; Holick; Krishnan and colleagues; and Takiishi and colleagues elsewhere in this issue for further exploration of this topic.

Intrauterine Effects of Maternal Vitamin D Deficiency

Conflicting results have been obtained concerning the effect of season on neonatal bone mass. In South Korea, where there are marked seasonal variations in neonatal 25-OHD, infants born in summer have higher bone mineral content than infants born in winter. Furthermore, there is a significant positive correlation between neonatal 25-OHD and bone mass and an inverse relationship between 25-OHD and a marker of bone resorption.[71] However in a study from the United States, where no seasonal variation in cord 25-OHD concentrations was found, the reverse seasonal relationships were noted, with neonates born in summer having lower bone mass than their peers born in winter.[72,73] An explanation for these differences is not readily apparent, although it has been suggested that differences in the degree of maternal vitamin D deficiency might play a role. Low maternal 25-OHD levels in late pregnancy (but not during the first trimester) have been associated with reduced intrauterine long bone growth, slightly shorter duration of gestation,[74] and possibly reduced limb lean tissue.[75] An association has also been found between vitamin D status during pregnancy and bone mass in the offspring at 9 years of age.[76]

Birth weight has been associated with maternal vitamin D status in several studies[77–79]; the birth-weight effect being approximately 200 g between those infants born to vitamin D deficient mothers and those born to sufficient mothers.[80] Infants born during the summer months, when 25-OHD levels are at the nadir during the months preceding their birth, had lower birth weights when compared with infants born in winter or spring months, when 25-OHD concentrations are highest in the months of pregnancy before delivery.[81] These effects on birth weight may have consequences as birth weight is associated with a wide range of cognitive and behavioral outcomes,[82] with superior neurocognitive outcomes being associated with heavier birth weights.[83]

RECOMMENDATIONS FOR THE PREVENTION OF VITAMIN D DEFICIENCY IN MOTHER AND CHILD

Vitamin D deficiency in the neonate and infant can be prevented by supplementing all at-risk pregnant and lactating women with vitamin D, by exposing pregnant and lactating women and their infants to sufficient sunlight, or by supplementing exclusively breastfed infants with vitamin D.

There are obstacles to the implementation of each of these preventive strategies. The lack of adequate training of physicians in a supposedly rickets-free era coupled with the lack of adequate recommendations (appropriate time frame and dosage) for vitamin D supplementation by professional organizations have contributed to the development of rickets in exclusively breastfed babies. Reluctance of health care providers to prescribe vitamin D supplements to breastfed infants has been documented from several locations.[84–87] However, the predominant reason is probably the belief that supplemental vitamin D is not needed by breastfed infants, perhaps based on misperceptions regarding the effectiveness of sunlight exposure at northern latitudes during winter[25] and that "breast is best." Furthermore, where effective guidelines are set in place, they are not consistently implemented.[26]

Previous studies have suggested implementing screening and education programs for at-risk immigrant groups or populations and for their medical attendants.[12,27] However, it may be more cost-effective to supplement all pregnant mothers and their infants in communities where vitamin D insufficiency is prevalent rather than assessing vitamin D levels in mothers and siblings in screening programs.

Ward and colleagues[26] are concerned that rickets continues to be a health issue in Canada despite simple measures for its prevention. Health Canada[88] and the Canadian Pediatric Society[89] recommend that all breastfed infants receive supplemental vitamin D (400 IU/d). Furthermore, they recommend that those breastfed infants who reside above 55° N latitude in Canada or in areas at lower latitudes that have a high incidence of vitamin D deficiency should receive 800 IU/d during the winter months.[89] Another concern raised by Ward and colleagues[26] was the inconsistent implementation of current recommended guidelines and the unawareness among health care providers and the general public on the prevention of vitamin D deficiency.

Preventative Strategies for Vitamin D Deficiency in the Pregnant Mother

Despite there being additional demands from the fetus on maternal vitamin D stores during pregnancy, there is no consensus on the optimal serum 25-OHD levels in pregnancy or on supplementation dosages during pregnancy that are needed to maintain adequate fetal growth and well-being.[80] Studies have documented low vitamin D status among pregnant women.[32,36,80,90,91] Bodnar[36] and Holmes and colleagues[91] found that despite the use of prenatal vitamins containing vitamin D, mother-infant pairs were at risk of developing vitamin D insufficiency. This evidence implies that current formulations of vitamins and minerals for pregnant women probably do not contain adequate doses of vitamin D and that separate vitamin D supplements are required for all pregnant women in at-risk communities/countries, as antenatal screening of 25-OHD levels is likely not to be a cost-effective measure compared with prophylactic preventative measures. A recent study from the United Kingdom among pregnant ethnic minorities found that the daily dose of 800 to 1600 IU/d of vitamin D was insufficient to normalize circulating 25-OHD concentrations at the time of delivery in some of the patients.[92]

Large research trials are required to determine the dose of vitamin D supplementation required to maintain vitamin D sufficiency during pregnancy.

A summary of the suggested recommendations for vitamin D supplementation during pregnancy in those communities where sunlight exposure is not adequate to maintain vitamin D sufficiency is as follows:

- Pregnant mothers should ingest at least 2000 IU/d of vitamin D, as there is growing evidence that adequate maternal vitamin D status is essential during pregnancy, not only for maternal well-being but also for fetal development.
- Health care professionals who provide obstetric care should consider vitamin D supplementation as part of routine antenatal care.

Preventative Strategies for Vitamin D Deficiency in Infants

The current American Academy of Pediatrics (AAP) guidelines[93] suggest that infants younger than 6 months should be kept out of direct sunlight and the Canadian Dermatology Association and Health Canada recommend that children younger than 1 year of age avoid direct sunlight and also use sunscreens.[88] By following these guidelines to protect against the risk of developing skin cancers, there is an added imperative for vitamin D supplementation during infancy.

There are conflicting recommendations as to what constitutes an adequate dosage of vitamin D supplementation to maintain vitamin D sufficiency during infancy. Further, there is no clear understanding of what defines vitamin D sufficiency; most pediatricians would accept that vitamin D sufficiency can be defined as levels of serum 25-OHD greater than 20 ng/mL, insufficiency as levels between 12 and 20 ng/mL, and deficiency as less than 12 ng/mL.[13]

Pittard and colleagues[94] compared supplementation with daily doses of 400 and 800 IU of vitamin D in preterm and term infants whose mothers had normal 25-OHD levels, and they concluded that a daily dose of 400 IU was sufficient to achieve normal serum 25-OHD levels of greater than 12 ng/mL. Recently the AAP has recommended a minimum daily intake of 400 IU beginning soon after birth. This recommendation replaces the previous recommendation of a minimum daily intake of 200 IU of vitamin D supplementation beginning in the first 2 months after birth and continuing through adolescence.[95] In the United Kingdom, 400 IU is recommended for all breastfeeding infants.[96]

To summarize the suggested recommendations for vitamin D supplementation during infancy:

- Breastfed infants should receive at least 400 IU/d of vitamin D supplementation within the first few days of life, regardless of whether they are being supplemented with formula.
- Although most formula-fed infants achieve a vitamin D intake of 400 IU/d by ingesting nearly 1 L formula per day after the first month of life, all nonbreastfed infants who are ingesting less than 1 L/d (400 IU D/L) of vitamin D-fortified formula should receive a vitamin D supplement of 400 IU/d.
- All infants living in communities above 37° latitude should receive 400 IU/d of vitamin D supplementation during the winter months.
- When compliance with a daily supplementation regimen might be problematic, monthly or 3-monthly large oral doses of vitamin D might be administered through the Integrated Management of Childhood Illnesses programs in countries with at-risk populations or groups.

Vitamin D Supplementation for the Lactating Mother and Her Infant

Studies conducted in the 1980s have shown that supplementation of lactating mothers with 2000 IU rather than 1000 IU of vitamin D had a significant effect on the breastfeeding infant's vitamin D status as measured by infant serum 25-OHD levels.[62]

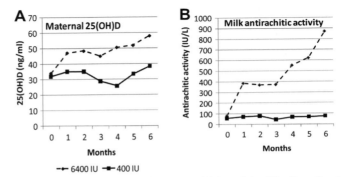

Fig. 6. Maternal 25-OHD levels (A) and milk antirachitic activity (B) after vitamin D₃ supplements during lactation. (*Modified from* Wagner CL, Hulsey TC, Fanning D, et al. High-dose vitamin D3 supplementation in a cohort of breastfeeding mothers and their infants: a 6-month follow-up pilot study. Breastfeed Med 2006;1(2):66–7; with permission.)

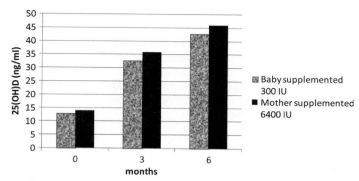

Fig. 7. Comparison of 25-OHD levels when supplementing mother and infant with vitamin D₃. (*Modified from* Wagner CL, Hulsey TC, Fanning D, et al. High-dose vitamin D3 supplementation in a cohort of breastfeeding mothers and their infants: a 6-month follow-up pilot study. Breastfeed Med 2006;1(2):67; with permission.)

Recent work by Wagner and colleagues[97] found that daily maternal supplements of 6400 IU/d of vitamin D during lactation raised the antirachitic activity of breast milk to 500 to 800 IU/L (**Fig. 6**) and that this level was sufficient to maintain adequate circulating levels of 25-OHD in the nursing infant. The effect on infant 25-OHD concentrations of maternal supplementation at this level was similar to that found in infants receiving a supplement of 300 IU/d of vitamin D (**Fig. 7**).[97] However, such large doses of supplementation in lactating women need to be validated in larger population studies from different ethnic groups and in dark- and light-skinned mothers to ensure the safety of these doses over prolonged periods, before being recommended for general use.

Breastfed babies require vitamin D 400 IU/d to maintain vitamin D status. If breastfed babies do not receive supplements, then mothers should possibly receive 4000 to 6000 IU/d to maintain the vitamin D status of their infants. The double effect of preventing vitamin D deficiency in the infant and mother through maternal supplementation seems to be the way forward; however, until further studies have verified the long-term safety in mothers and their infants of these high doses, a lower maternal dose of 2000 IU/d is recommended, with possible continued supplementation of the infant with 200 to 400 IU/d.

SUMMARY

The mother is the major source of circulating 25-OHD concentrations in the young infant. Thus maternal vitamin D status is an important factor in determining the vitamin D status of the infant and their risk of developing vitamin D deficiency and infantile nutritional rickets. As a result, breastfed infants of mothers with vitamin D deficiency who are unsupplemented and who receive little sunlight exposure are at high risk of developing vitamin D deficiency or rickets. Despite food fortification policies in many countries and recommendations for vitamin D supplementation of at-risk groups, vitamin D deficiency and infantile rickets remain major public health challenges in many developed and developing countries. There is evidence that the current supplementation recommendations, particularly for pregnant and lactating women, are inadequate to ensure vitamin D sufficiency in these groups. A widespread and concerted effort is needed to ensure daily supplementation of breastfed and other infants at high risk with vitamin D 400 IU from birth and pregnant women in high risk communities with 2000 IU; awareness needs to be developed among the public and medical practitioners of the urgent need to improve the vitamin D status of pregnant and lactating mothers and their infants. Further studies are required to determine the optimal doses of vitamin D supplementation in pregnancy and during lactation, and for normalizing vitamin D stores in infancy to reduce the prevalence of infantile nutritional rickets. Operational research studies also need to be conducted to understand the best methods of implementing supplementation programs and the factors that are likely to impede their success.

REFERENCES

1. Welch TR, Bergstrom WH, Tsang RC. Vitamin D-deficient rickets: the reemergence of a once-conquered disease. J Pediatr 2000;137(2):143–5.
2. Pettifor JM. Rickets and vitamin D deficiency in children and adolescents. Endocrinol Metab Clin North Am 2005;34(3):537–53.
3. Matsuoka LY, Ide L, Wortsman J, et al. Sunscreens suppress cutaneous vitamin D3 synthesis. J Clin Endocrinol Metab 1987;64(6):1165–8.
4. Taha SA, Dost SM, Sedrani SH. 25-Hydroxyvitamin D and total calcium: extraordinarily low plasma concentrations in Saudi mothers and their neonates. Pediatr Res 1984;18(8):739–41.
5. Agarwal KS, Mughal MZ, Upadhyay P, et al. The impact of atmospheric pollution on vitamin D status of infants and toddlers in Delhi, India. Arch Dis Child 2002; 87(2):111–3.
6. Dunn PM. Francis Glisson (1597-1677) and the "discovery" of rickets. Arch Dis Child Fetal Neonatal Ed 1998;78(2):F154–5.
7. Balasubramanian S, Shivbalan S, Kumar PS. Hypocalcemia due to vitamin D deficiency in exclusively breastfed infants. Indian Pediatr 2006;43(3):247–51.
8. Hatun S, Ozkan B, Orbak Z, et al. Vitamin D deficiency in early infancy. J Nutr 2005;135(2):279–82.
9. Beck-Nielsen SS, Brock-Jacobsen B, Gram J, et al. Incidence and prevalence of nutritional and hereditary rickets in southern Denmark. Eur J Endocrinol 2009; 160(3):491–7.
10. Cosgrove L, Dietrich A. Nutritional rickets in breast-fed infants. J Fam Pract 1985; 21(3):205–9.
11. Weisberg P, Scanlon KS, Li R, et al. Nutritional rickets among children in the United States: review of cases reported between 1986 and 2003. Am J Clin Nutr 2004;80(6 Suppl):1697S–705S.
12. Robinson PD, Hogler W, Craig ME, et al. The re-emerging burden of rickets: a decade of experience from Sydney. Arch Dis Child 2006;91(7):564–8.
13. Misra M, Pacaud D, Petryk A, et al. Vitamin D deficiency in children and its management: review of current knowledge and recommendations. Pediatrics 2008;122(2):398–417.
14. Ladhani S, Srinivasan L, Buchanan C, et al. Presentation of vitamin D deficiency. Arch Dis Child 2004;89(8):781–4.
15. Pal BR, Shaw NJ. Rickets resurgence in the United Kingdom: improving antenatal management in Asians. J Pediatr 2001;139(2):337–8.
16. Holick MF. Vitamin D: importance in the prevention of cancers, type 1 diabetes, heart disease, and osteoporosis. Am J Clin Nutr 2004;79(3):362–71.
17. Holick MF. Sunlight and vitamin D for bone health and prevention of autoimmune diseases, cancers, and cardiovascular disease. Am J Clin Nutr 2004;80(6 Suppl): 1678S–88S.

18. Kimlin MG. Geographic location and vitamin D synthesis. Mol Aspects Med 2008; 29(6):453–61.
19. Holick MF. Vitamin D and the underappreciated D-lightful hormone that is important for skeletal and cellular health. Curr Opin Endocrinol Diabetes 2002;9: 87–98.
20. Specker BL, Valanis B, Hertzberg V, et al. Sunshine exposure and serum 25-hydroxyvitamin D concentrations in exclusively breast-fed infants. J Pediatr 1985; 107(3):372–6.
21. Clemens TL, Adams JS, Henderson SL, et al. Increased skin pigment reduces the capacity of skin to synthesise vitamin D3. Lancet 1982;1(8263):74–6.
22. Holick MF. The vitamin D epidemic and its health consequences. J Nutr 2005; 135(11):2739S–48S.
23. Strand MA, Perry J, Guo J, et al. Doing the month: rickets and post-partum convalescence in rural China. Midwifery 2009;25(5):588–96.
24. Baroncelli GI, Bereket A, El KM, et al. Rickets in the Middle East: role of environment and genetic predisposition. J Clin Endocrinol Metab 2008;93(5):1743–50.
25. Ziegler EE, Hollis BW, Nelson SE, et al. Vitamin D deficiency in breastfed infants in Iowa. Pediatrics 2006;118(2):603–10.
26. Ward LM, Gaboury I, Ladhani M, et al. Vitamin D-deficiency rickets among children in Canada. CMAJ 2007;177(2):161–6.
27. Thomson K, Morley R, Grover SR, et al. Postnatal evaluation of vitamin D and bone health in women who were vitamin D-deficient in pregnancy, and in their infants. Med J Aust 2004;181(9):486–8.
28. Challa A, Ntourntoufi A, Cholevas V, et al. Breastfeeding and vitamin D status in Greece during the first 6 months of life. Eur J Pediatr 2005;164(12):724–9.
29. Callaghan AL, Moy RJ, Booth IW, et al. Incidence of symptomatic vitamin D deficiency. Arch Dis Child 2006;91(7):606–7.
30. Heckmatt JZ, Peacock M, Davies AE, et al. Plasma 25-hydroxyvitamin D in pregnant Asian women and their babies. Lancet 1979;2(8142):546–8.
31. Brooke OG, Brown IR, Cleeve HJ, et al. Observations on the vitamin D state of pregnant Asian women in London. Br J Obstet Gynaecol 1981;88(1):18–26.
32. Sachan A, Gupta R, Das V, et al. High prevalence of vitamin D deficiency among pregnant women and their newborns in northern India. Am J Clin Nutr 2005;81(5): 1060–4.
33. Bishop N, Fewtrell M. Metabolic bone disease of prematurity. In: Glorieux FH, Pettifor JM, Juppner H, editors. Pediatric bone; biology and diseases. San Diego (CA): Elsevier Science; 2003. p. 567–81.
34. Rothberg AD, Pettifor JM, Cohen DF, et al. Maternal-infant vitamin D relationships during breast-feeding. J Pediatr 1982;101(4):500–3.
35. Prentice A, Jarjou LMA, Stirling DM, et al. Biochemical markers of calcium and bone metabolism during 18 months of lactation in Gambian women accustomed to a low calcium intake and in those consuming a calcium supplement. J Clin Endocrinol Metab 1998;83(4):1059–66.
36. Bodnar LM, Simhan HN, Powers RW, et al. High prevalence of vitamin D insufficiency in black and white pregnant women residing in the northern United States and their neonates. J Nutr 2007;137(2):447–52.
37. Dawodu A, Wagner CL. Mother-child vitamin D deficiency: an international perspective. Arch Dis Child 2007;92(9):737–40.
38. Andiran N, Yordam N, Ozon A. Risk factors for vitamin D deficiency in breast-fed newborns and their mothers. Nutrition 2002;18(1):47–50.

39. Ozkan B, Doneray H, Karacan M, et al. Prevalence of vitamin D deficiency rickets in the eastern part of Turkey. Eur J Pediatr 2009;168(1):95–100.
40. Kovacs CS, Kronenberg HM. Maternal-fetal calcium and bone metabolism during pregnancy, puerperium, and lactation. Endocr Rev 1997;18(6):832–72.
41. Kovacs CS. Vitamin D in pregnancy and lactation: maternal, fetal, and neonatal outcomes from human and animal studies. Am J Clin Nutr 2008;88(2):520S–8S.
42. Kovacs CS. Calcium and bone metabolism during pregnancy and lactation. J Mammary Gland Biol Neoplasia 2005;10(2):105–18.
43. Bass JK, Chan GM. Calcium nutrition and metabolism during infancy. Nutrition 2006;22(10):1057–66.
44. Greer FR, Tsang RC, Searcy JE, et al. Mineral homeostasis during lactation- relationship to serum 1,25-dihydroxyvitamin D, 25-hydroxyvitamin D, parathyroid hormone and calcitonin. Am J Clin Nutr 1982;36(3):431–7.
45. Steichen JJ, Gratton TL, Tsang RC. Osteopenia of prematurity: the cause and possible treatment. J Pediatr 1980;96(3 Pt 2):528–34.
46. Salle BL, Delvin EE, Lapillonne A, et al. Perinatal metabolism of vitamin D. Am J Clin Nutr 2000;71(5 Suppl):1317S–24S.
47. Seki K, Furuya K, Makimura N, et al. Cord blood levels of calcium-regulating hormones and osteocalcin in premature infants. J Perinat Med 1994;22(3):189–94.
48. Cooper LJ, Anast CS. Circulating immunoreactive parathyroid hormone levels in premature infants and the response to calcium therapy. Acta Paediatr Scand 1985;74(5):669–73.
49. Loughead JL, Mimouni F, Tsang RC. Serum ionized calcium concentrations in normal neonates. Am J Dis Child 1988;142(5):516–8.
50. Salimpour R. Rickets in Tehran. Study of 200 cases. Arch Dis Child 1975;50(1):63–6.
51. el Hag AI, Karrar ZA. Nutritional vitamin D deficiency rickets in Sudanese children. Ann Trop Paediatr 1995;15:69–76.
52. Molla AM, Badawi MH, al-Yaish S, et al. Risk factors for nutritional rickets among children in Kuwait. Pediatr Int 2000;42(3):280–4.
53. Fleischman AR, Rosen JF, Cole J, et al. Maternal and fetal serum 1,25-dihydroxyvitamin D levels at term. J Pediatr 1980;97(4):640–2.
54. Hillman LS, Haddad JG. Human perinatal vitamin D metabolism. I. 25-hydroxyvitamin D in maternal and cord blood. J Pediatr 1974;84(5):742–9.
55. Gertner JM, Glassman MS, Coutsan DR, et al. Fetomaternal vitamin D relationships at term. J Pediatr 1980;1980(97):637–40.
56. Reeve LE, Chesney RW, DeLuca HF. Vitamin D of human milk: identification of biologically active forms. Am J Clin Nutr 1982;36(1):122–6.
57. Taylor SN, Wagner CL, Hollis BW. Vitamin D supplementation during lactation to support infant and mother. J Am Coll Nutr 2008;27(6):690–701.
58. Heaney RP, Armas LA, Shary JR, et al. 25-Hydroxylation of vitamin D3: relation to circulating vitamin D3 under various input conditions. Am J Clin Nutr 2008;87(6):1738–42.
59. Specker BL, Tsang RC, Hollis BW. Effect of race and diet on human-milk vitamin D and 25-hydroxyvitamin D. Am J Dis Child 1985;139(11):1134–7.
60. Greer FR, Hollis BW, Cripps DJ, et al. Effects of maternal ultraviolet B irradiation on vitamin D content of human milk. J Pediatr 1984;105(3):431–3.
61. Hollis BW, Roos BA, Draper HH, et al. Vitamin D and its metabolites in human and bovine milk. J Nutr 1981;111(7):1240–8.
62. Ala-Houhala M, Koskinen T, Terho A, et al. Maternal compared with infant vitamin D supplementation. Arch Dis Child 1986;61(12):1159–63.

63. Heaney RP, Davies KM, Chen TC, et al. Human serum 25-hydroxycholecalciferol response to extended oral dosing with cholecalciferol. Am J Clin Nutr 2003;77(1): 204–10.

64. Armas LA, Dowell S, Akhter M, et al. Ultraviolet-B radiation increases serum 25-hydroxyvitamin D levels: the effect of UVB dose and skin color. J Am Acad Dermatol 2007;57(4):588–93.

65. Parikh SJ, Edelman M, Uwaifo GI, et al. The relationship between obesity and serum 1,25-dihydroxy vitamin D concentrations in healthy adults. J Clin Endocrinol Metab 2004;89(3):1196–9.

66. Dawodu A, Agarwal M, Hossain M, et al. Hypovitaminosis D and vitamin D deficiency in exclusively breast-feeding infants and their mothers in summer: a justification for vitamin D supplementation of breast-feeding infants. J Pediatr 2003; 142(2):169–73.

67. Atiq M, Suria A, Nizami SQ, et al. Maternal vitamin-D deficiency in Pakistan. Acta Obstet Gynecol Scand 1998;77(10):970–3.

68. Specker BL, Tsang RC. Vitamin D in infancy and childhood: factors determining vitamin D status. Adv Pediatr 1986;33:1–22.

69. Javaid MK, Cooper C. Prenatal and childhood influences on osteoporosis. Best Pract Res Clin Endocrinol Metab 2002;16(2):349–67.

70. Mathieu C, Adorini L. The coming of age of 1,25-dihydroxyvitamin D(3) analogs as immunomodulatory agents. Trends Mol Med 2002;8(4):174–9.

71. Namgung R, Tsang RC. Bone in the pregnant mother and newborn at birth. Clin Chim Acta 2003;333(1):1–11.

72. Namgung R, Mimouni F, Campaigne BN, et al. Low bone mineral content in summer-born compared with winter-born infants. J Pediatr Gastroenterol Nutr 1992;15(3):285–8.

73. Namgung R, Tsang RC, Specker BL, et al. Low bone mineral content and high serum osteocalcin and 1,25-dihydroxyvitamin D in summer- versus winter-born newborn infants: an early fetal effect? J Pediatr Gastroenterol Nutr 1994;19(2): 220–7.

74. Morley R, Carlin JB, Pasco JA, et al. Maternal 25-hydroxyvitamin D and parathyroid hormone concentrations and offspring birth size. J Clin Endocrinol Metab 2006;91(3):906–12.

75. Pasco JA, Wark JD, Carlin JB, et al. Maternal vitamin D in pregnancy may influence not only offspring bone mass but other aspects of musculoskeletal health and adiposity. Med Hypotheses 2008;71(2):266–9.

76. Javaid MK, Crozier SR, Harvey NC, et al. Maternal vitamin D status during pregnancy and childhood bone mass at age 9 years: a longitudinal study. Lancet 2006;367(9504):36–43.

77. Morley R, Carlin JB, Pasco JA, et al. Maternal 25-hydroxyvitamin D concentration and offspring birth size: effect modification by infant VDR genotype. Eur J Clin Nutr 2009;63(6):802–4.

78. Scholl TO, Chen X. Vitamin D intake during pregnancy: association with maternal characteristics and infant birth weight. Early Hum Dev 2009;85(4):231–4.

79. Mannion CA, Gray-Donald K, Koski KG. Association of low intake of milk and vitamin D during pregnancy with decreased birth weight. CMAJ 2006;174(9): 1273–7.

80. Bowyer L, Catling-Paull C, Diamond T, et al. Vitamin D, PTH and calcium levels in pregnant women and their neonates. Clin Endocrinol (Oxf) 2009;70(3):372–7.

81. Wohlfahrt J, Melbye M, Christens P, et al. Secular and seasonal variation of length and weight at birth. Lancet 1998;352(9145):1990.

82. Kimball S, Fuleihan G, Vieth R. Vitamin D: a growing perspective. Crit Rev Clin Lab Sci 2008;45(4):339–414.

83. Richards M, Hardy R, Kuh D, et al. Birth weight and cognitive function in the British 1946 birth cohort: longitudinal population based study. BMJ 2001; 322(7280):199–203.

84. Hayward I, Stein MT, Gibson MI. Nutritional rickets in San Diego. Am J Dis Child 1987;141(10):1060–2.

85. Shaikh U, Alpert PT. Practices of vitamin D recommendation in Las Vegas, Nevada. J Hum Lact 2004;20(1):56–61.

86. Gessner BD, Plotnik J, Muth PT. 25-Hydroxyvitamin D levels among healthy children in Alaska. J Pediatr 2003;143(4):434–7.

87. Davenport ML, Uckun A, Calikoglu AS. Pediatrician patterns of prescribing vitamin supplementation for infants: do they contribute to rickets? Pediatrics 2004;113(1 Pt 1):179–80.

88. Health Canada Vitamin D supplementation for breastfed infants: 2004 Health Canada recommendation. http://www.hc-sc.gc.ca/fn-an/alt_formats/hpfb-dgpsa/pdf/nutrition/vita_d_supp-eng.pdf. 2009. Accessed June 6, 2009.

89. Canadian Paediatric Society. Vitamin D supplementation in northern Native communities. Paediatr Child Health 2002;7:459–63.

90. Nicolaidou P, Hatzistamatiou Z, Papadopoulou A, et al. Low vitamin D status in mother-newborn pairs in Greece. Calcif Tissue Int 2006;78(6):337–42.

91. Holmes VA, Barnes MS, Denis AH, et al. Vitamin D deficiency and insufficiency in pregnant women: a longitudinal study. Br J Nutr 2009;102(6):876–81.

92. Datta S, Alfaham M, Davies DP, et al. Vitamin D deficiency in pregnant women from a non-European ethnic minority population–an interventional study. BJOG 2002;109(8):905–8.

93. Ultraviolet light: a hazard to children. American Academy of Pediatrics. Committee on Environmental Health. Pediatrics 1999;104(2 Pt 1):328–33.

94. Pittard WB III, Geddes KM, Hulsey TC, et al. How much vitamin D for neonates? Am J Dis Child 1991;145(10):1147–9.

95. Wagner CL, Greer FR. Prevention of rickets and vitamin D deficiency in infants, children, and adolescents. Pediatrics 2008;122(5):1142–52.

96. Shaw NJ, Pal BR. Vitamin D deficiency in UK Asian families: activating a new concern. Arch Dis Child 2002;86(3):147–9.

97. Wagner CL, Hulsey TC, Fanning D, et al. High-dose vitamin D3 supplementation in a cohort of breastfeeding mothers and their infants: a 6-month follow-up pilot study. Breastfeed Med 2006;1(2):59–70.

Osteomalacia as a Result of Vitamin D Deficiency

Arti Bhan, MBBS[a], Ajay D. Rao, MD[b], D. Sudhaker Rao, MBBS[c],*

KEYWORDS

- Osteomalacia • Vitamin D deficiency
- Secondary hyperparathyroidism • Treatment

Among the metabolic bone diseases with known pathogenic mechanisms, osteoporosis is the most common and osteomalacia is the least common disorder. Nevertheless, osteomalacia occurs with regular frequency such that it may escape recognition especially in its early stages because of the often indefinite symptoms such as vague bone pain and muscle weakness. In reality, however, osteomalacia is an end-stage bone disease of severe vitamin D or phosphate depletion of any cause with characteristic biochemical, radiological, and bone histologic features. The descriptive term osteomalacia originally referred to a generalized softening of bone leading to crippling deformities, and is almost always caused by vitamin D deficiency, and rarely by phosphate and calcium depletion.[1] The cardinal histologic bone feature of osteomalacia is an excessive accumulation of unmineralized or poorly mineralized bone matrix.[1] In contrast, rickets (see the article by Thandrayen and Pettifor elsewhere in this issue for further exploration of this topic) is a disease of impaired mineralization of cartilage resulting in defective enchondral bone formation. By definition, therefore, rickets occurs only in children and adolescents before epiphyseal fusion, whereas osteomalacia occurs in children and in adults. Although this is an important clinical distinction, the pathogenesis of rickets and osteomalacia is similar.

HISTORICAL PERSPECTIVE AND SCOPE OF THE PROBLEM

The first description of osteomalacia was by Gustav Pommer, a German pathologist, in the late nineteenth century who discussed the histologic differences between osteomalacia, osteoporosis, and osteitis fibrosa.[1] One of the earliest reports of osteomalacia studied by tetracycline-based bone histomorphometry of the ribs was reported from Henry Ford Hospital in 1966.[2] Based on current concepts of bone

[a] Division of Endocrinology, Diabetes and Bone & Mineral Disorders, Henry Ford Hospital, Detroit, MI 48202, USA
[b] Division of Endocrinology, Diabetes, and Hypertension, Brigham and Women's Hospital, 221 Longwood Avenue, Boston, MA 02115, USA
[c] Bone & Mineral Research Laboratory, Henry Ford Hospital, E&R Building 7th Floor, 2799 West Grand Boulevard, Detroit, MI 48202, USA
* Corresponding author.
E-mail address: srao1@hfhs.org

Endocrinol Metab Clin N Am 39 (2010) 321–331
doi:10.1016/j.ecl.2010.02.001
0889-8529/10/$ – see front matter © 2010 Elsevier Inc. All rights reserved.

remodeling, Pommer's observations can be restated as replacement of resorbed bone by the same amount of bone in healthy adults, by a lesser amount of bone in age-related osteoporosis, and by unmineralized bone matrix (or osteoid) in osteomalacia. With the realization of the critical role of vitamin D in bone and mineral metabolism in general and bone mineralization in particular, it became apparent that almost all cases of bone softening were the result of vitamin D deficiency, and osteomalacia was synonymous with bone disease that could be cured by vitamin D repletion. However, it is now clear that not all cases of osteomalacia are cured by vitamin D therapy and similarly not all individuals with vitamin D depletion develop osteomalacia. Nevertheless, it is important to bear in mind that almost all individuals with prolonged severe vitamin D depletion will eventually develop osteomalacia with irreversible cortical bone loss and increased risk of fractures for the rest of their lives.[3] Osteomalacia manifests as a distinct metabolic bone disease with its characteristic clinical, biochemical, radiographic, and histologic bone features,[4] that can be distinguished unambiguously from osteoporosis or any other metabolic bone disease.

Because of the lack of any systematic studies on osteomalacia it is difficult to estimate the precise prevalence of osteomalacia. A MEDLINE search from 1950 to 2009 using the MeSH term "osteomalacia" reveals several articles, but all are concerned with individual case reports or case series. Nevertheless, vitamin D deficiency is the most common cause of osteomalacia worldwide, but in the United States, gastrointestinal disorders causing vitamin D deficiency and hypophosphatemic osteomalacia are the most common. Gastric bypass surgery for morbid obesity is now emerging as the leading cause of vitamin D deficiency osteomalacia in this country. Other uncommon causes of vitamin D deficiency osteomalacia are summarized in **Box 1**.

Evolution of Hypovitaminosis D Osteopathy and Osteomalacia

In its early stages, vitamin D deficiency is associated with increased serum alkaline phosphatase and parathyroid hormone (PTH) levels, increased bone turnover without mineralization defect, and irreversible cortical bone loss, which the authors defined as hypovitaminosis D osteopathy stage I (HVO-I) or preosteomalacia.[4] Recognition of this preclinical stage is important to prevent PTH-mediated cortical bone loss and progression to frank osteomalacia.[3] In the next stage, hypovitaminosis D osteopathy stage II (HVO-II), there is progressive accumulation of unmineralized matrix (or osteoid) with some preservation of mineralization. In the last stage, hypovitaminosis D osteopathy stage III (HVO-III), there is complete cessation of mineralization with no tetracycline uptake, conforming to the traditional descriptions of osteomalacia.[4] The distinguishing histologic bone features of osteomalacia and osteoporosis along with reference ranges are summarized in **Table 1**. Osteoporosis is characterized by a quantum decrease in bone volume without mineralization defect, whereas osteomalacia is associated with a decrease in bone volume and excess osteoid accumulation.[5] The extent of bone mineralization is either near normal or slightly reduced in osteoporosis, whereas it is always absent in osteomalacia. Secondary hyperparathyroidism, an inevitable consequence of chronic vitamin D deficiency, in rare cases is associated with bone marrow fibrosis, similar to that found in primary hyperparathyroidism. In osteomalacia, osteoid volume, thickness, and surface are all increased, whereas in osteitis fibrosa, only the osteoid volume and surface but not the thickness are increased and usually not to the same extent as in osteomalacia (see **Table 1**). A mineralization lag time (MLT) of more than 100 days separates osteomalacia unambiguously from all other conditions with increased osteoid indices as a result of increased bone turnover, such as

---

Box 1
Common causes of vitamin D deficiency osteomalacia

Extrinsic

Decreased exposure to sunlight

Use of sunscreens (especially >8 SPF)

Use of a veil (or hijab)

Increased or dark skin pigmentation

Inadequate dietary intake

Morbid obesity

Intrinsic

Advancing age with decreased cutaneous production of vitamin D

Malabsorption caused by various gastrointestinal disorders

    Gastrectomy (partial, total, or bypass procedure)

    Small intestinal disease, resection, or bypass

    Gluten enteropathy (celiac sprue)

    Biliary cirrhosis (uncommon)

    Pancreatic insufficiency including cystic fibrosis (uncommon)

Acquired vitamin D deficiency

(as a result of increased catabolism or metabolic clearance)

    Anticonvulsants

    Calcium deficiency with secondary hyperparathyroidism

    Primary hyperaparathyroidism

    Paget's disease of bone (depletion caused by excess consumption)

---

hyperparathyroidism, hyperthyroidism, and Paget disease of bone (see **Table 1**). Thus a combination of increased osteoid thickness greater than 15 μm and an MLT more than 100 days should be used as diagnostic criteria for osteomalacia of any cause including vitamin D deficiency osteomalacia.[1,4]

CLINICAL MANIFESTATIONS OF OSTEOMALACIA

Osteomalacia in its classic form manifests with a constellation of symptoms and signs that can be collectively referred to as osteomalcic syndrome. Some symptoms are vague and nonspecific and can easily escape the attention of the clinician, whereas others are highly specific and often diagnostic. Between these 2 extremes a patient may present with a combination of symptoms and signs. Therefore, a high degree of suspicion in the right clinical context is necessary to diagnose osteomalacia especially in the early stages. Because of the increase in serum alkaline phosphatase levels and dramatic appearance on bone scans, metastatic disease is often suspected leading to exhaustive, expensive, and often unnecessary testing. A recent case seen by the senior author illustrates the problem. A 59-year-old white woman with no previous history of cancer or gastrointestinal surgery was seen for a high serum alkaline phosphatase level (890–950 IU/L) that had progressively increased over

Table 1
Representative bone histomorphometric and bone density measurements in patients with osteoporosis and osteomalacia

Measurement	Normal Postmenopausal White Women[a]	Osteoporosis (With Fractures)[a]	Osteomalacia
Bone Histomorphometry			
Osteoid surface/bone surface (%)	20.3 (4.35–39.7)	15.7 (2.78–34.5)	69 ± 13
Osteoid thickness (μm)	8.49 (5.75–12.2)	7.63 (4.74–11.5)	27 ± 9
Mineralization lag time (MLT; days)	71.2 (18.6–158)	73.8 (17.1–132)	>100
Bone formation rate/bone surface ($\mu m^3/\mu m^2/y$)	15.9 (1.00–33.9)	13.0 (0.436–33.7)	0
Bone Mineral Density			
Spine T-score	Referrent	−2.3 ± 1.8	−3.0 ± 1.6
Spine Z-score	Referrent	−1.2 ± 0.8	−2.0 ± 1.4
Femoral neck T-score	Referrent	−2.1 ± 1.6	−4.1 ± 1.0
Femoral neck Z-score	Referrent	−1.1 ± 0.6	−2.7 ± 0.7
Forearm Z-score	Referrent	−1.1 ± 1.0	−6.0 ± 2.3
Forearm T-score	Referrent	−0.85 ± 0.5	−3.8 ± 0.8

Note the magnitude and pattern of bone mineral deficits with more trabecular bone deficit (spine and hip) in postmenopausal osteoporosis and predominant cortical bone deficit (forearm bone mineral density) in osteomalacia.

[a] Representative data from the authors' laboratory (published and unpublished).

Data from Basha B, Rao DS, Han Z-H, Parfitt AM. Osteomalacia due to vitamin D depletion in the US. Am J Med 2000;108:296–300.

a period of 1 to 2 years during which she developed vague musculoskeletal symptoms, which she described as aches and pains of getting old. A whole body bone scan showed multiple bilateral rib fractures without increased uptake elsewhere in the skeleton (**Fig. 1**), an unusual finding in malignancy, but nevertheless referred to an oncologist for further evaluation. She underwent an exhaustive investigation for cancer and myeoloproliferative diseases including a bone marrow examination that was normal. Only when a house officer ordered measurement of serum PTH, because that was the only test that had not yet been performed, and found to be 879 pg/mL was the patient referred to a bone and mineral specialist. The house officer did not consider measurement of 25-hydroxyvitamin D. She had profound proximal myopathy, diffuse bone pain, and an undetectable level of serum 25-hydroxyvitamin D (<4 ng/mL). Bone biopsy confirmed severe osteomalacia (**Fig. 2**) and all her symptoms improved dramatically within 3 to 4 months of vitamin repletion. This case illustrates the problems with diagnosis of osteomalacia even though much has been written on vitamin D deficiency recently.

Clinical manifestations of osteomalacia are primarily related to a variety of underlying pathogenetic mechanisms that are poorly understood. The classic symptoms are bone pain and tenderness, muscle weakness, and difficulty in walking, all of which can often be vague and unremitting but less in severity during the summer months. Consequently patients are labeled with varied diagnoses ranging from fibromyalgia, severe myopathy,[6] unusual pain syndrome,[7] or neurologic disorders of unknown cause. In patients with the genetic forms of osteomalacia and those with childhood

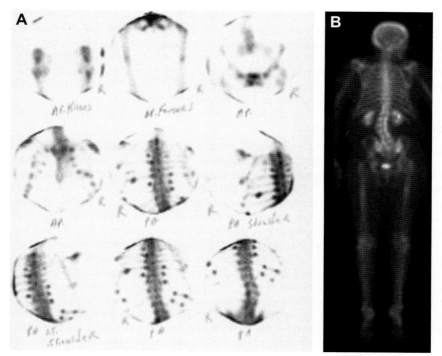

Fig. 1. A whole body bone scan before (*A*) and after (*B*) vitamin D therapy in the patient described in the text. Complete and thorough evaluation did not reveal any cause for vitamin D deficiency other than nutritional deficiency. Note multiple bilateral hot spots in the ribs without any other discrete foci elsewhere in the body, characteristic of osteomalacia, but not of metastatic disease as was thought initially in this patient. Also, note a decreased uptake in the kidney in the absence of renal insufficiency suggesting an avid uptake and retention in the skeleton.

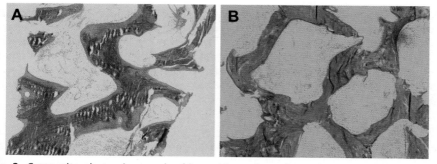

Fig. 2. Composite photomicrograph of bone biopsy from the patient with vitamin D deficiency osteomalacia. (*A*) Low-power view showing increased osteoid (*magenta or red color*) surface covering the entire bone surfaces with poorly mineralized trabecular bone (*green with red areas within*), thick osteoid seams, and relatively well-preserved trabecular architecture. (*B*) After vitamin D repletion there was complete healing of osteomalacia with substantial decrease in osteoid surface and thickness.

celiac disease, residual deformities of rickets with associated short stature may be seen, but are not usually seen in patients with nutritional rickets. Deformities related to the softening of the adult skeleton include kyphosis, coxa vara, pigeon breast, protrusio acetabuli, and triradiate pelvis with a narrow pubic arch; the latter can lead to difficulty in labor and vaginal delivery. However, such extreme skeletal abnormalities are uncommon in contemporary practice in the United States,[8] but are not uncommon in parts of the world where vitamin D depletion is endemic.[9]

Bone Pain and Tenderness

Pain in osteomalacia is dull and poorly localized but clearly felt in the bones rather than in the joints and is distinct from muscle pain. The pain is believed to be caused by hydration of the unmineralized bone matrix underneath the periosteum that stretches causing throbbing pain.[10] Patients are often able to distinguish between muscle and bone pain on carefully directed questioning. The bone pain is usually persistent, made worse by weight-bearing or contraction of the muscles during locomotion, and is rarely relieved completely by rest. Pain is usually symmetric and diffuse, beginning in the lower back, later spreading to the pelvic girdle, hips and upper thighs, and ribs. It is almost never of a radicular nature and in the absence of fracture there is tenderness on percussion of bones, especially over the tibial shins. Lateral compression of the ribs or of the pelvic girdle and compression of the sternum are useful clinical maneuvers to elicit pain in mild to moderate cases. The anatomic location of the pain to the axial rather than appendicular skeleton is most likely as a result of a higher proportion of cancellous bone in the spine, which accumulates relatively more osteoid than the cortical bones in the long bones of the extremities. A few patients are completely asymptomatic despite severe hypocalcemia,[11] whereas others suffer from excruciating pain with the least movement; the reasons for such dichotomy are not clear.

Muscle Weakness

Proximal limb muscle weakness is characteristic of osteomalacia. The severity varies from a subtle abnormality detectable only on careful physical examination to severe disability verging on complete paralysis.[12] Muscle atrophy is mild in relation to the severity of weakness, tone is reduced, and fasciculation is absent, but deep tendon reflexes are preserved or increased. In mild cases, true weakness must be distinguished from unwillingness to tense the muscle because of pain. Specific symptoms include difficulty in rising from a chair, walking up or down stairs, and the characteristic gait described as waddling gait caused by inability to lift the leg off the ground because of quadriceps weakness or flex the hip or the knee joints. A more recent meta-analysis suggests a close relationship between muscle strength and serum 25-hydroxyvitamin D level particularly when the serum levels decrease to less than 20 ng/mL.[13]

Difficulty in Walking

Abnormal gait can be the result of either pain or weakness, but usually both contribute to the problem. A change in gait discriminates more reliably between young adults with and without osteomalacia than any other symptoms. Many patients feel pain only when walking, which they consequently avoid. Because of weakness, the legs may feel heavy and the patient tires easily, walks more slowly with flatfooted springless gait, and is more likely to stumble. A waddling gait is characteristic of osteomalacia.

RADIOLOGICAL FEATURES OF OSTEOMALACIA

Many structural and pathologic changes in bone can be detected on radiograph examination and are the result of increased PTH secretion or of impaired matrix mineralization (**Figs. 3–6**). Secondary hyperparathyroidism, an inevitable consequence of vitamin D depletion, leads to thinning of cortical bone. Increased cortical porosity is manifested as cortical striations in the metacarpals and phalanges on high-resolution radiographs of the hands. Rarely, generalized osteitis fibrosa cystica may be present.[14] The most common radiographic manifestation of impaired mineralization in cancellous bone is osteopenia. Changes in bone shape such as protrusio acetabuli (see **Fig. 6**) can be seen, although rare in this country.

The best known and the characteristic radiographic feature of osteomalacia is the Looser's zone (see **Figs. 3–6**), a lucent band adjacent to the periosteum that represents an unhealed insufficiency-type stress fracture. Stress fractures are incomplete fissures without displacement that occur as a result of repetitive trauma. Looser's zones occur most commonly in ribs, pubic rami, and outer borders of scapulae (see **Figs. 3–6**), and less commonly on the inferior aspect of the femoral necks, medial aspect of proximal femur, metatarsals, and medial aspect of the shafts of long bones. This is in contrast to the fissure fractures that occur on the outer convex border of the long bones in Paget disease of bone. Occasionally pseudofractures can occur without osteomalacia.[15,16]

Radionuclide bone scans are most useful in evaluating patients with suspected osteomalacia. This imaging method can present in many different ways ranging

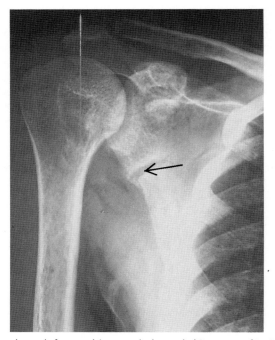

Fig. 3. Looser's zone (pseudofracture) in scapula (*arrow*). (*Courtesy of* Dr Sanjay K. Bhadada, Post Graduate Institute of Medical Education and Research, Chandigarh, India.)

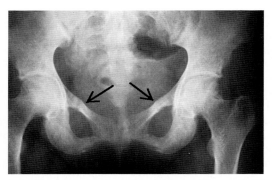

Fig. 4. Looser zone (pseudofracture) in superior pubic rami (*arrows*). (*Courtesy of* Dr Sanjay K. Bhadada, Post Graduate Institute of Medical Education and Research, Chandigarh, India.)

from the so-called super scan, in which no discrete focal abnormalities are seen, to many discrete foci of increased radionuclide uptake mimicking metastatic cancer.[1]

Bone mineral density as assessed by dual-energy x-ray absorptiometry (DXA) is always reduced at all relevant skeletal sites (spine, hip, and forearm) with the greatest deficits at the cortical-rich bone in the forearms.[1,8,17] The contrasting features of the pattern of bone mineral deficits in osteoporosis and osteomalacia are summarized in **Table 1**.

SKELETAL FRACTURES

Several types of fractures occur in patients with osteomalacia with the pseudofractures that can progress to a complete fracture, usually in the subtronchanteric region of the femur or metatarsals, the greatest load-bearing bones. Rib fractures also occur commonly. When osteomalacia begins in childhood, the adult bones tend to be soft rather than brittle. Conversely, when osteomalacia begins later in adult life, the usual type fractures are more common. Spontaneous fractures of the sternum in the absence of trauma are almost always a result of adult onset osteomalacia.

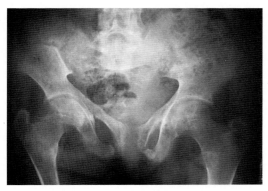

Fig. 5. Late effects of osteomalacia leading to triradiate pelvis. (*Courtesy of* Dr Sanjay K. Bhadada, Post Graduate Institute of Medical Education and Research, Chandigarh, India.)

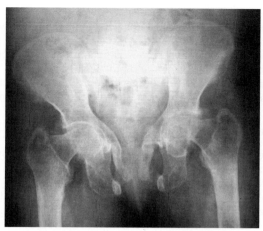

Fig. 6. Advanced osteomalacia with protrusioacetabuli and triradiate pelvis. (*Courtesy of* Dr Sanjay K. Bhadada, Post Graduate Institute of Medical Education and Research, Chandigarh, India.)

BIOCHEMICAL CHANGES IN OSTEOMALACIA

In its classic presentation, hypocalcemia, hypophosphatemia, and increased serum alkaline phosphatase level are the classic biochemical triad of osteomalacia,[1,8] but increased serum alkaline phosphatase level is the most frequent and the earliest biochemical manifestation.[8] As the vitamin D depletion advances, so does PTH hypersecretion leading to increased bone remodeling, endocortical bone resorption, and cortical thinning, which collectively results in irreversible cortical bone loss and increased fracture risk.[3] Most patients at this earliest stage of hypovitaminosis D osteopathy are asymptomatic and recognition at this stage is of paramount importance to prevent fractures and progression of preosteomalacia to frank osteomalacia.[3,4,8] Because of the associated secondary hyperparathyroidism, biochemical markers of bone turnover are increased.[1]

DIAGNOSTIC APPROACH TO OSTEOMALACIA

In the right clinical setting, a careful history and physical examination and a high degree of suspicion should facilitate the diagnosis of osteomalacia. However, despite many advances in biochemical measurements none of them are specific and most have moderate to low sensitivity. A reduced serum calcium × phosphate product and high alkaline phosphatase level in the presence of low 25-hydroxyvitamin D and high PTH makes the diagnosis of osteomalacia highly likely. On the other hand, a low serum 25-hydroxyvitamin D level is a poor predictor of osteomalacia, just as a low serum vitamin B_{12} level is a poor predictor of bone marrow findings. Skeletal radiographs and bone scans might reveal pseudofractures and the bone scan might suggest only a super scan. An in vivo tetracycline-labeled transiliac bone biopsy may help to diagnose osteomalacia in challenging cases.[2,4]

The authors routinely recommend in vivo tetracycline-labeled bone biopsy in all patients with gastrointestinal-related vitamin D depletion with increased alkaline phosphatase and PTH levels.[8] A bone biopsy for detailed bone histomorphometry can be accomplished with a simple 11G or 8G Jamshidi needle using the same approach as transiliac trephine biopsy used in the evaluation of bone quality measurements in patients with osteoporosis. The small Jamshidi needle biopsy provides an adequate quantity of cancellous bone sample for diagnostic purposes. The procedure can be performed in less than 30 minutes in the outpatient setting under local anesthesia with minimal discomfort to the patient and practically no morbidity.[18] The undecalcified bone biopsy specimen should be preserved in 70% alcohol (not formalin) and can be sent to one of several specialized laboratories for detailed bone histomorphometry.

TREATMENT OF OSTEOMALACIA

Depending on the urgency with which vitamin D replenishment is needed, several dose regimens can be used.[19] Although each has some advantages the authors routinely prescribe ergocalciferol (vitamin D_2) or cholecalciferol (vitamin D_3) 50,000 IU (1.25 mg) once a week for 8 weeks followed by dose adjustments based on serum 25-hydroxyvitamin D and PTH levels. In our experience, there are no distinct differences between the vitamin D preparations except perhaps a shorter half-life of vitamin D_2 and consequently the need for more frequent dosing during the maintenance phase. Most patients need longer duration of the weekly doses and many with intestinal disorders need daily doses as high as 150,000 IU/d in the first 1 to 3 months with dose reduction based on biochemical responses. Bone biopsy findings often help to decide on the dose and duration of high-dose therapy if the osteoid indices are high and if marrow fibrosis is also present. This is somewhat analogous to hungry-bone syndrome following parathyroidectomy in patients with severe primary or secondary hyperparathyroidism.

Careful and close follow-up is necessary during the first few months (1–3 months) of therapy to avoid therapy-related problems, although it is extremely uncommon to see hypercalcemia or renal dysfunction. More problematic is the risk of long-bone and hip fractures as the patient's muscle weakness improves and bone pain remits before bone mass and strength is restored. Long-term maintenance therapy is largely dictated by clinical and biochemical responses; the latter might take months and at times years to resolve. The authors routinely repeat Jamshidi needle biopsy to document healing of osteomalacia before recommending antiresorptive or anabolic therapy for the associated residual osteoporosis. Almost all patients with gastrointestinal-related vitamin D deficiency osteomalacia require life-long follow-up to avoid recurrence of osteomalacia caused by lapses in therapy, treatment of associated osteoporosis, and for the rare development of hypercalcemic autonomous secondary hyperparathyroidism. Despite these demanding needs, treatment of osteomalacia is most gratifying to the patient and the clinician, similar to that of myxedema or pernicious anemia.

REFERENCES

1. Parfitt AM. Osteomalacia and related disorders. In: Avioli LV, Krane SM, editors. Metabolic bone disease and clinically related disorders. Philadelphia: WB Saunders; 1990. p. 329–96.
2. Ramser JR, Frost HM, Frame B, et al. Tetracycline-based studies of bone dynamics in rib of 6 cases of osteomalacia. Clin Orthop Relat Res 1966;46: 219–36.
3. Parfitt AM, Rao DS, Stanciu J, et al. Irreversible bone loss in osteomalacia: comparison of radial photon absorptiometry with iliac bone histomorphometry during treatment. J Clin Invest 1985;76:2403–12.

4. Rao DS, Villanueva AR, Mathews M. Histologic evolution of vitamin D depletion in patients with intestinal malabsorption or dietary deficiency. In: Frame B, Potts JTJ, editors. Clinical disorders of bone and mineral metabolism. Amsterdam: Excerpta Medica; 1983. p. 224–6.

5. McKenna MJ, Freaney R, Casey OM, et al. Osteomalacia and osteoporosis: evaluation of a diagnostic index. J Clin Pathol 1983;36:245–52.

6. Prabhala A, Garg R, Dandona P. Severe myopathy associated with vitamin D deficiency in western New York. Arch Intern Med 1999;160:1199–203.

7. Gloth FM, Lindsay JM, Zelesnick LB, et al. Can vitamin D deficiency produce an unusual pain syndrome? Arch Intern Med 1991;151:1662–4.

8. Basha B, Rao DS, Han ZH, et al. Osteomalacia due to vitamin D depletion in the US. Ame J Med 2000;108:296–300.

9. Mathew JT, Seshadri MS, Thomas K, et al. Osteomalacia: fifty five patients seen in a teaching institution over a 4 year period. J Assoc Physicians India 1994;42: 692–4.

10. Holick MF. Vitamin D deficiency. N Engl J Med 2007;357:266–81.

11. Rao DS, Parfitt AM, Kleerekoper M, et al. Dissociation between the effects of endogenous parathyroid hormone on adenosine 3′,5′-monophosphate generation and phosphate reabsorption in hypocalcemia due to vitamin D depletion: an acquired disorder resembling pseudohypoparathyroidism type II. J Clin Endocrinol Metab 1985;61:285–90.

12. Russell JA. Osteomalacic myopathy. Muscle Nerve 1994;17:578–80.

13. Bischoff-Ferrari HA, Dawson-Hughes B, Willett WC, et al. Effect of vitamin D on falls: a meta-analysis. JAMA 2004;291:1999–2006.

14. Hajjar ET, Vincenti F, Salti CS. Gluten-induced enteropathy; osteomalacia as a principal manifestation. Arch Intern Med 1974;134:565–7.

15. Perry HM, Weinstein RS, Teitelbaum SL, et al. Pseudofractures in the absence of osteomalacia. Skeletal Radiol 1982;8:17–9.

16. McKenna MJ, Kleerekoper M, Ellis BI, et al. Atypical insufficiency fractures confused with Looser zones of osteomalacia. Bone 1987;8:71–8.

17. Parfitt AM. Accelerated cortical bone loss: primary and secondary hyperparathyroidism. In: Uhthoff HK, Stahl E, editors. Current concepts of bone fragility. Berlin: Springer-Verlag; 1986. p. 279–85.

18. Rao DS, Matkovic V, Duncan H. Transiliac bone biopsy: complications and diagnostic value. Henry Ford Hosp Med J 1980;28:112–5.

19. Pepper KJ, Judd SE, Nanes MS, et al. Evaluation of vitamin D repletion regimens to correct vitamin D status in adults. Endocr Pract 2009;15:95–103.

Genetic Disorders and Defects in Vitamin D Action

Peter J. Malloy, PhD*, David Feldman, MD

KEYWORDS

- 1α-Hydroxylase deficiency
- Hereditary vitamin D–resistant rickets
- Vitamin D receptor • Mutations • Rickets • Alopecia

Vitamin D is an inactive precursor, requiring 2 hydroxylation steps, first in the liver and then the kidney, to be converted to $1\alpha,25$-dihydroxyvitamin D_3 (calcitriol), the active hormone. The details of this metabolic conversion are described in other articles in this issue. Calcitriol then binds to the vitamin D receptor (VDR) to mediate the actions of the hormone. As described in other articles in this issue, calcitriol/VDR complexes regulate multiple target genes throughout the body. Most obvious are genes that regulate calcium and phosphate metabolism and that are responsible for normal mineralization of bone. In the absence of either the active hormone (calcitriol) or a functional receptor (VDR), calcium absorption is impaired and bones become inadequately mineralized. When this occurs in children, the disease rickets develops, when it happens in adults, osteomalacia develops. The most common cause of rickets and osteomalacia is vitamin D deficiency as described in articles by Thandrayen and Pettifor; and Bhan and colleagues elsewhere this issue for children and adults.

However, 2 rare genetic diseases can also cause rickets in children. These diseases, and the knockout mouse models of the 2 human diseases, have provided exceptional insight into the metabolism and mechanism of action of calcitriol. The critical enzyme to synthesize calcitriol from 25-hydroxyvitamin D [25(OH)D], the circulating hormone precursor, is 25-hydroxyvitamin D-1α-hydroxylase (1α-hydroxylase). When this enzyme is defective and calcitriol can no longer be synthesized, the disease 1α-hydroxylase deficiency develops. The disease is also known as vitamin D–dependent rickets type 1 (VDDR-1) or pseudovitamin D deficiency rickets. When the VDR is defective, the disease hereditary vitamin D–resistant rickets (HVDRR), also known as vitamin D–dependent rickets type 2 (VDDR-2), develops. Both diseases are rare autosomal

This work was supported by Grant No. DK042482 from the National Institutes of Health.
Division of Endocrinology, Gerontology and Metabolism, Stanford University School of Medicine, Stanford University, S-025 Endocrinology, 300 Pasteur Drive, Stanford, CA 94305-5103, USA
* Corresponding author.
E-mail address: pjmalloy@stanford.edu

recessive disorders characterized by hypocalcemia, secondary hyperparathyroidism, and early onset severe rickets. As discussed later in more detail, a crucial difference between the 2 diseases is that 1α-hydroxylase deficiency is characterized by extremely low to absent serum calcitriol levels, whereas HVDRR, characteristic of a target organ resistance disease, is distinguished by exceedingly high levels of calcitriol. In this article, these 2 genetic childhood diseases, which present similarly with hypocalcemia and rickets in infancy, are discussed and compared. However, the focus is on HVDRR, a more complex and serious disease, because affected children do not usually respond to treatment with calcitriol, whereas 1α-hydroxylase deficiency does.

1α-HYDROXYLASE DEFICIENCY IN CHILDREN

In 1973 Fraser and colleagues[1] postulated that VDDR-1 was an inborn error of vitamin D metabolism involving defective conversion of 25(OH)D to 1α,25(OH)$_2$D$_3$. Approximately 25 years later in 1997 the gene (CYP27B1) encoding the 1α-hydroxylase enzyme was cloned by several groups[2–6] and it was immediately demonstrated that VDDR-1 was caused by mutations in the CYP27B1 gene.[2]

Children with 1α-hydroxylase deficiency present with a clinical picture of joint pain and deformity, hypotonia, muscle weakness, growth failure, and sometimes hypocalcemic seizures or fractures in early infancy.[7–9] Laboratory analysis reveals hypocalcemia, secondary hyperparathyroidism, increased alkaline phosphatase activity and low or undetectable calcitriol in the presence of adequate 25(OH)D levels (**Table 1**). Radiographic findings show characteristic changes of rickets. The children have no clinical response to high doses of cholecalciferol but respond to physiologic doses of calcitriol or 1α-hydroxyvitamin D.[10] Although it is a rare inborn error, 1α-hydroxylase deficiency is more frequently found in the French Canadian population.[11]

MUTATIONS IN THE CYP27B1 GENE AS THE MOLECULAR BASIS FOR 1α-HYDROXYLASE DEFICIENCY

VDDR-1 is caused by heterogeneous mutations in the CYP27B1 gene that abolish or reduce 1α-hydroxylase enzymatic activity. A recent review by the Miller and Portale group[12] catalogs the many different mutations in the CYP27B1 gene that have been described including missense mutations, deletions, duplications, and splice site changes. To date, 48 patients have been described with mutations in the CYP27B1 gene including both genders of children from multiple ethnic backgrounds often in the setting of consanguinity.

The 1α-hydroxylase is a type 1 mitochondrial P450 enzyme that functions as an oxidase. The reaction uses electrons from reduced nicotinamide adenine dinucleotide

Table 1
Comparison of genetic defect in vitamin D action

	1α-Hydroxylase Deficiency	HVDRR
Gene	CYP27B1	VDR
1,25(OH)$_2$D$_3$	Low	High
Parathyroid hormone	High	High
Calcium	Low	Low
Phosphate	Low	Low
Alopecia	No	Yes
Response to calcitriol	Yes	No

phosphate and molecular oxygen. The P450 moiety binds the 25(OH)D substrate, receives electrons and molecular oxygen, and catalyzes the reaction using the heme group iron to coordinate oxygen.[12,13] Deletions, premature termination as a result of splice site mutations and insertions, are the commonest defects that disrupt or eliminate the heme-binding domain and thereby inactivate the enzyme.[12] In some cases of 1α-hydroxylase deficiency, missense mutations have been identified in the CYP27B1 gene that disrupt α helical structures, the meander sequence, the cysteine pocket that binds the heme group and the substrate recognition sites (**Fig. 1**).

The major site in the body of 1α-hydroxylase activity is the kidney. 1α-Hydroxylase is also expressed in many tissues of the body including breast, prostate, colon, placenta, and macrophages.[14] These regions of local production are hypothesized to be of considerable importance for the expanded role of calcitriol in reducing cancer risk, fighting infection, and mediating antiinflammatory actions, and so forth. However, it is the renal enzyme that determines the circulating 1α,25(OH)$_2$D$_3$ concentration. The renal enzyme is under careful regulation by parathyroid hormone (PTH), calcium status, and calcitriol levels so that calcium homeostasis is tightly controlled by complex feedback loops.

Children with 1α-hydroxylase deficiency caused by mutations in the CYP27B1 gene present for medical attention with metabolic abnormalities in early infancy usually before 2 years of age. In utero development is considered to be normal as a result of maternal normocalcemia. When the infants come to medical attention they characteristically show growth retardation, bone and joint deformities, and bone pain. Teeth may show marked hypoplasia of the enamel. Serum levels show hypocalcemia, hypophosphatemia, secondary hyperparathyroidism, and increased alkaline phosphatase activity. Radiographs show the classic features of rickets. Since the availability of 1α-hydroxylated vitamin D metabolites such as calcitriol or 1α-hydroxyvitamin D, therapeutic responses and complete remission of the disease can be routinely achieved. Dosages of calcitriol of 1 to 3 μg/d are adequate to heal the rickets and return serum chemistries to normal. Calcium levels improve within days and radiologic improvement in bones can be seen within 2 to 3 months. Healing of rickets has been reported in 9 to 10 months.[10]

MOUSE MODELS OF 1α-HYDROXYLASE DEFICIENCY

Several groups have developed mouse models of 1α-hydroxylase deficiency using targeted disruption of the CYP27B1 gene.[15,16] The targeted region of the gene has been the hormone-binding and heme-binding domains of the protein. After weaning, the 1α-hydroxylase null mice develop the classic features of human 1α-hydroxylase deficiency with hypocalcemia, secondary hyperparathyroidism, retarded growth, and skeletal changes of rickets. Many of the nonskeletal changes seen, including reproductive and immune function abnormalities, were probably at least partly caused by severe hypocalcemia. It was subsequently discovered that feeding the mice a rescue diet high in calcium, phosphorus, and lactose could normalize the hypocalcemia present in these mice as well as the VDR null mice and seemed to heal the rickets.[17,18] The Goltzman group went on to compare findings in 1α-hydroxylase null mice with VDR null mice and the double mutant that combines disruption of both 1α-hydroxylase and VDR.[19,20] In addition, the investigators studied the effects of normalizing calcium homeostasis with the rescue diet and treatment with calcitriol. They concluded that normalization of calcium cannot entirely substitute for 1,25(OH)$_2$D$_3$ action in skeletal and mineral homeostasis and that the 2 agents have discrete and overlapping functions. Both are required to maintain normal osteoclastic

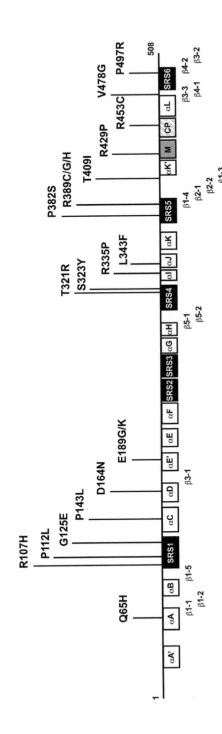

Fig. 1. Missense mutations identified in patients with 1α-hydroxylase deficiency. The human 1α-hydroxylase enzyme is composed of 508 amino acids. The locations of the missense mutations are shown above the line. The names of the α helices (open boxes), the meander sequence (M, gray box), the cysteine pocket (CP, hatched box), substrate recognition sites (SRS, black boxes), and the β turns are shown below the line.

bone resorption and osteoblastic bone formation. The widened cartilaginous growth plates characteristic of rickets could only be completely normalized by a combination of calcium and $1,25(OH)_2D_3$. These issues are discussed further in the sections on HVDRR and VDR mutations.

HVDRR IN CHILDREN

Children with HVDRR develop hypocalcemia and severe rickets usually within months of birth. Affected children have bone pain, muscle weakness, hypotonia, and occasionally have convulsions caused by the hypocalcemia. They are often growth retarded and in some cases develop severe dental caries or hypoplasia of the teeth.[21,22] The laboratory findings include low serum concentrations of calcium and phosphate and increased serum alkaline phosphatase activity. The children have secondary hyperparathyroidism with markedly increased PTH levels. Serum 25(OH)D values are usually normal and $1,25(OH)_2D$ levels are substantially increased. This clinical finding distinguishes HVDRR from 1α-hydroxylase deficiency in which serum $1,25(OH)_2D$ values are low or absent (see **Table 1**). Many children with HVDRR also have sparse body hair and some have total scalp and body alopecia including eyebrows and in some cases eyelashes. This feature also helps distinguish HVDRR from 1α-hydroxylase deficiency. Most affected children are resistant to therapy with supraphysiologic doses of all forms of vitamin D including calcitriol.

HVDRR is an autosomal recessive disease with males and females equally affected. The parents of patients, who are heterozygous carriers of the genetic trait, usually show no symptoms of the disease and have normal bone development. These findings indicate that a single defective allele is not sufficient to cause disease. In most cases, consanguinity is associated with the disease with each parent contributing a defective gene.

MUTATIONS IN THE VDR GENE AS THE MOLECULAR BASIS FOR HVDRR

More than 100 cases of HVDRR have been recorded and many of these have been analyzed at the biochemical and molecular level.[21–23] Presently, 34 heterogeneous mutations have been identified in the VDR gene as the cause of HVDRR (**Fig. 2**). Mutations in the DNA-binding domain (DBD) prevent the VDR from binding to DNA causing total $1,25(OH)_2D_3$ resistance even though $1,25(OH)_2D_3$ binding to the VDR is normal. On the other hand, mutations in the ligand-binding domain (LBD) may disrupt ligand binding, or heterodimerization with retinoid X receptor (RXR), or prevent coactivators from binding to the VDR and cause partial or total hormone resistance. Other mutations that have been identified in the VDR that cause $1,25(OH)_2D_3$ resistance include nonsense mutations, insertions/substitutions, insertions/duplications, deletions, and splice site mutations. Some of these VDR mutations are described in this article.

To date, 9 missense mutations have been identified in the VDR DBD as the cause of HVDRR (**Fig. 2A**). These mutant VDRs have normal ligand binding but defective DNA binding.[21,22] A common feature of patients with mutations in the DBD is that they all have alopecia. The heterozygotic parents with a single mutant allele are asymptomatic.

Several nonsense mutations have been identified in the VDR gene that truncate the VDR protein.[21,22] Fibroblasts from patients with VDR nonsense mutations exhibit no ligand binding and often the truncated VDR protein cannot be detected by immunoblotting. One particular mutation, a single base change in exon 8 that introduced a premature termination codon (Y295X), was identified in several families in a large kindred where consanguineous marriages were common.[24] The VDR mRNA was

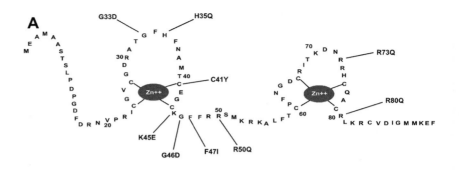

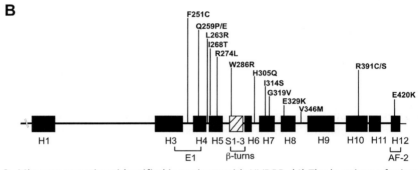

Fig. 2. Missense mutations identified in patients with HVDRR. (*A*) The locations of missense mutations in the VDR DNA-binding domain depicted as a 2-zinc finger structure. (*B*) The locations of the missense mutations in the VDR LBD are shown above the line. The filled rectangles represent α helices (H1–H12) and the hatched box represents the β sheet structure. The location of the E1 and AF-2 domains are also indicated.

undetectable by Northern blot analysis indicating that the Y295X mutation led to nonsense-mediated mRNA decay. In 1 family with an R30X mutation, the parents of the affected child had somewhat increased serum 1,25(OH)$_2$D levels indicating some resistance to 1,25(OH)$_2$D.[25] All of the affected children with nonsense mutations had alopecia.

Splice site mutations in the VDR gene have also been identified as the cause of HVDRR. These mutations usually cause a frameshift and eventually introduce a downstream premature stop signal resulting in a nonfunctional VDR. Splice site mutations in the VDR gene cause exons to be skipped[26,27] or cause incorporation of an intron into the VDR mRNA.[28] In 1 case, a cryptic 5′ donor splice site was generated in exon 6 that deleted 56 nucleotide bases and led to a frameshift in exon 7.[29]

To date, 15 missense mutations have been identified in the VDR LBD (see **Fig. 2**).[30,31] One patient had an R274L mutation that altered the contact point for the 1α-hydroxyl group of 1,25(OH)$_2$D$_3$.[30,32] The mutation lowered the binding affinity of the VDR for 1,25(OH)$_2$D$_3$. A second patient had an H305Q mutation that altered the contact point for the 25-hydroxyl group of 1,25(OH)$_2$D$_3$.[32,33] This mutation also lowered the binding affinity of the VDR for 1,25(OH)$_2$D$_3$. These cases illustrate the importance of critical amino acids as contact points for 1,25(OH)$_2$D$_3$ and demonstrate that mutations of these residues can be the basis for HVDRR.

Mutations have also been identified in the VDR that disrupt VDR:RXR protein interaction as a cause of HVDRR. For example, an R391C mutation in the VDR LBD had no affect on ligand binding but reduced its transactivation activity. R391 is located in helix H10 where the RXR dimer interface is formed from helix H9 and helix H10 and the interhelical loops between H7-H8 and H8-H9 in VDR.[32] R391 was also mutated to serine (R391S).[34] Several other mutations have been identified in the VDR that affect RXR heterodimerization including Q259P and F251C.[29,35] Q259 was also mutated to glutamic acid (Q259E).[36] A V346M mutation was identified in a patient with HVDRR and may be important in RXR heterodimerization.[37] All of the patients with defects in RXR heterodimerization had alopecia.

A mutation has also been identified in the VDR that prevented coactivator recruitment that is critical for transcriptional activity.[38] An E420K mutation located in helix H12 had no effect on ligand binding, VDR-RXR heterodimerization, or DNA binding. However, the E420K mutation abolished binding by the coactivators SRC-1 and DRIP205. The child with the E420K mutation did not have alopecia[38] suggesting that ligand-mediated transactivation and coactivator recruitment by the VDR is not required for hair growth.

Several compound heterozygous mutations in the VDR gene have been identified in children with HVDRR. In these cases each heterozygotic parent harbored a different mutant VDR and consanguinity was not involved. One patient was heterozygous for an E329K mutation and had a second mutation on the other allele that deleted a single nucleotide 366 (366delC) in exon 4.[39] The single base deletion resulted in a frameshift creating a premature termination signal that truncated most of the LBD. The E329K mutation in helix H8, which is important in heterodimerization with RXR, likely disrupts this activity. L263R and R391S compound heterozygous mutations were also identified in the VDR gene in a child with HVDRR and early childhood-onset type 1 diabetes.[34] The mutant VDRs in this case had differential effects on 24-hydroxylase and RelB promoters. The 24-hydroxylase responses were abolished in the L263R mutant but only partially altered in the R391S mutant. On the other hand, RelB responses were normal for the L263R mutant but the R391S mutant was defective in this response.[34] The reason for the differential activities of these VDR mutants is unknown. Compound heterozygous mutations were also found in the VDR gene in a patient with HVDRR and alopecia.[40] The patient was heterozygous for a nonsense mutation R30X and a 3-bp deletion in exon 6 that deleted the codon for lysine at amino acid 246 (ΔK246). The ΔK246 mutation did not affect ligand binding but abolished heterodimerization with RXR and binding to coactivators.[40] All of the patients with compound heterozygous mutations had alopecia.

Two cases of insertions/duplications in the VDR gene causing HVDRR have been reported. In 1 case a unique 5-bp deletion/8-bp insertion was found in the VDR gene.[41] The mutation deleted amino acids H141 and Y142 and inserted 3 amino acids (L141, W142, and A143). Only the laboratory engineered A143 insertion into the wild-type (WT) VDR disrupted transactivation to the same extent as the natural mutation. The patient with this mutation did not have alopecia. In the second case, a 102-bp insertion/duplication was found in the VDR gene that introduced a premature stop (Y401X) and deleted helix H12.[42] The truncated VDR was able to heterodimerize with RXR, bind to DNA, and interact with the corepressor hairless (HR) but failed to bind coactivators and was transactivation defective. The patient with this mutation had patchy alopecia.

There is only a single reported case where investigators failed to detect a mutation in the VDR as the basis of HVDRR.[43] In this case the investigators speculated that the resistance to the action of $1,25(OH)_2D_3$ was caused by abnormal expression of hormone response element–binding proteins belonging to the hnRNP family that prevented the VDR-RXR complex from binding to vitamin D response elements in target genes.[44]

MOUSE MODELS OF HVDRR

Mouse models of HVDRR have been created by targeted ablation of the VDR.[45,46] The targeted region has been the DBD domain. The VDR null mice (VDRKO) recapitulate the findings in children with HVDRR. The VDRKO mice appear normal at birth and become hypocalcemic and their parathyroid hormone (PTH) levels increase sometime after weaning. Bone mineralization is severely impaired and the changes of rickets develop over time. The VDRKO mice have normal hair at birth but develop progressive alopecia, thickened skin, enlarged sebaceous glands and epidermal cysts.[45,46] In 1 VDRKO mouse model, uterine hypoplasia with impaired folliculogenesis was found in female reproductive organs.[46] When the VDRKO mice are fed a rescue diet, their calcium can be normalized and the rickets reversed or prevented as was described for children with HVDRR successfully treated with intravenous or oral calcium. Many nonskeletal abnormalities seen in the hypocalcemic mice are prevented by the rescue diet indicating the abnormalities resulted from the hypocalcemia and were not directly caused by the absence of a functional VDR. However, again as in children with HVDRR, the alopecia is not reversed or prevented by normalization of calcium homeostasis.

THERAPY FOR HVDRR

Mutations in the VDR that cause HVDRR result in partial or total resistance to $1,25(OH)_2D_3$ action. The patients become hypocalcemic predominately because of a lack of VDR signaling in the intestine to promote calcium absorption. The hypocalcemia leads to a decrease in bone mineralization and causes rickets. Some patients with HVDRR improved clinically and radiologically when treated with pharmacologic doses of vitamin D ranging from 5000 to 40,000 IU/d, 20 to 200 μg/d of $25(OH)D_3$, and 17 to 20 μg/d of $1,25(OH)_2D_3$.[21,22] Some patients also responded to $1\alpha(OH)D_3$.[21,22] The patient with the H305Q mutation, a contact point for the 25-hydroxyl group of $1,25(OH)_2D_3$, showed improvement with 12.5 μg/d calcitriol treatment.[33,47] On the other hand, the patient with the R274L mutation, a contact point for the 1α-hydroxyl group of $1,25(OH)_2D_3$, was unresponsive to treatment with 600,000 IU vitamin D, up to 24 μg/d of $1,25(OH)_2D_3$, or 12 μg/d $1\alpha(OH)D_3$.[48]

When patients fail to respond to vitamin D or $1,25(OH)_2D_3$, intensive calcium therapy is used. Oral calcium can be absorbed in the intestine by vitamin D–dependent and vitamin D–independent pathways. In children with nonfunctional VDR, the vitamin D-independent pathway becomes critical. When oral calcium therapy is successful, the calcium levels in the gut have been increased enough so that passive diffusion or other non-vitamin D–dependent absorption is adequate to maintain normocalcemia. Intravenous (IV) calcium infusions are used to treat children with HVDRR who fail previous treatments with large doses of vitamin D derivatives and/or oral calcium.[49–53] IV calcium therapy bypasses the calcium absorption defect in the intestine caused by the lack of action of the mutant VDR. However, in affected children receiving IV calcium, when the IV therapy is discontinued the syndrome recurs slowly over time. Some children have been managed with intermittent IV calcium regimens using oral calcium in the intervals.[27] Once the child is older, perhaps when the skeleton has finished major growth, oral calcium often suffices to maintain normocalcemia and the IV calcium regimen can be discontinued.[52] Oral calcium alone has sometimes been used successfully as a therapy for patients with HVDRR.[54] Spontaneous healing of rickets has been observed in some patients with HVDRR as they get older and sometimes all therapy can be discontinued.[55–57] In all of the cases regardless of the therapy, if alopecia is present, it is unchanged by the treatment despite normalization of calcium and healing of rickets.

A most unexpected finding is that raising the serum calcium level to normal by IV or oral calcium administration reversed all aspects of HVDRR including hypocalcemia, hypophosphatemia, secondary hyperparathyroidism, rickets, increased alkaline phosphatase activity, and so forth, except for alopecia (discussed later). Correcting the hypocalcemia often corrects the hypophosphatemia without the need for phosphate supplements. This finding indicates that the low phosphate level was caused by the secondary hyperparathyroidism, which normalizes with correction of the hypocalcemia even in the absence of VDR action. The inescapable conclusion is that the most important actions of $1,25(OH)_2D_3$ on calcium and bone homeostasis occur in the intestine on calcium absorption and not in the bone. The ability of the rachitic bone abnormality to normalize in the absence of VDR-mediated vitamin D action was surprising. The data are incomplete in patients about whether the bones are entirely normal and Panda and colleagues,[20] using VDR knockout mice, has data suggesting that subtle defects remain in the bones of VDR null mice whose serum calcium level had been corrected by a rescue diet. However, the reversal of all clinical aspects of HVDRR with IV calcium does indicate that healing of bone and reversal of secondary hyperparathyroidism and hypophosphatemia can take place without normal VDR-mediated vitamin D action. There is no doubt that vitamin D has important actions on bone and parathyroid cells. However, these actions can apparently be compensated for in vivo if the calcium level is normalized.

In recent years there have been many new actions attributed to vitamin D that mediate important and widespread effects that are unrelated to calcium and bone homeostasis.[58,59] These include actions to reduce the risk of cancer, autoimmune disease, infection, neurodegeneration, and so forth. At this time, the authors have not detected a trend toward an increased risk for any of these potential problems in children with HVDRR. However, there are very few cases of HVDRR and most of the cases are detected in infants and young children so that it may be too early in their life to detect an increased tendency toward any of these potential health problems.

ALOPECIA

The molecular analysis of the VDR from patients with HVDRR with and without alopecia has provided several clues to the functions of the VDR that are important for hair growth. For example, patients with premature stop mutations and VDR knockout mice have alopecia indicating that the intact VDR protein is critical for renewed hair growth after birth.[45,46] Expression of the WT VDR in keratinocytes of VDR knockout mice prevented alopecia, a finding that further supports a role for the VDR in regulating hair growth.[60] Patients with DBD mutations also have alopecia indicating that VDR binding to DNA is critical to prevent alopecia. Patients with VDR mutations that inhibit RXR heterodimerization have alopecia indicating an essential role for VDR-RXR heterodimers in hair growth.[29,31,35] Inactivation of RXRα in keratinocytes in mice also caused alopecia clearly demonstrating a role for RXR in hair growth.[61]

On the other hand, patients with VDR mutations that abolish ligand binding or patients with 1α-hydroxylase deficiency and other forms of vitamin D deficiency do not have alopecia suggesting that a ligand-independent action of the VDR is critical to regulate the normal hair cycle.[38,62–64] The patient with the E420K mutation that abolished coactivator binding (but not ligand binding or RXR heterodimerization) did not have alopecia indicating that VDR actions to regulate hair growth were independent of coactivator interactions.[38] Also, when ligand-binding defective or coactivator-binding defective mutant VDRs were specifically expressed in keratinocytes in VDR knockout mice that have alopecia, hair growth was fully or partially restored.[64]

The alopecia associated with HVDRR is clinically and pathologically indistinguishable from the generalized disease atrichia with papular lesions (APL) found in patients with mutations in the *hairless* (*hr*) gene.[39,65,66] The *hr* gene product, HR acts as a corepressor and directly interacts with the VDR and suppresses $1,25(OH)_2D_3$-mediated transactivation.[62,66,67] It has been hypothesized that the role of the VDR in the hair cycle is to repress the expression of a gene(s) in a ligand-independent manner.[38,62,64,66] The ligand-independent activity requires that the VDR heterodimerize with RXR and bind to DNA.[38,63] The corepressor actions of HR may also be required in order for the unliganded VDR to repress gene transcription during the hair cycle. Mutations in the VDR that disrupt the ability of the unliganded VDR to suppress gene transcription are hypothesized to lead to the derepression of a gene(s) whose product, when expressed inappropriately, disrupts the hair cycle that ultimately leads to alopecia.[38,62,64,66] Inhibitors of the Wnt signaling pathway are possible candidates.[68,69] Thus far, there have been no reports of mutations in the VDR that affect interactions with HR. The role of HR in regulating the unliganded action of the VDR during the hair cycle remains to be discovered.

SUMMARY

The biochemical and genetic analysis of the VDR in patients with HVDRR has yielded important insights into the structure and function of the receptor in mediating $1,25(OH)_2D_3$ action. Similarly, study of children affected by HVDRR continues to provide a more complete understanding of the biologic role of $1,25(OH)_2D_3$ in vivo. A concerted investigative approach to HVDRR at the clinical, cellular, and molecular levels has proved valuable in gaining knowledge of the functions of the domains of the VDR and elucidating the detailed mechanism of action of $1,25(OH)_2D_3$. These studies have been essential to promote the well-being of the families with HVDRR and in improving the diagnostic and clinical management of this rare genetic disease.

REFERENCES

1. Fraser D, Kooh SW, Kind HP, et al. Pathogenesis of hereditary vitamin-D-dependent rickets. An inborn error of vitamin D metabolism involving defective conversion of 25-hydroxyvitamin D to 1 alpha,25-dihydroxyvitamin D. N Engl J Med 1973;289:817–22.
2. Fu GK, Lin D, Zhang MY, et al. Cloning of human 25-hydroxyvitamin D-1 alpha-hydroxylase and mutations causing vitamin D-dependent rickets type 1. Mol Endocrinol 1997;11:1961–70.
3. Monkawa T, Yoshida T, Wakino S, et al. Molecular cloning of cDNA and genomic DNA for human 25-hydroxyvitamin D_3 1 alpha-hydroxylase. Biochem Biophys Res Commun 1997;239:527–33.
4. Shinki T, Shimada H, Wakino S, et al. Cloning and expression of rat 25-hydroxyvitamin D_3-1alpha-hydroxylase cDNA. Proc Natl Acad Sci U S A 1997;94: 12920–5.
5. St-Arnaud R, Messerlian S, Moir JM, et al. The 25-hydroxyvitamin D 1-alpha-hydroxylase gene maps to the pseudovitamin D-deficiency rickets (PDDR) disease locus. J Bone Miner Res 1997;12:1552–9.

6. Takeyama K, Kitanaka S, Sato T, et al. 25-Hydroxyvitamin D_3 1alpha-hydroxylase and vitamin D synthesis. Science 1997;277:1827–30.
7. Arnaud C, Maijer R, Reade T, et al. Vitamin D dependency: an inherited postnatal syndrome with secondary hyperparathyroidism. Pediatrics 1970;46:871–80.
8. Glorieux FH, St-Arnaud R. Vitamin D pseudodeficiency. In: Feldman D, Pike JW, Glorieux FH, editors. Vitamin D. 2nd edition. San Diego (CA): Elsevier Academic Press; 2005. p. 1197–205.
9. Marx SJ, Spiegel AM, Brown EM, et al. A familial syndrome of decrease in sensitivity to 1,25-dihydroxyvitamin D. J Clin Endocrinol Metab 1978;47:1303–10.
10. Delvin EE, Glorieux FH, Marie PJ, et al. Vitamin D dependency: replacement therapy with calcitriol? J Pediatr 1981;99:26–34.
11. De Braekeleer M, Larochelle J. Population genetics of vitamin D-dependent rickets in northeastern Quebec. Ann Hum Genet 1991;55:283–90.
12. Kim CJ, Kaplan LE, Perwad F, et al. Vitamin D 1alpha-hydroxylase gene mutations in patients with 1alpha-hydroxylase deficiency. J Clin Endocrinol Metab 2007;92:3177–82.
13. Miller WL. Minireview: regulation of steroidogenesis by electron transfer. Endocrinology 2005;146:2544–50.
14. Hewison M, Zehnder D, Chakraverty R, et al. Vitamin D and barrier function: a novel role for extra-renal 1 alpha-hydroxylase. Mol Cell Endocrinol 2004;215:31–8.
15. Dardenne O, Prud'homme J, Arabian A, et al. Targeted inactivation of the 25-hydroxyvitamin D(3)-1(alpha)-hydroxylase gene (CYP27B1) creates an animal model of pseudovitamin D-deficiency rickets. Endocrinology 2001;142:3135–41.
16. Panda DK, Miao D, Tremblay ML, et al. Targeted ablation of the 25-hydroxyvitamin D 1alpha -hydroxylase enzyme: evidence for skeletal, reproductive, and immune dysfunction. Proc Natl Acad Sci U S A 2001;98:7498–503.
17. Amling M, Priemel M, Holzmann T, et al. Rescue of the skeletal phenotype of vitamin D receptor-ablated mice in the setting of normal mineral ion homeostasis: formal histomorphometric and biomechanical analyses. Endocrinology 1999;140:4982–7.
18. Li YC, Amling M, Pirro AE, et al. Normalization of mineral ion homeostasis by dietary means prevents hyperparathyroidism, rickets, and osteomalacia, but not alopecia in vitamin D receptor-ablated mice. Endocrinology 1998;139:4391–6.
19. Goltzman D, Miao D, Panda DK, et al. Effects of calcium and of the Vitamin D system on skeletal and calcium homeostasis: lessons from genetic models. J Steroid Biochem Mol Biol 2004;89-90:485–9.
20. Panda DK, Miao D, Bolivar I, et al. Inactivation of the 25-hydroxyvitamin D 1alpha-hydroxylase and vitamin D receptor demonstrates independent and interdependent effects of calcium and vitamin D on skeletal and mineral homeostasis. J Biol Chem 2004;279:16754–66.
21. Malloy PJ, Pike JW, Feldman D. Hereditary 1,25-dihydroxyvitamin D resistant rickets. In: Feldman D, Pike JW, Glorieux F, editors. Vitamin D. 2nd edition. San Diego (CA): Elsevier; 2005. p. 1207–38.
22. Malloy PJ, Pike JW, Feldman D. The vitamin D receptor and the syndrome of hereditary 1,25-dihydroxyvitamin D-resistant rickets. Endocr Rev 1999;20:156–88.
23. Malloy PJ, Feldman D. Molecular defects in the vitamin D receptor associated with hereditary 1,25-dihydroxyvitamin D resistant rickets. In: Holick MF, editor. Vitamin D: physiology, molecular biology, and clinical applications. Totowa (NJ): Humana Press; 1999. p. 317–36.

24. Malloy PJ, Hochberg Z, Tiosano D, et al. The molecular basis of hereditary 1,25-dihydroxyvitamin D_3 resistant rickets in seven related families. J Clin Invest 1990; 86:2071–9.
25. Mechica JB, Leite MO, Mendonca BB, et al. A novel nonsense mutation in the first zinc finger of the vitamin D receptor causing hereditary 1,25-dihydroxyvitamin D_3-resistant rickets. J Clin Endocrinol Metab 1997;82:3892–4.
26. Hawa NS, Cockerill FJ, Vadher S, et al. Identification of a novel mutation in hereditary vitamin D resistant rickets causing exon skipping. Clin Endocrinol 1996;45: 85–92.
27. Ma NS, Malloy PJ, Pitukcheewanont P, et al. Hereditary vitamin D resistant rickets: identification of a novel splice site mutation in the vitamin D receptor gene and successful treatment with oral calcium therapy. Bone 2009;45:743–6.
28. Katavetin P, Wacharasindhu S, Shotelersuk V. A girl with a novel splice site mutation in VDR supports the role of a ligand-independent VDR function on hair cycling. Horm Res 2006;66:273–6.
29. Cockerill FJ, Hawa NS, Yousaf N, et al. Mutations in the vitamin D receptor gene in three kindreds associated with hereditary vitamin D resistant rickets. J Clin Endocrinol Metab 1997;82:3156–60.
30. Rut AR, Hewison M, Rowe P, et al. A novel mutation in the steroid binding region of the vitamin D receptor (VDR) gene in hereditary vitamin D resistant rickets (HVDRR). In: Norman AW, Bouillon R, Thomasset M, editors. Vitamin D: gene regulation, structure-function analysis, and clinical application eighth workshop on vitamin D. New York: Walter de Gruyter; 1991. p. 94–5.
31. Whitfield GK, Selznick SH, Haussler CA, et al. Vitamin D receptors from patients with resistance to 1,25-dihydroxyvitamin D_3: point mutations confer reduced transactivation in response to ligand and impaired interaction with the retinoid X receptor heterodimeric partner. Mol Endocrinol 1996;10:1617–31.
32. Rochel N, Wurtz JM, Mitschler A, et al. The crystal structure of the nuclear receptor for vitamin D bound to its natural ligand. Mol Cell 2000;5:173–9.
33. Malloy PJ, Eccleshall TR, Gross C, et al. Hereditary vitamin D resistant rickets caused by a novel mutation in the vitamin D receptor that results in decreased affinity for hormone and cellular hyporesponsiveness. J Clin Invest 1997;99: 297–304.
34. Nguyen M, d'Alesio A, Pascussi JM, et al. Vitamin D-resistant rickets and type 1 diabetes in a child with compound heterozygous mutations of the vitamin D receptor (L263R and R391S): dissociated responses of the CYP-24 and rel-B promoters to 1,25-dihydroxyvitamin D3. J Bone Miner Res 2006;21:886–94.
35. Malloy PJ, Zhu W, Zhao XY, et al. A novel inborn error in the ligand-binding domain of the vitamin D receptor causes hereditary vitamin D-resistant rickets. Mol Genet Metab 2001;73:138–48.
36. Macedo LC, Soardi FC, Ananias N, et al. Mutations in the vitamin D receptor gene in four patients with hereditary 1,25-dihydroxyvitamin D-resistant rickets. Arq Bras Endocrinol Metabol 2008;52:1244–51.
37. Arita K, Nanda A, Wessagowit V, et al. A novel mutation in the VDR gene in hereditary vitamin D-resistant rickets. Br J Dermatol 2008;158:168–71.
38. Malloy PJ, Xu R, Peng L, et al. A novel mutation in helix 12 of the vitamin D receptor impairs coactivator interaction and causes hereditary 1,25-dihydroxyvitamin D-resistant rickets without alopecia. Mol Endocrinol 2002;16:2538–46.
39. Miller J, Djabali K, Chen T, et al. Atrichia caused by mutations in the vitamin D receptor gene is a phenocopy of generalized atrichia caused by mutations in the hairless gene. J Invest Dermatol 2001;117:612–7.

40. Zhou Y, Wang J, Malloy PJ, et al. Compound heterozygous mutations in the vitamin D receptor in a patient with hereditary 1,25-dihydroxyvitamin D-resistant rickets with alopecia. J Bone Miner Res 2009;24:643–51.

41. Malloy PJ, Xu R, Cattani A, et al. A unique insertion/substitution in helix H1 of the vitamin D receptor ligand binding domain in a patient with hereditary 1,25-dihydroxyvitamin D-resistant rickets. J Bone Miner Res 2004;19:1018–24.

42. Malloy PJ, Wang J, Peng L, et al. A unique insertion/duplication in the VDR gene that truncates the VDR causing hereditary 1,25-dihydroxyvitamin D-resistant rickets without alopecia. Arch Biochem Biophys 2007;460:285–92.

43. Hewison M, Rut AR, Kristjansson K, et al. Tissue resistance to 1,25-dihydroxyvitamin D without a mutation of the vitamin D receptor gene. Clin Endocrinol 1993;39:663–70.

44. Chen H, Hewison M, Hu B, et al. Heterogeneous nuclear ribonucleoprotein (hnRNP) binding to hormone response elements: a cause of vitamin D resistance. Proc Natl Acad Sci U S A 2003;100:6109–14.

45. Li YC, Pirro AE, Amling M, et al. Targeted ablation of the vitamin D receptor: an animal model of vitamin D-dependent rickets type II with alopecia. Proc Natl Acad Sci U S A 1997;94:9831–5.

46. Yoshizawa T, Handa Y, Uematsu Y, et al. Mice lacking the vitamin D receptor exhibit impaired bone formation, uterine hypoplasia and growth retardation after weaning. Nat Genet 1997;16:391–6.

47. Van Maldergem L, Bachy A, Feldman D, et al. Syndrome of lipoatrophic diabetes, vitamin D resistant rickets, and persistent Müllerian ducts in a Turkish boy born to consanguineous parents. Am J Med Genet 1996;64:506–13.

48. Fraher LJ, Karmali R, Hinde FR, et al. Vitamin D-dependent rickets type II: extreme end organ resistance to 1,25-dihydroxy vitamin D_3 in a patient without alopecia. Eur J Pediatr 1986;145:389–95.

49. Balsan S, Garabedian M, Larchet M, et al. Long-term nocturnal calcium infusions can cure rickets and promote normal mineralization in hereditary resistance to 1,25-dihydroxyvitamin D. J Clin Invest 1986;77:1661–7.

50. Balsan S, Garabedian M, Liberman UA, et al. Rickets and alopecia with resistance to 1,25-dihydroxyvitamin D: two different clinical courses with two different cellular defects. J Clin Endocrinol Metab 1983;57:803–11.

51. Bliziotes M, Yergey AL, Nanes MS, et al. Absent intestinal response to calciferols in hereditary resistance to 1,25-dihydroxyvitamin D: documentation and effective therapy with high dose intravenous calcium infusions. J Clin Endocrinol Metab 1988;66:294–300.

52. Hochberg Z, Tiosano D, Even L. Calcium therapy for calcitriol-resistant rickets. J Pediatr 1992;121:803–8.

53. Weisman Y, Bab I, Gazit D, et al. Long-term intracaval calcium infusion therapy in end-organ resistance to 1,25-dihydroxyvitamin D. Am J Med 1987;83:984–90.

54. Sakati N, Woodhouse NJ, Niles N, et al. Hereditary resistance to 1,25-dihydroxyvitamin D: clinical and radiological improvement during high-dose oral calcium therapy. Horm Res 1986;24:280–7.

55. Chen TL, Hirst MA, Cone CM, et al. 1,25-Dihydroxyvitamin D resistance, rickets, and alopecia: analysis of receptors and bioresponse in cultured fibroblasts from patients and parents. J Clin Endocrinol Metab 1984;59:383–8.

56. Hirst MA, Hochman HI, Feldman D. Vitamin D resistance and alopecia: a kindred with normal 1,25-dihydroxyvitamin D binding, but decreased receptor affinity for deoxyribonucleic acid. J Clin Endocrinol Metab 1985;60:490–5.

57. Hochberg Z, Benderli A, Levy J, et al. 1,25-Dihydroxyvitamin D resistance, rickets, and alopecia. Am J Med 1984;77:805–11.
58. Feldman D, Malloy PJ, Krishnan AV, et al. Vitamin D: biology, action, and clinical implications. In: Marcus R, Feldman D, Nelson DA, et al, editors. Osteoporosis. 3rd edition. San Diego (CA): Academic Press; 2007. p. 317–82.
59. Feldman D, Pike JW, Glorieux FH, editors. Vitamin D. 2nd edition. San Diego (CA): Elsevier Academic Press; 2005. p. 1892.
60. Chen CH, Sakai Y, Demay MB. Targeting expression of the human vitamin D receptor to the keratinocytes of vitamin D receptor null mice prevents alopecia. Endocrinology 2001;142:5386–9.
61. Li M, Chiba H, Warot X, et al. RXR-alpha ablation in skin keratinocytes results in alopecia and epidermal alterations. Development 2001;128:675–88.
62. Hsieh JC, Sisk JM, Jurutka PW, et al. Physical and functional interaction between the vitamin D receptor and hairless corepressor, two proteins required for hair cycling. J Biol Chem 2003;278:38665–74.
63. Malloy PJ, Feldman D. Hereditary 1,25-dihydroxyvitamin D-resistant rickets. Endocr Dev 2003;6:175–99.
64. Skorija K, Cox M, Sisk JM, et al. Ligand-independent actions of the vitamin D receptor maintain hair follicle homeostasis. Mol Endocrinol 2005;19:855–62.
65. Ahmad W, Faiyaz ul Haque M, Brancolini V, et al. Alopecia universalis associated with a mutation in the human hairless gene. Science 1998;279:720–4.
66. Wang J, Malloy PJ, Feldman D. Interactions of the vitamin D receptor with the corepressor hairless: analysis of hairless mutants in atrichia with papular lesions. J Biol Chem 2007;282:25231–9.
67. Xie Z, Chang S, Oda Y, et al. Hairless suppresses vitamin D receptor transactivation in human keratinocytes. Endocrinology 2006;147:314–23.
68. Beaudoin GM 3rd, Sisk JM, Coulombe PA, et al. Hairless triggers reactivation of hair growth by promoting Wnt signaling. Proc Natl Acad Sci U S A 2005;102:14653–8.
69. Thompson CC, Sisk JM, Beaudoin GM 3rd. Hairless and Wnt signaling: allies in epithelial stem cell differentiation. Cell Cycle 2006;5:1913–7.

Vitamin D and Fracture Prevention

Heike A. Bischoff-Ferrari, MD, DrPH[a,b,c],*

KEYWORDS

- Vitamin D - Falls - Bone density - Fractures
- Supplementation - 25-Hydroxyvitamin D

Vitamin D modulates fracture risk in 2 ways: by decreasing falls and increasing bone density. Two most recent meta-analyses of double-blind randomized controlled trials (RCTs) came to the conclusion that vitamin D reduces the risk of falls by 19%, the risk of hip fracture by 18%, and the risk of any nonvertebral fracture by 20%. However, this benefit was dose-dependent. Fall prevention was only observed in trials of at least 700 IU vitamin D per day, and fracture prevention required a received dose (treatment dose multiplied by adherence) of more than 400 IU vitamin D per day. Antifall efficacy started with achieved 25-hydroxyvitamin D levels of at least 60 nmol/L (24 ng/mL) and antifracture efficacy started with achieved 25-hydroxyvitamin D levels of at least 75 nmol/L (30 ng/mL). Both end points improved further with higher achieved 25-hydroxyvitamin D levels. Based on these evidence-based data derived from the general older population, vitamin D supplementation should be at least 700 to 1000 IU per day and taken with good adherence to cover the needs for fall and fracture prevention. Desirable 25-hydroxyvitamin D for optimal fracture prevention may be at least 75 nmol/L for both end points. Further work is needed to better define the doses that will achieve optimal blood levels in most of the population.

GOING BEYOND BONE

Antiresorptive treatment alone may not reduce fractures among individuals 80 years and older in the presence of nonskeletal risk factors for fractures despite an improvement in bone metabolism.[1] This is explained by a close relationship between fracture risk and muscle weakness[2] and falling[3,4] at an older age, and falls being the primary risk factor for hip fractures.[5] Moreover, falling may affect bone density through

[a] Centre on Aging and Mobility, University of Zurich, Gloriastrasse 25, CH-8091 Zurich, Switzerland
[b] Department of Rheumatology and Institute of Physical Medicine, University Hospital Zurich, Gloriastrasse 25, CH-8091 Zurich, Switzerland
[c] Jean Mayer USDA Human Nutrition Research Center on Aging, Tufts University, Boston, MA, USA
* Department of Rheumatology and Institute of Physical Medicine, University Hospital Zurich, Gloriastrasse 25, CH-8091 Zurich, Switzerland.
E-mail address: Heike.Bischoff@usz.ch

Endocrinol Metab Clin N Am 39 (2010) 347–353
doi:10.1016/j.ecl.2010.02.009
0889-8529/10/$ – see front matter © 2010 Published by Elsevier Inc.

endo.theclinics.com

increased immobility from self-restriction of activities.[6] After their first fall, about 30% of persons develop a fear of falling resulting in self-restriction of activities and decreased quality of life.[6] Based on new evidence, vitamin D reduces nonvertebral fractures, including those at the hip, irrespective of prevalent nonskeletal risk factors and offers an inexpensive and comprehensive primary fracture prevention strategy at higher age.[7] Nonvertebral fracture prevention by vitamin D may be largely modulated by its effect on muscle strength and fall prevention.[8] Thus, if antiresorptive treatment is initiated at an older age, it should be partnered with vitamin D in a dose of at least 700–1000 IU per day for fall prevention.[8]

VITAMIN D: ITS ROLE IN MUSCLE HEALTH

In humans, 4 lines of evidence support a role of vitamin D in muscle health. First, proximal muscle weakness is a prominent feature of the clinical syndrome of vitamin D deficiency.[9] Vitamin D deficiency myopathy includes proximal muscle weakness, diffuse muscle pain, and gait impairments such as a waddling way of walking.[10] Second, vitamin D receptor (VDR) is expressed in human muscle tissue,[11] and VDR activation may promote de novo protein synthesis in muscle.[12] Mice lacking VDR show a skeletal muscle phenotype with smaller and variable muscle fibers and persistence of immature muscle gene expression during adult life, which suggests a role of vitamin D in muscle development.[13,14] These abnormalities persist after correction of systemic calcium metabolism by a rescue diet.[14] Third, several observational studies suggest a positive association between 25-hydroxyvitamin D and muscle strength or lower extremity function in older persons.[15,16] Four, in several double-blind RCTs, vitamin D supplementation increased muscle strength and balance,[17,18] and reduced the risk of falling in community-dwelling individuals,[18–20] as well as in institutionalized individuals.[17,21] A study by Glerup and colleagues[9] suggested that vitamin D deficiency may cause muscular impairment even before adverse effects on bone occur.

A dose-response relationship between vitamin D status and muscle health was examined in NHANES III (The Third National Health and Nutrition Examination Survey), which included 4100 ambulatory adults aged 60 years and older. Muscle function measured as the 8-ft walk test and the repeated sit-to-stand test was poorest in subjects with the lowest level of 25-hydroxyvitamin D (<20 nmol/L). Similar results were found in a Dutch cohort of older individuals.[15] A threshold of 50 nmol/L has been suggested for optimal function from the smaller Dutch cohort.[15] A threshold beyond which function would not further improve was not identified in the larger NHANES III survey, even beyond the upper end of the reference range (>100 nmol/L).[16] In NHANES III, a similar benefit of higher 25-hydroxyvitamin D status was documented by gender, level of physical activity, and level of calcium intake.

These associations between higher 25-hydroxyvitamin D status and better function observed in epidemiologic studies in the United States and Europe were confirmed by 3 recent double-blind RCTs with 800 IU vitamin D_3 resulting in a 4% to 11% gain in lower extremity strength or function,[17,18] and up to 28% improvement in body sway[18,20] in older adults aged 65+ years, within 2 to 12 months of treatment.

A dose-dependent benefit of vitamin D with regard to fall prevention was suggested by a 2004 meta-analysis[22] and a recent multidose double-blind RCT among 124 nursing home residents receiving 200, 400, 600, or 800 IU vitamin D compared with placebo for a 5-month period.[21] Participants in the 800 IU group had a 72% lower rate of falls than those taking placebo or a lower dose of vitamin D (rate ratio 0.28; 95% confidence interval [CI] 0.11–0.75).[21] Including this trial, a most recent meta-analysis of 8 high-quality double-blind RCTs (n = 2426) found significant heterogeneity by dose (low dose <700 IU/d versus higher dose 700–1000 IU/d; P = .02) and achieved 25-hydroxyvitamin D level (<60 nmol/L versus $\geq$60 nmol/L; P = .005).[8] Higher-dose supplemental vitamin D between 700 and 1000 IU per day reduced fall risk by 19% (pooled relative risk (RR) 0.81; 95% CI 0.71–0.92; n = 1921 from 7 trials) versus a lower dose that did not (pooled RR = 1.10, 95% CI 0.89–1.35 from 2 trials). Achieved serum 25-hydroxyvitamin D concentrations less than 60 nmol/L did not reduce the risk of falling (pooled RR = 1.35, 95% CI, 0.98–1.84). At the higher dose, this meta-analysis documented a 38% significant reduction in the risk of falling with treatment duration of 2 to 5 months and a sustained significant effect of 17% fall reduction with treatment duration of 12 to 36 months. Thus, the benefits of vitamin D on fall prevention are rapid and sustained provided a high enough dose is given. Subgroup analyses for the prevention of falls at a dose of 700 to 1000 IU per day suggested a benefit in all subgroups of the older population, and possibly better fall reduction with D_3 compared with D_2.

VITAMIN D: ITS ROLE IN BONE HEALTH

A threshold for optimal 25-hydroxyvitamin D and hip bone mineral density (BMD) has been addressed among 13,432 individuals in NHANES III including younger (20–49 years) and older (50+ years) individuals with different ethnic and racial backgrounds.[23] In the regression plots, higher serum 25-hydroxyvitamin D levels were associated with higher BMD throughout the reference range of 22.5 to 94 nmol/L in all subgroups. In younger whites and younger Mexican Americans, higher 25-hydroxyvitamin D level was associated with higher BMD even beyond 100 nmol/L.

A 2009 meta-analysis of 12 double-blind RCTs for nonvertebral fractures (n = 42,279) and 8 RCTs for hip fractures (n = 40,886) consistently found that antifracture efficacy of vitamin D is dose dependent and increases significantly with a higher achieved level of 25-hydroxyvitamin D in the treatment group starting at 75 nmol/L.[7] No fracture reduction was observed for a received dose of 400 IU or less per day, whereas a higher received dose (dose multiplied by adherence) of 482 to 770 IU supplemental vitamin D per day reduced nonvertebral fractures by 20% (pooled RR 0.80; 95% CI 0.72–0.89; n = 33,265 from 9 trials) and hip fractures by 18% (pooled RR 0.82; 95% CI 0.69–0.97; n = 31,872 from 5 trials). Subgroup analyses for the prevention of nonvertebral fractures with the higher received dose suggested a benefit in all subgroups of the older population, and possibly better fracture reduction with D_3 compared with D_2. Additional calcium did not further improve antifracture efficacy (**Table 1**).

In August 2007, a review and meta-analysis commissioned by the US Department of Health and Human Services (HHS) addressed the effect of vitamin D supplementation on all fractures in postmenopausal women and men aged 50 yearsand older.[5] The pooled results for all fractures included 10 double-blind and 3 open-design trials (n = 58,712) and did not support a significant reduction of fractures with vitamin D (pooled odds ratio 0.90; 95% CI 0.81–1.02). The report suggested that the benefit of vitamin D may depend on additional calcium and may be seen primarily in institutionalized individuals, which is consistent with the meta-analysis of Boonen and colleagues[24] in the same year. However, in both reports heterogeneity by dose may have been missed because of the inclusion of open-design trials plus a dose evaluation that did not incorporate adherence. Biologically, the exclusion of heterogeneity by dose seems implausible even if a formal test of heterogeneity is not statistically significant.

Table 1
Nonvertebral fracture reduction with vitamin D based on evidence from double-blind RCTs

Subgroups by Received Dose of Vitamin D	Fracture Reduction	
Pooled analysis from 3 trials with low-dose vitamin D (340–380 IU/d)	+2%	Non-significant
Pooled analysis from 9 trials with higher dose vitamin D (482–770 IU/d)	−20%	Significant
Pooled subgroup analysis from trials with higher dose vitamin D (482–770 IE/Tag)		
Vitamin D_2	−10%	Non-significant
Vitamin D_3	−23%	Significant
Age 65–74 years	−33%	Significant
Age >75 years	−17%	Significant
Institutionalized >65 years	−15%	Significant
Community-dwelling >65 years	−29%	Significant
Vitamin D plus calcium	−21%	Significant
Vitamin D main effect	−21%	Significant

Adapted from Bischoff-Ferrari HA, Willett WC, Wong JB, et al. Prevention of nonvertebral fractures with oral vitamin D and dose dependency: a meta-analysis of randomized controlled trials. Arch Intern Med 2009;169(6):551–61; with permission. Copyright © (2009), American Medical Association.

In 2007, Tang and colleagues[25] suggested in their meta-analysis that together with calcium supplementation a daily intake of 800 IU vitamin D reduces total fracture by 3% compared with calcium supplementation together with a lower dose of vitamin D. However, with their focus on calcium, the investigators excluded 4 high-quality trials of vitamin D alone compared with placebo.[4,22,23,26]

ADDING CALCIUM TO VITAMIN D

The pooled RR reduction was 21% with or without additional calcium for the higher dose of vitamin D based on the 2009 meta-analysis (see **Table 1**). Previous meta-analyses may have missed this finding because their analyses included all doses of vitamin D. Physiologically, the calcium-sparing effect of vitamin D may explain why there was no additional benefit of calcium supplementation at a higher dose of vitamin D in the 2009 meta-analysis.[27,28]

The calcium-sparing effect of vitamin D is supported by 2 recent epidemiologic studies suggesting that parathyroid suppression[29] and hip bone density[30] may only depend on a higher calcium intake if serum 25-hydroxyvitamin D levels are low.

Thus, as calcium absorption is improved with higher serum 25-hydroxyvitamin D levels,[29,31] future studies may need to evaluate whether current calcium intake recommendations may require downward adjustment, especially with higher doses of vitamin D.[31] If dietary calcium is a threshold nutrient, as suggested by Heaney,[32] then that threshold for optimal calcium absorption may be at a lower calcium intake when vitamin D supplementation is adequate.

SUMMARY

Based on evidence from double-blind RCTs, vitamin D supplementation reduces falls and nonvertebral fractures, including those at the hip. However, this benefit is dose-dependent. According to 2 meta-analysis in 2009 of double-blind RCTs, no fall reduction was observed for a dose of less than 700 IU per day. A higher dose of 700 to 1000 IU supplemental vitamin D per day reduced falls by 19%.[8] Similarly, no fracture reduction was observed for a received dose of 400 IU or less per day. A higher received dose of 482 to 770 IU supplemental vitamin D per day reduced nonvertebral fractures by 20% and hip fractures by 18%. The antifracture effect was present in all subgroups of the older population and was most pronounced among community-dwellers (−29%) and those ages 65 to 74 years (−33%).

Consistently, fall prevention and nonvertebral fracture prevention increased significantly with higher achieved 25-hydroxyvitamin D levels in the 2009 meta-analyses. Fall prevention occurred with 25-hydroxyvitamin D levels of 60 to 95 nmol/L[8]; levels of 75 to 112 nmol/L were required for nonvertebral fracture prevention.[7] Given the absence of data beyond this beneficial range, these recent meta-analyses do not preclude the possibility that higher doses or higher achieved 25-hydroxyvitamin D concentrations would have been even more efficient in reducing falls and nonvertebral fractures.

REFERENCES

1. McClung MR, Geusens P, Miller PD, et al. Effect of risedronate on the risk of hip fracture in elderly women. Hip Intervention Program Study Group. N Engl J Med 2001;344:333–40.
2. Cummings SR, Nevitt MC, Browner WS, et al. Risk factors for hip fracture in white women. Study of Osteoporotic Fractures Research Group. N Engl J Med 1995; 332:767–73.
3. Centers for Disease Control and Prevention (CDC). Fatalities and injuries from falls among older adults–United States, 1993–2003 and 2001–2005. MMWR Morb Mortal Wkly Rep 2006;55:1221–4.
4. Schwartz AV, Nevitt MC, Brown BW Jr, et al. Increased falling as a risk factor for fracture among older women: the study of osteoporotic fractures. Am J Epidemiol 2005;161:180–5.
5. Cummings SR, Nevitt MC. Non-skeletal determinants of fractures: the potential importance of the mechanics of falls. Study of Osteoporotic Fractures Research Group. Osteoporos Int 1994;4(Suppl 1):67–70.
6. Vellas BJ, Wayne SJ, Romero LJ, et al. Fear of falling and restriction of mobility in elderly fallers. Age Ageing 1997;26:189–93.
7. Bischoff-Ferrari HA, Willett WC, Wong JB, et al. Prevention of nonvertebral fractures with oral vitamin D and dose dependency: a meta-analysis of randomized controlled trials. Arch Intern Med 2009;169:551–61.
8. Bischoff-Ferrari HA, Dawson-Hughes B, Staehelin HB, et al. Fall prevention with supplemental and active forms of vitamin D: a meta-analysis of randomized controlled trials. BMJ 2009;339:b3692. DOI:10.1136/bmj.b3692.
9. Glerup H, Mikkelsen K, Poulsen L, et al. Hypovitaminosis D myopathy without biochemical signs of osteomalacic bone involvement. Calcif Tissue Int 2000;66: 419–24.
10. Schott GD, Wills MR. Muscle weakness in osteomalacia. Lancet 1976;1:626–9.
11. Bischoff-Ferrari HA, Borchers M, Gudat F, et al. Vitamin D receptor expression in human muscle tissue decreases with age. J Bone Miner Res 2004;19:265–9.
12. Sorensen OH, Lund B, Saltin B, et al. Myopathy in bone loss of ageing: improvement by treatment with 1 alpha-hydroxycholecalciferol and calcium. Clin Sci (Lond) 1979;56:157–61.

13. Bouillon R, Bischoff-Ferrari H, Willett W. Vitamin D and health: perspectives from mice and man. J Bone Miner Res 2008;23:974–9.

14. Endo I, Inoue D, Mitsui T, et al. Deletion of vitamin D receptor gene in mice results in abnormal skeletal muscle development with deregulated expression of myoregulatory transcription factors. Endocrinology 2003;144:5138–44.

15. Wicherts IS, van Schoor NM, Boeke AJ, et al. Vitamin D status predicts physical performance and its decline in older persons. J Clin Endocrinol Metab 2007;6:6.

16. Bischoff-Ferrari HA, Dietrich T, Orav EJ, et al. Higher 25-hydroxyvitamin D concentrations are associated with better lower-extremity function in both active and inactive persons aged >=60 y. Am J Clin Nutr 2004;80:752–8.

17. Bischoff HA, Stahelin HB, Dick W, et al. Effects of vitamin D and calcium supplementation on falls: a randomized controlled trial. J Bone Miner Res 2003;18: 343–51.

18. Pfeifer M, Begerow B, Minne HW, et al. Effects of a long-term vitamin D and calcium supplementation on falls and parameters of muscle function in community-dwelling older individuals. Osteoporos Int 2008;16:16.

19. Bischoff-Ferrari HA, Orav EJ, Dawson-Hughes B. Effect of cholecalciferol plus calcium on falling in ambulatory older men and women: a 3-year randomized controlled trial. Arch Intern Med 2006;166:424–30.

20. Pfeifer M, Begerow B, Minne HW, et al. Effects of a short-term vitamin D and calcium supplementation on body sway and secondary hyperparathyroidism in elderly women. J Bone Miner Res 2000;15:1113–8.

21. Broe KE, Chen TC, Weinberg J, et al. A higher dose of vitamin D reduces the risk of falls in nursing home residents: a randomized, multiple-dose study. J Am Geriatr Soc 2007;55:234–9.

22. Bischoff-Ferrari HA, Dawson-Hughes B, Willett CW, et al. Effect of vitamin D on falls: a meta-analysis. JAMA 2004;291:1999–2006.

23. Bischoff-Ferrari HA, Dietrich T, Orav EJ, et al. Positive association between 25-hydroxy vitamin D levels and bone mineral density: a population-based study of younger and older adults. Am J Med 2004;116:634–9.

24. Boonen S, Lips P, Bouillon R, et al. Need for additional calcium to reduce the risk of hip fracture with vitamin d supplementation: evidence from a comparative metaanalysis of randomized controlled trials. J Clin Endocrinol Metab 2007; 92(4):1415–23.

25. Tang BM, Eslick GD, Nowson C, et al. Use of calcium or calcium in combination with vitamin D supplementation to prevent fractures and bone loss in people aged 50 years and older: a meta-analysis. Lancet 2007;370(9588): 657–66.

26. Heaney RP, Barger-Lux MJ, Dowell MS, et al. Calcium absorptive effects of vitamin D and its major metabolites. J Clin Endocrinol Metab 1997;82:4111–6.

27. Giovannucci E, Liu Y, Hollis BW, et al. 25-Hydroxyvitamin D and risk of myocardial infarction in men: a prospective study. Arch Intern Med 2008; 168:1174–80.

28. Dobnig H, Pilz S, Scharnagl H, et al. Independent association of low serum 25-hydroxyvitamin D and 1,25-dihydroxyvitamin D levels with all-cause and cardiovascular mortality. Arch Intern Med 2008;168:1340–9.

29. Steingrimsdottir L, Gunnarsson O, Indridason OS, et al. Relationship between serum parathyroid hormone levels, vitamin D sufficiency, and calcium intake. JAMA 2005;294:2336–41.

30. Bischoff-Ferrari HA, Kiel DP, Dawson-Hughes B, et al. Dietary calcium and serum 25-hydroxyvitamin D status in relation to BMD among U.S. adults. J Bone Miner Res 2009;24:935–42.
31. Heaney RP, Dowell MS, Hale CA, et al. Calcium absorption varies within the reference range for serum 25-hydroxyvitamin D. J Am Coll Nutr 2003;22:142–6.
32. Heaney RP. The vitamin D requirement in health and disease. J Steroid Biochem Mol Biol 2005;15:15.

Vitamin D in Kidney Disease: Pathophysiology and the Utility of Treatment

Rizwan A. Qazi, MD*, Kevin J. Martin, MB, BCh

KEYWORDS

- Vitamin D • Hyperphosphatemia
- Hyperparathyroidism • Survival

Vitamin D physiology has gained more importance and publicity than any of its counterparts in the water- and fat-soluble vitamin groups combined. This is partly because vitamin D deficiency is still widely prevalent in the developed world and the beneficial effects are thought to extend beyond the regulation of calcium and phosphorus homeostasis alone. Vitamin D deficiency becomes even more important in the various stages of chronic kidney disease (CKD); CKD itself is also on the increase. How vitamin D physiology is altered in CKD and how the various treatment modalities can alter the morbidity and mortality associated with CKD is the topic of discussion for this article. Chronic kidney disease, mineral and bone disorder (CKD-MBD) is the broad term used to describe the disease complex of hyperphosphatemia, secondary hyperparathyroidism, low levels of vitamin D, and their associated complications.[1] The National Kidney Foundation, Kidney Disease Outcomes and Quality Initiative (KDOQI), and subsequently, Kidney Disease: Improving Global Outcomes (KDIGO), has endeavored to provide evidence-based clinical practice guidelines for various stages of CKD and has set certain target levels for the major factors involved in CKD-MBD.[2,3] These factors include calcium, phosphorus, vitamin D, and parathyroid hormone (PTH). Whether achieving and maintaining these targets will provide any benefit for the overall survival of patients with kidney disease remains to be demonstrated.

CALCIUM

Calcium in present abundantly in the body. The skeleton acts as reservoir and buffer for calcium such that when a large oral load of calcium is ingested and absorbed, it gets buffered in the skeleton and when calcium is acutely needed, it is mobilized

---

Division of Nephrology, Saint Louis University, 3635 Vista Avenue FDT 9, Saint Louis, MO 63110, USA
* Corresponding author.
E-mail address: qazir@SLU.EDU

Endocrinol Metab Clin N Am 39 (2010) 355–363
doi:10.1016/j.ecl.2010.02.005
0889-8529/10/$ – see front matter © 2010 Elsevier Inc. All rights reserved.
endo.theclinics.com

from the skeleton. Regulation of serum calcium is under complex control with short-term and long-term regulation. This regulatory control is governed by vitamin D metabolism, phosphorus metabolism, fibroblast growth factor 23 (FGF-23), and PTH. These regulators of calcium homeostasis are heavily dependent on each other, and there are continuous positive and negative feedback mechanisms. For various reasons that are discussed later, these regulatory mechanisms of calcium homeostasis become disrupted in CKD and result in the presentation of CKD-MBD.

CKD-MBD

Patients with kidney disease are at a many fold higher risk of bone fracture than their age-matched controls. Hyperphosphatemia and hyperparathyroidism are virtually universal in patients with advanced kidney disease. Vascular calcification can be debilitating and is strongly associated with the increased cardiovascular morbidity and mortality associated with CKD.[4–6] Many patients in CKD stage 4 (estimated glomerular filtration rate [eGFR] 15–29) never seem to progress to CKD stage 5 (eGFR<15), and mortality from cardiovascular disease may be a contributing factor. CKD-MBD starts early, usually by CKD stage 3 (eGFR 30–59) and, for the most part, is a silent problem that only becomes manifest as CKD advances. Vitamin D deficiency is widely prevalent in the general population and even more so in patients with kidney disease.

NORMAL VITAMIN D PHYSIOLOGY

Vitamin D is crucial for calcium and phosphorus homeostasis and the regulation of parathyroid function. In addition to obtaining vitamin D from diet, a significant amount is formed in the skin (**Fig. 1**). Ultraviolet rays of the correct wavelength (UVB) in sunlight convert 7-dehydrocholesterol in the skin to previtamin D. This is then transported to the liver where it is hydroxylated at carbon 25 to form 25-hydroxyvitamin D [25(OH)D]. This is the main storage form of vitamin D in the human body and is the

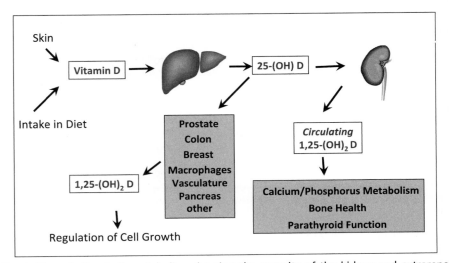

Fig. 1. Normal vitamin D metabolism showing the capacity of the kidney and extrarenal sites to produce the active vitamin D sterol, 1,25-dihydroxyvitamin D.

vitamin D metabolite that reflects the state of vitamin D nutrition. Almost all 25(OH)D is bound to circulating vitamin D–binding protein (DBP) and is then filtered by the kidney and taken up by the proximal convoluted tubule by an endocytic receptor, megalin. The 25(OH)D-DBP complex is degraded in proximal tubule lysosomes, releasing 25(OH)D, which then translocates to the mitochondria. In the mitochondria, 25(OH)D is converted to 1,25-dihydroxyvitamin D by the enzyme 1α-hydroxylase and returned to the circulation as the active form of vitamin D.[7–11] New research has shown the presence of this enzyme in organs other than the kidney, such as pancreas, brain, lymph nodes, heart, gastrointestinal tract, adrenal glands, and prostate gland, such that 1,25-dihydroxyvitamin D may be made locally in these tissues. The biologic role of the extrarenal 1α-hydroxylase and the local effects of 1,25-dihydroxyvitamin D in extrarenal sites is the subject of ongoing studies.[12]

The actions of 1,25-dihydroxyvitamin D are mediated by binding to the vitamin D receptor (VDR) and result in the alteration of the transcription of many genes in the various target organs.

VITAMIN D METABOLISM IN KIDNEY DISEASE

Kidney disease seems to be a risk factor for vitamin D deficiency[13] and as many as 70% to 85% of patients with CKD are found to have low levels of 25(OH)D.[14,15] Many factors may contribute, including lack of sunlight, loss of 25(OH)D-DBP with heavy proteinuria, diabetes, chronic illness, decreased production of previtamin D in the skin,[16] and other unknown factors. Thus, the concentration of substrate for conversion to 1,25-dihydroxyvitamin D is decreased. This is further complicated by the fact that with decreases in glomerular filtration rate (GFR) and decreased renal mass, there is decreased delivery of substrate to the renal 1α-hydroxylase, which limits the ability of the diseased kidney to produce the active 1,25-dihydroxyvitamin D. In addition, as CKD develops, phosphate retention occurs decreasing 1α-hydroxylase activity, directly[12] and leading to increases in the levels of FGF-23, which in turn, can directly decrease the activity of 1α-hydroxylase.[17,18] FGF-23 is a recently discovered phosphaturic hormone that is regulated by dietary phosphate, serum phosphate, and 1,25-dihydroxyvitamin D. FGF-23 levels increase early in CKD, presumably in response to phosphate retention, in an effort to increase phosphate excretion in conjunction with increases in PTH. Although PTH stimulates the activity of 1α-hydroxylase, the suppressive effect of FGF-23 on 1α-hydroxylase activity seems to dominate in this clinical situation. In addition, it has been suggested that accumulation of N-terminally truncated PTH peptides of C-terminal PTH fragments may decrease 1α-hydroxylase.[19] Thus, because of these abnormalities (**Fig. 2**), it is not surprising that the levels of 1,25-dihydroxyvitamin D are reduced in CKD and progressively decline with advancing stages of CKD.[20] In addition to decreased production of 1,25-dihydroxyvitamin D, there is also evidence for resistance to the actions of vitamin D as kidney disease progresses in that there may be decreased concentrations of the VDR, impaired binding of the 1,25-dihydroxyvitamin D binding to the VDR, and possibly impaired binding of the VDR complex to the vitamin D response elements in the nuclei.[21] This altered vitamin D physiology in patients with renal disease contributes to subclinical or less commonly overt hypocalcemia and leads to the need for increased levels of PTH, which mobilizes minerals from the skeleton by stimulation of osteoclastic-mediated bone resorption. This process leads to the loss of lamellar bone and replacement with the woven and structurally weaker bone, increased propensity for fractures, and overall decreased quality of bone.

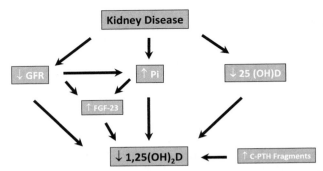

Fig. 2. The mechanisms contributing to the progressive decrease in the levels of 1,25-dihydroxyvitamin D in kidney disease. (*Modified from* Al-Badr W, Martin KJ. Vitamin D and kidney disease. Clin J Am Soc Nephrol 2008;3(5):1555–60; with permission.)

PHOSPHORUS

Abnormal phosphorus metabolism is a major factor in CKD-MBD. Phosphate retention, as a consequence of decreased GFR, is thought to be a major factor in the pathogenesis of CKD-MBD. Phosphorus retention can lead to increased PTH directly[22] and indirectly by increasing the levels of FGF-23, which, in turn, decreases the activity of 1α-hydroxylase.[17,18] High levels of phosphorus have been shown to promote vascular calcification in animal models and are associated with vascular calcification in experiments in vitro.[23–25]

ROLE OF VITAMIN D TREATMENT IN CKD-MBD

Because of the major role of abnormal vitamin D metabolism in the disturbances of calcium and phosphorus homeostasis and in the pathogenesis of secondary hyperparathyroidism in the setting of CKD, use of vitamin D sterols is an important aspect of the therapy of patients with CKD. Current practice guidelines suggest evaluation for the presence of hyperparathyroidism early in the course of CKD, and if PTH values are elevated, vitamin D deficiency should be evaluated by measurement of 25(OH)D levels. If 25(OH)D levels are less than 30 ng/mL then vitamin D supplementation should be initiated. This is most often accomplished by the administration of ergocalciferol or cholecalciferol. Although the KDOQI guidelines suggest a dosage regimen for ergocalciferol, this is not always effective in achieving correction of the low levels of 25(OH)D in this patient group.[26] The reasons for this are currently unclear. However, if the levels of 25(OH)D are increased then PTH values are seen to decrease in CKD stage 3. The decrease in PTH in patients with CKD stage 4 seems to be less, but again, there is marked heterogeneity in response to ergocalciferol.[26,27] Accordingly, the use of active vitamin D sterols can be considered. The preparations available in North America are: calcitriol (1,25-dihydroxyvitamin D_3), doxercalciferol (1α-25-hydroxyvitamin D_2), and paricalcitol (19-nor-1,25-dihydroxyvitamin D_3). All are effective in reducing the secondary hyperparathyroidism associated with CKD, consistent with the finding that activation of the VDR in parathyroid glands results in decreased PTH gene transcription. Dosing should be monitored carefully to avoid toxicity, which is mainly manifested by hypercalcemia. In studies in animals, the analogue, paricalcitol, has been shown to be less calcemic and less phosphatemic than the native hormone.[28,29] There are limited data on head-to-head studies of the active vitamin D sterols in patients, but paricalcitol seems to have the widest therapeutic window. It is likely that early recognition of secondary hyperparathyroidism and initiation of therapy early in the course of CKD may lead to effective control of hyperparathyroidism and prevent parathyroid growth.

EFFECTS OF VITAMIN D ON THE CARDIOVASCULAR SYSTEM

Studies have shown that VDR knockout mice have an overactive renin-angiotensin-aldosterone system (RAAS) and develop hypertension and left ventricular hypertrophy (LVH).[30] Similarly, Dahl salt-sensitive rats develop vitamin D deficiency and LVH with diastolic dysfunction, and the administration of paricalcitol has been shown to be associated with decreased LVH in these rats.[31] Similarly, 1α-hydroxylase knockout mice develop hypertension, cardiac hypertrophy, and depressed cardiac function.[32] These effects are not corrected by correction of calcium and phosphorus alone. Calcitriol, however, seems to ameliorate hypertension and improve cardiac function in this animal group.[32] Therefore, it seems that the vitamin D system is a regulator of the renin-angiotensin system. These observations, coupled with other animal studies that have shown improved cardiac function and decreased LVH and the suggestion that 1,25-dihydroxyvitamin D may actually suppress the RAAS axis, have led to the initiation of 2 prospective trials in patients to evaluate this possibility. The Paricalcitol benefits in Renal Failure Induced Cardiac Morbidity (PRIMO) trials, PRIMO I and PRIMO II will evaluate the beneficial effects of paricalcitol in patients predialysis and those on dialysis, respectively (clinicaltrials.gov NCT00497146 and NCT00616902).

VITAMIN D AND OVERALL SURVIVAL

Some observational studies have shown decreased overall mortality in patients with end-stage renal disease (ESRD) who are being treated with an active vitamin D sterol. In 1 study there was a 26%, 2-year reduction in mortality in the patient groups who received some form of vitamin D versus those who received none.[33] In another observational study by Teng and colleagues,[34] in 60,000 patients undergoing hemodialysis there were lower rates of mortality in those treated with paricalcitol versus calcitriol. Other studies have also shown similar survival benefits with the use of paricalcitol. Melamed and colleagues[35] (KI2006) noted a 26% reduction in mortality with injectable vitamin D as part of the Choices for Health Outcomes in Caring for ESRD (CHOICE) study. Tentori and colleagues[36] showed a similar survival benefit irrespective of the formulation of the active vitamin D sterol (calcitriol, paricalcitol, or doxercalciferol). Similarly, Kalantar-Zadeh and colleagues[37] showed paricalcitol administration to be associated with improved survival compared with those receiving no vitamin D in patients with ESRD. Similar apparent survival benefits associated with the use of active vitamin D sterols are now being presented in predialysis patients.[38,39] Indeed, low levels of 25(OH)D have been associated with greater mortality in patients with cardiovascular disease as well as in patients with hypertension, and even in apparently normal people.[40] These observational studies warrant the need for prospective, randomized trials to evaluate any survival benefit of vitamin D therapy in patients with CKD.

OTHER POTENTIALLY BENEFICIAL EFFECTS OF VITAMIN D TREATMENT IN CKD

Vitamin D metabolism has a role in immune function, which was elucidated by Liu and colleagues[41] in studies evaluating the response of human macrophages to activation of toll-like receptors. These studies demonstrated that the antimicrobial protein cathelicidin was regulated by the generation of 1,25-dihydroxyvitamin D by the macrophage 1α-hydroxylase. This pathway may be important in CKD, which has a high incidence of infections. Indeed, an association between low levels of the cathelicidin, hCAP18, and death from infectious causes in patients on hemodialysis has been observed.[42]

It is also possible that the vitamin D system may affect the progression of CKD. Several studies in animals show that administration of active vitamin D sterols can favorably affect the processes that lead to progression of kidney disease.[43-50] Recently, studies have shown that paricalcitol seems to reduce proteinuria in patients with CKD,[51] and this has been confirmed in a randomized controlled trial.[52]

SUMMARY

CKD is associated with decreased vitamin D metabolites, both the storage form 25(OH)D and the active form 1,25-dihydroxyvitamin D. This contributes to hyperparathyroidism, and increased levels of PTH mobilize minerals from the skeleton and increase the risk for fractures. Treatment with vitamin D sterols efficiently reduces secondary hyperparathyroidism of CKD. Observational studies suggest survival and other potential benefits of vitamin D treatment in the CKD population. These observations need to be verified with controlled prospective trials.

REFERENCES

1. Moe S, Drueke T, Cunningham J, et al. Definition, evaluation, and classification of renal osteodystrophy: a position statement from kidney disease: improving global outcomes (KDIGO). Kidney Int 2006;69(11):1945–53.
2. Kidney Disease: Improving Global Outcomes (KDIGO) CKD-MBD Work Group. KDIGO clinical practice guideline for the diagnosis, evaluation, prevention, and treatment of chronic kidney disease-mineral and bone disorder (CKD-MBD). Kidney Int Suppl 2009;76(113):S1–130.
3. National Kidney Foundation. K/DOQI clinical practice guidelines for bone metabolism and disease in chronic kidney disease. Am J Kidney Dis 2003;42:S1–201.
4. Blacher J, Guerin AP, Pannier B, et al. Arterial calcifications, arterial stiffness, and cardiovascular risk in end-stage renal disease. Hypertension 2001;38(4):938–42.
5. Goodman WG, Goldin J, Kuizon BD, et al. Coronary-artery calcification in young adults with end-stage renal disease who are undergoing dialysis. N Engl J Med 2000;342(20):1478–83.
6. Moe SM. Vascular calcification and renal osteodystrophy relationship in chronic kidney disease. Eur J Clin Invest 2006;36(Suppl 2):51–62.
7. Hilpert J, Wogensen L, Thykjaer T, et al. Expression profiling confirms the role of endocytic receptor megalin in renal vitamin D3 metabolism. Kidney Int 2002; 62(5):1672–81.
8. Willnow TE, Nykjaer A. Pathways for kidney-specific uptake of the steroid hormone 25-hydroxyvitamin D3. Curr Opin Lipidol 2002;13(3):255–60.
9. Nykjaer A, Fyfe JC, Kozyraki R, et al. Cubilin dysfunction causes abnormal metabolism of the steroid hormone 25(OH) vitamin D(3). Proc Natl Acad Sci U S A 2001;98(24):13895–900.
10. Leheste JR, Rolinski B, Vorum H, et al. Megalin knockout mice as an animal model of low molecular weight proteinuria. Am J Pathol 1999;155(4):1361–70.
11. Nykjaer A, Dragun D, Walther D, et al. An endocytic pathway essential for renal uptake and activation of the steroid 25-(OH) vitamin D3. Cell 1999;96(4):507–15.
12. Dusso AS, Brown AJ, Slatopolsky E. Vitamin D. Am J Physiol Renal Physiol 2005; 289(1):F8–28.

13. Thomas MK, Lloyd-Jones DM, Thadhani RI, et al. Hypovitaminosis D in medical inpatients. N Engl J Med 1998;338(12):777–83.

14. Gonzalez EA, Sachdeva A, Oliver DA, et al. Vitamin D insufficiency and deficiency in chronic kidney disease. A single center observational study. Am J Nephrol 2004;24(5):503–10.

15. LaClair RE, Hellman RN, Karp SL, et al. Prevalence of calcidiol deficiency in CKD: a cross-sectional study across latitudes in the United States. Am J Kidney Dis 2005;45(6):1026–33.

16. Jacob AI, Sallman A, Santiz Z, et al. Defective photoproduction of cholecalciferol in normal and uremic humans. J Nutr 1984;114(7):1313–9.

17. Perwad F, Azam N, Zhang MY, et al. Dietary and serum phosphorus regulate fibroblast growth factor 23 expression and 1,25-dihydroxyvitamin D metabolism in mice. Endocrinology 2005;146(12):5358–64.

18. Shimada T, Hasegawa H, Yamazaki Y, et al. FGF-23 is a potent regulator of vitamin D metabolism and phosphate homeostasis. J Bone Miner Res 2004; 19(3):429–35.

19. Usatii M, Rousseau L, Demers C, et al. Parathyroid hormone fragments inhibit active hormone and hypocalcemia-induced 1,25(OH)2D synthesis. Kidney Int 2007;72(11):1330–5.

20. Levin A, Bakris GL, Molitch M, et al. Prevalence of abnormal serum vitamin D, PTH, calcium, and phosphorus in patients with chronic kidney disease: results of the study to evaluate early kidney disease. Kidney Int 2007;71(1):31–8.

21. Patel SR, Ke HQ, Vanholder R, et al. Inhibition of calcitriol receptor binding to vitamin D response elements by uremic toxins. J Clin Invest 1995;96(1):50–9.

22. Slatopolsky E, Finch J, Denda M, et al. Phosphorus restriction prevents parathyroid gland growth. High phosphorus directly stimulates PTH secretion in vitro. J Clin Invest 1996;97(11):2534–40.

23. Giachelli CM, Jono S, Shioi A, et al. Vascular calcification and inorganic phosphate. Am J Kidney Dis 2001;38(4 Suppl 1):S34–7.

24. Jono S, McKee MD, Murry CE, et al. Phosphate regulation of vascular smooth muscle cell calcification. Circ Res 2000;87(7):E10–7.

25. Moe SM, Chen NX. Mechanisms of vascular calcification in chronic kidney disease. J Am Soc Nephrol 2008;19(2):213–6.

26. Al-Aly Z, Qazi R, Gonzalez EA, et al. Changes in serum 25-hydroxyvitamin D and plasma intact PTH levels following treatment with ergocalciferol in patients with CKD. Am J Kidney Dis 2007;50(1):59–68.

27. Zisman AL, Hristova M, Ho LT, et al. Impact of ergocalciferol treatment of vitamin D deficiency on serum parathyroid hormone concentrations in chronic kidney disease. Am J Nephrol 2007;27(1):36–43.

28. Finch JL, Brown AJ, Slatopolsky E. Differential effects of 1,25-dihydroxy-vitamin D3 and 19-nor-1,25-dihydroxy-vitamin D2 on calcium and phosphorus resorption in bone. J Am Soc Nephrol 1999;10(5):980–5.

29. Slatopolsky E, Finch J, Ritter C, et al. A new analog of calcitriol, 19-nor-1,25-$(OH)_2D_2$, suppresses parathyroid hormone secretion in uremic rats in the absence of hypercalcemia. Am J Kidney Dis 1995;26(5):852–60.

30. Xiang W, Kong J, Chen S, et al. Cardiac hypertrophy in vitamin D receptor knockout mice: role of the systemic and cardiac renin-angiotensin systems. Am J Physiol Endocrinol Metab 2005;288(1):E125–32.

31. Bodyak N, Ayus JC, Achinger S, et al. Activated vitamin D attenuates left ventricular abnormalities induced by dietary sodium in Dahl salt-sensitive animals. Proc Natl Acad Sci U S A 2007;104(43):16810–5.

32. Zhou C, Lu F, Cao K, et al. Calcium-independent and 1,25(OH)2D3-dependent regulation of the renin-angiotensin system in 1alpha-hydroxylase knockout mice. Kidney Int 2008;74(2):170–9.

33. Teng M, Wolf M, Ofsthun MN, et al. Activated injectable vitamin D and hemodialysis survival: a historical cohort study. J Am Soc Nephrol 2005;16(4):1115–25.

34. Teng M, Wolf M, Lowrie E, et al. Survival of patients undergoing hemodialysis with paricalcitol or calcitriol therapy. New Engl J Med 2003;349(5):446–56.

35. Melamed ML, Eustace JA, Plantinga L, et al. Changes in serum calcium, phosphate, and PTH and the risk of death in incident dialysis patients: a longitudinal study. Kidney Int 2006;70(2):351–7.

36. Tentori F, Hunt WC, Stidley CA, et al. Mortality risk among hemodialysis patients receiving different vitamin D analogs. Kidney Int 2006;70(10):1858–65.

37. Kalantar-Zadeh K, Kuwae N, Regidor DL, et al. Survival predictability of time-varying indicators of bone disease in maintenance hemodialysis patients. Kidney Int 2006;70(4):771–80.

38. Kovesdy CP, Ahmadzadeh S, Anderson JE, et al. Association of activated vitamin D treatment and mortality in chronic kidney disease. Arch Intern Med 2008;168(4):397–403.

39. Shoben AB, Rudser KD, de Boer IH, et al. Association of oral calcitriol with improved survival in nondialyzed CKD. J Am Soc Nephrol 2008;19(8):1613–9.

40. Dobnig H, Pilz S, Scharnagl H, et al. Independent association of low serum 25-hydroxyvitamin D and 1,25-dihydroxyvitamin D levels with all-cause and cardiovascular mortality. Arch Inter Med 2008;168(12):1340–9.

41. Liu PT, Stenger S, Li H, et al. Toll-like receptor triggering of a vitamin D-mediated human antimicrobial response. Science 2006;311(5768):1770–3..

42. Gombart AF, Bhan I, Borregaard N, et al. Low plasma level of cathelicidin antimicrobial peptide (hCAP18) predicts increased infectious disease mortality in patients undergoing hemodialysis. Clin Infect Dis 2009;48(4):418–24.

43. Aschenbrenner JK, Sollinger HW, Becker BN, et al. 1,25-(OH(2))D(3) alters the transforming growth factor beta signaling pathway in renal tissue. J Surg Res 2001;100(2):171–5.

44. Kruger S, Kreft B. 1,25-Dihydroxyvitamin D3 differentially regulates IL-1alpha-stimulated IL-8 and MCP-1 mRNA expression and chemokine secretion by human primary proximal tubular epithelial cells. Exp Nephrol 2001;9(3):223–8.

45. Kuhlmann A, Haas CS, Gross ML, et al. 1,25-Dihydroxyvitamin D3 decreases podocyte loss and podocyte hypertrophy in the subtotally nephrectomized rat. Am J Physiol Renal Physiol 2004;286(3):F526–33.

46. Mizobuchi M, Morrissey J, Finch JL, et al. Combination therapy with an angiotensin-converting enzyme inhibitor and a vitamin D analog suppresses the progression of renal insufficiency in uremic rats. J Am Soc Nephrol 2007;18(6):1796–806.

47. Schwarz U, Amann K, Orth SR, et al. Effect of 1,25 (OH)2 vitamin D3 on glomerulosclerosis in subtotally nephrectomized rats. Kidney Int 1998;53(6):1696–705.

48. Subramaniam N, Leong GM, Cock TA, et al. Cross-talk between 1,25-dihydroxyvitamin D3 and transforming growth factor-beta signaling requires binding of VDR and Smad3 proteins to their cognate DNA recognition elements. J Biol Chem 2001;276(19):15741–6.

49. Zhang Z, Sun L, Wang Y, et al. Renoprotective role of the vitamin D receptor in diabetic nephropathy. Kidney Int 2008;73(2):163–71.

50. Zhu KJ, Shen QY, Zheng M, et al. Effects of calcitriol and its analogues on interaction of MCP-1 and monocyte derived dendritic cells in vitro. Acta Pharmacol Sin 2001;22(1):62–5.
51. Agarwal R, Acharya M, Tian J, et al. Antiproteinuric effect of oral paricalcitol in chronic kidney disease. Kidney Int 2005;68(6):2823–8.
52. Fishbane S, Chittineni H, Packman M, et al. Oral paricalcitol in the treatment of patients with CKD and proteinuria: a randomized trial. Am J Kidney Dis 2009; 54(4):647–52.

Vitamin D and the Immune System: New Perspectives on an Old Theme

Martin Hewison, PhD

KEYWORDS

- Vitamin D • CYP27b1 • Toll-like receptor • Macrophage
- Cathelicidin • Regulatory T cells

HISTORICAL PERSPECTIVE

Nonclassic actions of vitamin D were first recognized 30 years ago when receptors for active 1,25-dihydroxyvitamin D_3 (1,25(OH)$_2$D$_3$) were detected in various neoplastic cells lines.[1,2] Other studies immediately following this showed that binding of 1,25(OH)$_2$D$_3$ to the vitamin D receptor (VDR) promoted antiproliferative and prodifferentiation responses in cancer cells,[3,4] highlighting an entirely new facet of vitamin D action. The spectrum of nonclassic responses to vitamin D was then extended to include actions on cells from the immune system.[5,6] This interaction was further endorsed by the observation that some patients with the granulomatous disease sarcoidosis present with increased circulating levels of 1,25(OH)$_2$D$_3$ and associated hypercalcemia.[7,8] In these patients the high serum level of 1,25(OH)$_2$D$_3$ is caused by increased activity of the enzyme 25-hydroxyvitamin D-1α-hydrooxylase (1α-hydroxylase). However, in contrast to normal subjects in whom 1α-hydroxylase is classically localized in the kidney, the increased synthesis of 1,25(OH)$_2$D$_3$ in patients with sarcoidosis involves 1α-hydroxylase activity in disease-associated macrophages.[9-11] Thus, it was concluded that the immune system had the potential to synthesize 1,25(OH)$_2$D$_3$ and elicit autocrine or paracrine responses from immune cells expressing the VDR.[12]

Despite these early advances, the precise nature of the interaction between vitamin D and the immune system remained unresolved for many years. Some pieces of the puzzle were easier to complete than others. For example, it became evident that dysregulation of 1,25(OH)$_2$D$_3$ was not restricted to sarcoidosis but was a common feature of many granulomatous disorders and some forms of cancer.[13] Likewise, at least in

This work was supported by NIH grant RO1AR050626 to M.H.

Department of Orthopaedic Surgery, Molecular Biology Institute, David Geffen School of Medicine at UCLA, 615 Charles East Young Drive South, Los Angeles, CA 90095, USA

E-mail address: mhewison@mednet.ucla.edu

Endocrinol Metab Clin N Am 39 (2010) 365–379

doi:10.1016/j.ecl.2010.02.010

endo.theclinics.com

0889-8529/10/$ – see front matter © 2010 Elsevier Inc. All rights reserved.

vitro, it was possible to potently regulate a range of immune cell functions using 1,25(OH)$_2$D$_3$ or its synthetic analogs.[14,15] However, the key remaining question was whether or not vitamin D could act as a physiologic regulator of normal immune responses. Answers to this question began to appear about 5 years ago and new information on the fundamental nature of vitamin D sufficiency/insufficiency has provided a fresh perspective on nonclassic actions of vitamin D. As a consequence, there is now a much broader acceptance that vitamin D plays an active role in regulating specific facets of human immunity. Details of this are reviewed and the possible effect of vitamin D insufficiency and vitamin D supplementation on normal immune function and human disease are discussed in this article.

VITAMIN D AND INNATE IMMUNITY
Macrophages, Vitamin D, and Cathelicidin

Consistent with the earlier seminal observations of extrarenal 1α-hydroxylase activity in patients with sarcoidosis, the effects of vitamin D on macrophage function have been central to many of the new observations implicating vitamin D in the regulation of immune responses. In common with natural killer cells (NK) and cytotoxic T lymphocytes (cytotoxic T cells), macrophages, and their monocyte precursors play a central role in initial nonspecific immune responses to pathogenic organisms or tissue damage, so-called cell-mediated immunity. Their role is to phagocytose pathogens or cell debris and then eliminate or assimilate the resulting waste material. In addition, macrophages can interface with the adaptive immune system by using phagocytic material for antigen presentation to T lymphocytes (T cells).

For many years, the key action of vitamin D on macrophages was believed to be its ability to stimulate differentiation of precursor monocytes to more mature phagocytic macrophages.[3,5,16,17] This concept was supported by observations showing differential expression of VDR and 1α-hydroxylase during the differentiation of human monocytes macrophages.[18] The latter report also emphasized early studies showing that normal human macrophages were able to synthesize 1,25(OH)$_2$D$_3$ when stimulated with interferon gamma (IFNγ).[19] Localized activation of vitamin D, coupled with expression of endogenous VDR was strongly suggestive of an autocrine or intracrine system for vitamin D action in normal monocytes/macrophages.

However, confirmation of such a mechanism was only obtained in 2006 when Liu and colleagues[20] carried out DNA array analyses to define innate immunity genes that were specifically modulated in monocytes by *Mycobacterium tuberculosis*. In a seminal investigation both the VDR and the gene for 1α-hydroxylase (CYP27B1) were shown to be induced following activation of the principal pathogen recognition receptor for *M tuberculosis*, toll-like receptor 2/1 (TLR2/1). Subsequent experiments confirmed that precursor 25-hydroxyvitamin D$_3$ (25OHD$_3$) was able to induce intracrine VDR responses in monocytes that had been treated with a TLR2/1 activator. In particular, the TLR2/1-25OHD$_3$ combination stimulated expression of the antibacterial protein cathelicidin, so that vitamin D was able to promote monocyte killing of *M tuberculosis*.[20] Notably, the ability to promote expression of the antibacterial protein following a TLR2/1 challenge was directly influenced by the 25OHD$_3$ status of the donor serum used for monocyte culture.[20] More recently, the authors have shown that vitamin D supplementation in vivo can also enhance TLR2/1-induced cathelicidin expression.[21] Cathelicidin was identified several years ago as a target for transcriptional regulation by 1,25(OH)$_2$D$_3$-liganded VDR, in that its gene promoter contains a functional vitamin D response element (VDRE).[22,23] This VDRE occurs within a small interchangeable nuclear element (SINE) sequence which only seems to be present in the cathelicidin gene promoter of higher primates, suggesting that vitamin D regulation of this facet of innate immunity is a relatively recent evolutionary development.[22]

Recent reports have underlined the importance of cathelicidin as a target for vitamin D but also suggest that this mechanism may be more complex than initially believed. As yet, the precise signal system by which TLR activation induces expression of VDR and 1α-hydroxylase remains unclear. Promoter-reporter analysis of the events involved in transcriptional regulation of CYP27B1 suggest that TLR4-mediated induction of the enzyme involves JAK-STAT, MAP kinase and nuclear factor kappaB (NF-κB) pathways, and that these synergize with IFNγ-mediated induction of CYP27B1.[24] However, other studies have proposed that TLR2/1 induction of 1α-hydroxylase occurs indirectly as a consequence of TLR2/1-induced interleukin (IL)-15, which is a potent inducer of CYP27B1 and 1α-hydroxylase activity.[25] In a similar fashion, IL-17A has been shown to enhance $1,25(OH)_2D_3$-mediated induction of cathelicidin, although this response does not seem to involve transcriptional regulation of 1α-hydroxylase or increased VDR sensitivity.[26] One pathway that has been poorly studied in this regard concerns the enzyme 24-hydroxylase, which is conventionally considered to function by inactivating $1,25(OH)_2D_3$. The gene for 24-hydroxylase (CYP24) is potently induced by $25OHD_3$ following TLR2/1 activation of monocytes[20] but, as yet, it is unclear whether this involves the nonmetabolic splice variant form of CYP24 known to be expressed by macrophages.[27]

Regulation of the antibacterial protein by $1,25(OH)_2D_3$ has been described for a wide variety of cell types other than macrophages, including keratinocytes,[23,28,29] lung epithelial cells,[30] myeloid cell lines,[22,23,29] and placental trophoblasts.[31] In some cases,[28,31] this seems to involve an intracrine response similar to that reported for monocytes. However, the mechanisms controlling local synthesis of $1,25(OH)_2D_3$ in these cells vary considerably. In keratinocytes, low baseline expression of 1α-hydroxylase is enhanced following epidermal wounding by transforming growth factor beta (TGFβ).[28] The resulting increase in $1,25(OH)_2D_3$ concentration up-regulates expression of TLR2 and TLR4 by keratinocytes, thereby priming these cells for further innate immune responses to pathogens or tissue damage.[28] By contrast, in trophoblasts, induction of cathelicidin and subsequent bacterial killing by $25OHD_3$ seems to be caused by constitutive 1α-hydroxylase activity, which is not further enhanced by TLR activation.[31] The latter may be a result of the rapid nonimmune induction of 1α-hydroxylase and VDR that occurs within the placenta during early gestation.[32]

Although most of the studies on vitamin D-mediated innate immunity have focused on the role of $1,25(OH)_2D_3$-bound VDR as a pivotal transcriptional regulator of cathelicidin, it is also important to recognize that other ligands may interact with the VDR.[33] For example, recent studies of biliary epithelial cells have shown that cathelicidin expression can be induced in a VDR-dependent fashion by bile salts.[34] This provides a mechanism for maintaining biliary sterility, although additive effects of $1,25(OH)_2D_3$ also highlight a novel therapeutic application for vitamin D in the treatment of primary biliary cirrhosis. Conversely, other compounds may act to disrupt normal $1,25(OH)_2D_3$-VDR-mediated immunity. The polycyclic aromatic hydrocarbon benzo[a]pyrene, a prominent product of cigarette smoking, has been shown to attenuate vitamin D-mediated induction of macrophage cathelcidin in a VDR-dependent fashion by stimulating expression of 24-hydroxylase and vitamin D catabolism.[35] The precise mechanism by which this occurs has yet to be determined but these data suggest that some toxic compounds are actively detrimental to vitamin D-mediated immunity.

The observations described earlier show clearly that vitamin D is a potent stimulator of mechanisms associated with pathogen elimination. In subsequent sections the clinical importance of this with respect to vitamin D insufficiency and immune-related diseases is discussed in more detail. However, 1 key question that immediately arises from the current observations is why there is a need to involve the vitamin D system in the TLR-induction of innate immunity. As previously described, VDR-mediated transcriptional regulation of cathelicidin is a relatively recent evolutionary change and was presumably advantageous when primates (including early *Homo sapiens*) were exposed to abundant sunlight, thereby priming high serum levels of vitamin D. Other benefits of incorporating vitamin D into innate immune regulation include the fact that it is associated with key feedback control pathways. As already mentioned, vitamin D has its own catabolic enzyme in the form of 24-hydroxylase, which sensitively attenuates responses to $1,25(OH)_2D_3$ and, in the case of the CYP24 splice variant, may also attenuate synthesis of this vitamin D metabolite.[27] However, vitamin D may also provide feedback regulation of immune activation pathways in that $1,25(OH)_2D_3$ has been shown to potently down-regulate expression of monocyte TLR2 and TLR4, thereby suppressing inflammatory responses that are normally activated by these receptors.[36] Thus, by using CYP24 and TLR regulatory mechanisms, vitamin D may help to promote appropriate innate immune responses while preventing an over elaboration of innate immune responses and the tissue damage frequently associated with this.

Dendritic Cells and Antigen Presentation

In addition to the phagocytic acquisition and elimination of pathogens and cell debris, innate immunity also involves the presentation of resultant antigen to cells involved in the adaptive arm of the immune system (**Fig. 1**). Although several cells are able to do this, the most well-recognized group of professional antigen-presenting cells (APCs) are dendritic cells (DCs). Expression of VDR by purified tissue DCs was first reported in 1987.[37] Subsequent studies using populations of DCs isolated from skin (Langerhans cells) provided evidence that $1,25(OH)_2D_3$ could act to attenuate antigen presentation.[38] However, it was not until the later advent of in vitro monocyte-derived DC models that the effects of vitamin D metabolites on antigen presentation were fully elucidated. In 2000, parallel studies by the Adorini and Kumar groups showed that $1,25(OH)_2D_3$[39] and its synthetic analogs[40] inhibited the maturation of monocyte-derived DCs, thereby suppressing their capacity to present antigen to T cells. Based on these observations, it was proposed that vitamin D could act to promote tolerance and this was endorsed by studies of pancreatic islet transplantation in which lower rejection rates were observed in $1,25(OH)_2D_3$-treated mice.[41] Crucially this response to $1,25(OH)_2D_3$ appeared to be caused by decreased DC maturation and concomitant enhancement of suppressor or regulatory T cells (Treg).[41] Further studies have underlined the importance of Treg generation[42] as part of the interaction between vitamin D and the immune system, and this is discussed in greater detail in later sections of this article.

Although regulation of DC maturation represents a potential target for $1,25(OH)_2D_3$ and its synthetic analogs as treatment of autoimmune disease and host-graft rejection, another perspective was provided by the observation that DCs express 1α-hydroxylase in a similar fashion to macrophages.[43,44] Data from monocyte-derived DCs showed that 1α-hydroxylase expression and activity increases as DCs differentiate towards a mature phenotype.[44] Functional analyses showed that treatment with $25OHD_3$ suppresses DC maturation and inhibits T-cell proliferation, confirming the existence of an intracrine pathway for vitamin D similar to that observed for macrophages.[44] Mature DCs showed lower levels of VDR than immature DCs or monocytes.[44] This reciprocal organization of 1α-hydroxylase and VDR expression may be advantageous in that mature antigen-presenting DCs may be relatively insensitive to $1,25(OH)_2D_3$, thereby allowing induction of an initial T-cell response. However, the

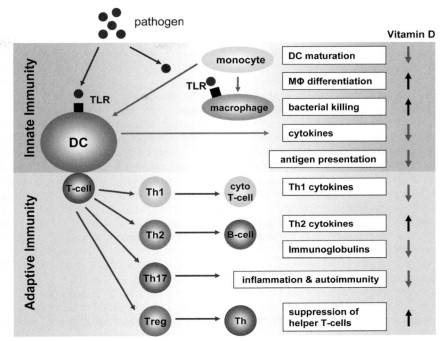

Fig. 1. Effects of vitamin D on innate and adaptive immunity. The principal innate and adaptive immune responses to a pathogenic challenge, and the positive or negative regulation of these responses by vitamin D. B-cell, B lymphocyte; cyto T-cell, cytotoxic T cell; DC, dendritic cell; MΦ, macrophage; T-cell, T lymphocyte; TLR, toll-like receptor; Treg, regulatory T cell.

high levels of $1,25(OH)_2D_3$ being synthesized by these cells can to act on VDR-expressing immature DCs and thus prevent their further development.[45] In this way, paracrine action of locally produced $1,25(OH)_2D_3$ allows initial presentation of antigen to T cells while preventing continued maturation of DCs and over stimulation of T cells.

Although DCs are heterogeneous in terms of their location, phenotype, and function, they are broadly divided into 2 groups based on their origin. Myeloid (mDCs) and plasmacytoid (pDCs) express different types of cytokines and chemokines and seem to exert complementary effects on T-cell responses, with mDCs being the most effective APCs[46] and pDCs being more closely associated with immune tolerance.[47] Therefore $1,25(OH)_2D_3$ preferentially regulates mDCs, suggesting that the key effect of vitamin D in this instance is to suppress activation of naive T cells. Although in this study pDCs showed no apparent immune response to $1,25(OH)_2D_3$, this does not preclude a role for vitamin D in the regulation of tolerogenic responses. One possibility is that local intracrine synthesis of $1,25(OH)_2D_3$ is more effective in achieving these responses. Alternatively, $1,25(OH)_2D_3$ synthesized by pDCs may regulate tolerance through paracrine effects on VDR-expressing T cells. This is discussed in further detail in the following section.

VITAMIN D AND ADAPTIVE IMMUNITY
Vitamin D and T-cell Function

Resting T cells express almost undetectable levels of VDR, but levels of the receptor increase as T cells proliferate following antigenic activation.[48–50] As a consequence, initial studies of the effects of vitamin D on T cells focused on the ability of 1,25(OH)$_2$D$_3$ to suppress T-cell proliferation.[48–50] However, the recognition that CD4$^+$ effector T cells were capable of considerable phenotypic plasticity, suggested that vitamin D might also influence the phenotype of T cells. Lemire and colleagues[51] first reported that 1,25(OH)$_2$D$_3$ preferentially inhibited T helper 1 (Th1) cells, which are a subset of CD4$^+$ effector T cells closely associated with cellular, rather than humoral, immune responses. Subsequent studies confirmed this observation and demonstrated that the cytokine profile of 1,25(OH)$_2$D$_3$-treated human T cells was consistent with Th2 cells, a subset of CD4$^+$ T cells associated with humoral (antibody)-mediated immunity.[52,53] The conclusion from these observations was that vitamin D promotes a T-cell shift from Th1 to Th2 and thus might help to limit the potential tissue damage associated with Th1 cellular immune responses. However, the validity of this generalization was called into question by studies using mouse T cells in which 1,25(OH)$_2$D$_3$ was shown to inhibit cytokines associated with Th1 (IFNγ) and Th2 (IL-4). Subsequent analysis of immune cells from the VDR gene knockout mouse added further confusion by showing that these animals had reduced (rather than the predicted increased) levels of Th1 cells.[54] Thus, although in vitro vitamin D seems to broadly support a shift from Th1 to Th2 in CD4$^+$ cells, it seems likely that in vivo its effects on T cells are more complex.

The T-cell repertoire has continued to expand with the characterization of another effector T-cell lineage distinct from Th1 or Th2 cells, termed Th17 cells because of their capacity to synthesize IL-17.[55,56] Th17 cells play an essential role in combating certain pathogens but they have also been linked to tissue damage and inflammation.[57,58] The precise role of vitamin D as a regulator of Th17 cells has yet to be fully elucidated but studies of animal models of the gastrointestinal inflammatory disease colitis have shown that treatment with 1,25(OH)$_2$D$_3$ reduces expression of IL-17,[59] and loss of 1,25(OH)$_2$D$_3$ as a result of CYP27b1 gene ablation leads to increased levels of this cytokine.[60] Thus, it possible that vitamin D exerts some of its effects on inflammation and autoimmune disease through the regulation of Th17 cells.

A fourth group of CD4$^+$ T cells exert suppressor rather than effector functions and are known as regulatory T cells or Tregs. In view of its early recognition as a suppressor of T-cell proliferation, it was anticipated that vitamin D would have effects on Tregs, and indeed in 2002 Barrat and colleagues[61] showed that 1,25(OH)$_2$D$_3$, in conjunction with glucocorticoids, potently stimulated the generation of IL-10–producing CD4$^+$/CD25$^+$ Tregs. Subsequent reports indicated that 1,25(OH)$_2$D$_3$ alone can induce Tregs,[62] and it seems that preferential differentiation of Tregs is a pivotal mechanism linking vitamin D and adaptive immunity, with potential beneficial effects for autoimmune disease and host-graft rejection.[63–65] This immunosuppressive mechanism is likely to be mediated by the induction of tolerogenic DCs as described in the previous section of the review,[41,66,67] but direct effects on T cells may also be important.[68] In this latter study, it was notable that 1,25(OH)$_2$D$_3$ increased IL-10 secretion and TLR9 expression by Tregs, suggesting a novel link between innate and adaptive immune responses.[68]

Relative to the amount of literature on CD4$^+$ effector cells, our understanding of the effects of vitamin D on CD8$^+$ suppressor T cells remains somewhat limited. In contrast to CD4$^+$ cells, CD8$^+$ cells show poor antiproliferative response to 1,25(OH)$_2$D$_3$.[50,69,70] However, VDR expression seems to be abundant in CD8$^+$ cells suggesting that they are still potential targets for 1,25(OH)$_2$D$_3$. Indeed subsequent reports have shown that 1,25(OH)$_2$D$_3$ actively regulates cytokine production by CD8$^+$ cells,[71] and can also regulate the proliferation of CD8$^+$ cells following specific immune stimuli.[72] Despite this, $1,25(OH)_2D_3$ does not seem to have a significant effect on animal disease models such as experimental autoimmune encephalomyelitis in which $CD8^+$ cells have been implicated.[73]

Although many of the studies linking $1,25(OH)_2D_3$ with adaptive immunity have focused on changes in T-cell proliferation and phenotype, it is important to recognize that other facets of T-cell function may also be affected by the hormone. In particular, recent studies have shown that vitamin D can exert powerful effects on the homing of T cells to specific tissues. Initial studies suggested that $1,25(OH)_2D_3$ acts to inhibit migration of T cells to lymph nodes.[74] However, more recent reports have shown an active role for vitamin D in promoting homing of T cells to the skin via up-regulation of chemokine receptor 10 (CCR10), the ligand for which, CCL27, is expressed by epidermal keratinocytes.[75] This T-cell homing response was induced by $25OHD_3$ as well as $1,25(OH)_2D_3$ and the author suggested that DCs and T cells were possible sources of the local 1α-hydroxylase activity.[75] In contrast to its positive effect on epidermal T-cell homing, vitamin D seems to exert a negative effect on chemokines and chemokine receptors associated with the gastrointestinal tract.[75] However, it seems likely that this is highly T-cell selective as newer studies using the VDR gene knockout mouse have shown aberrant gastrointestinal migration of a subset of $CD8^+$ cells, and this effect seems to be closely linked to the increased risk of colitis in VDR knockout mice.[76]

Vitamin D and B-cell Function

Like T cells, active but not inactive B cells express the VDR.[77] Consequently, initial studies indicated that $1,25(OH)_2D_3$ could directly regulate B-cell proliferation[78] and immunoglobulin (Ig) production.[77] Subsequent work contradicted this, suggesting instead that the ability of $1,25(OH)_2D_3$ to suppress proliferation and Ig production was caused by indirect effects mediated via helper T cells.[79] However, more recent reports have shown that $1,25(OH)_2D_3$ does indeed exert direct effects on B-cell homeostasis.[80] In addition to confirming direct VDR-mediated effects on B-cell proliferation and Ig production, this study also highlighted the ability of $1,25(OH)_2D_3$ to inhibit the differentiation of plasma cells and class-switched memory cells, suggesting a potential role for vitamin D in B-cell–related disorders such as systemic lupus erythematosus. Expression of CYP27b1 was also detected in B cells, indicating that B cells may be capable of autocrine/intracrine responses to vitamin D.[80] Indeed, this may be common to lymphocytes in general as CYP27b1 expression has also been detected in T cells.[75]

VITAMIN D, THE IMMUNE SYSTEM AND HUMAN HEALTH

For many years vitamin D status was defined simply by whether or not the patient had symptoms of the bone disease rickets (osteomalacia in adults). However, an entirely new perspective on vitamin D status has arisen from the observation that serum levels of the main circulating form of vitamin D ($25OHD_3$) as high as 75 nM correlate inversely with parathyroid hormone.[81] This, has prompted the introduction of a new term, vitamin D insufficiency, defined by serum levels of $25OHD_3$ that are suboptimal (<75 nM) but not necessarily rachitic (<20 nM).[82] Unlike serum concentrations of $1,25(OH)_2D_3$, which are primarily defined by the endocrine regulators of the vitamin D–activating enzyme, 1α-hydroxylase, circulating levels of $25OHD_3$ are a direct reflection of vitamin D status, which for any given individual depends on access to vitamin D either through exposure to sunlight or through dietary intake. The net effect of this is that vitamin D status can vary significantly in populations depending on geographic, social, or economic factors. As a result of these new parameters for vitamin D status, a consensus statement from the 13th Workshop on Vitamin D concluded that vitamin D insufficiency was a worldwide epidemic. Moreover, recent studies have shown that in the last 10 years alone, serum vitamin D levels have on average fallen by 20%.[83] The key question now being considered is what is the physiologic and clinical effect of global vitamin D insufficiency beyond classic bone diseases such as rickets? Epidemiologic studies have highlighted possible links between vitamin D insufficiency and a wide range of human diseases.[82] The final section of the article describes 4 of the key clinical problems that have been linked to the immunomodulatory properties of vitamin D.

Vitamin D and Tuberculosis

The observation that vitamin D acts to promote innate immune responses to TLR activation by *M tuberculosis*[20] has provided a new perspective on observations made many decades ago on the beneficial effects of ultraviolet light exposure on tuberculosis (TB). As a consequence this has become the most well-studied facet of the interaction between vitamin D and innate immunity.[84] Initial studies to assess the effects of 25OHD status on ex vivo macrophage function have shown that supplementation with a single oral dose of 2.5 mg of vitamin D enhances the ability of recipient macrophages to combat Bacille Calmette Guérin infection in vitro.[85] The potential benefits of vitamin D as treatment of TB have been further endorsed by a study that showed that adjunct vitamin D supplementation (0.25 mg vitamin D/d) of TB patients receiving conventional therapy for the disease reduced the time for sputum smear conversion from acid-fast bacteria (AFB)–positive to AFB-negative status.[86] A recent, double-blind, randomized, placebo-controlled trial showed that vitamin D supplementation had no effect on clinical outcomes or mortality amongst TB patients, although it should be emphasized that none of the supplemented patients in this study showed a significant increase in serum vitamin D levels.[87]

Vitamin D and Multiple Sclerosis

Several epidemiology studies have reported an association between vitamin D insufficiency and the incidence and/or severity of the autoimmune disease multiple sclerosis (MS) (reviewed in Ref.[88]). These observations have been supported by analysis of animal models, such as the experimental autoimmune encephalomyelitis (EAE) mouse, which show increased disease severity under dietary vitamin D restriction.[89] Conversely, administration of 1,25(OH)$_2$D$_3$ to EAE mice confers disease protection through effects on cytokine synthesis and apoptosis of inflammatory cells.[90,91] Some effects of 1,25(OH)$_2$D$_3$ on EAE seem to be dependent on IL-10 activity.[65]

Vitamin D and Type 1 Diabetes

In common with MS, published reports suggest that there is a link between vitamin D deficiency and another autoimmune disease, type 1 diabetes (reviewed in Ref.[92]). Low circulating levels of 25OHD$_3$ have been reported in adolescents at the time of diagnosis of type 1 diabetes,[93] and other data have documented the beneficial effects of vitamin D supplementation in protecting against type 1 diabetes.[94] Another strand of evidence linking vitamin D with type 1 diabetes stems from extensive genetic analyses on the physiologic effect of inherited variations in the genes for various components of the vitamin D metabolic and signaling system. Previous studies have indicated that some VDR gene haplotypes confer protection against diabetes,[95] and more recently this has been expanded to show that genetic variants of the CYP27b1 gene also affect susceptibility to type 1 diabetes.[96] Similar to animal model studies for MS, in vivo use of the nonobese diabetic (NOD) mouse as a model for type 1 diabetes has shown increased disease severity under conditions of dietary vitamin D restriction.[97]

Vitamin D and Crohn Disease

Several strands of evidence have linked vitamin D to the dysregulated immune responses observed with inflammatory bowel diseases such as Crohn disease. First, epidemiology suggests that patients with Crohn disease have decreased serum levels of 25OHD$_3$.[98–100] Second, studies in vivo using various animal models indicate that 1,25(OH)$_2$D$_3$ plays a crucial role in the pathophysiology of experimentally induced forms of inflammatory bowel disease.[60,101–103] Third, expression of 1α-hydroxylase has been detected in the human colon,[104] with the vitamin D–activating enzyme being up-regulated in disease-affected tissue from patients with Crohn disease.[105] In the case of the latter, dysregulated colonic expression of 1α-hydroxylase was associated with increased circulating levels of 1,25(OH)$_2$D$_3$ indicating that, as with sarcoidosis, localized synthesis of this vitamin D metabolite can spill over into the general circulation under conditions of persistent disease.[105] Current studies have implicated aberrant innate immune handling of enteric microbiota as an initiator of the adaptive immune damage associated with Crohn disease.[106] It is thus tempting to speculate that effects of vitamin D on this disease may involve the activation of innate immunity, together with the suppression of adaptive immunity and associated inflammation.

SUMMARY

It is almost 30 years since an interaction between vitamin D and the immune system was first documented. Although this was initially proposed as a nonclassic effect of vitamin D associated with granulomatous diseases, our current view is now changed considerably. Recent studies have shown a potential physiologic role for vitamin D in regulating normal innate and adaptive immunity. Future studies now need to focus on the clinical implications of vitamin D–mediated immunity and, in particular, the possible beneficial effects of supplementary vitamin D with respect to infectious and autoimmune diseases.

REFERENCES

1. Eisman JA, Martin TJ, MacIntyre I, et al. 1,25-Dihydroxyvitamin-D-receptor in breast cancer cells. Lancet 1979;2:1335.
2. Manolagas SC, Haussler MR, Deftos LJ. 1,25-Dihydroxyvitamin D3 receptors in cancer. Lancet 1980;1:828.
3. Abe E, Miyaura C, Sakagami H, et al. Differentiation of mouse myeloid leukemia cells induced by 1alpha,25-dihydroxyvitamin D3. Proc Natl Acad Sci U S A 1981;78:4990.
4. Colston K, Colston MJ, Feldman D. 1,25-Dihydroxyvitamin D3 and malignant melanoma: the presence of receptors and inhibition of cell growth in culture. Endocrinology 1981;108:1083.
5. Abe E, Miyaura C, Tanaka H, et al. 1 alpha,25-dihydroxyvitamin D3 promotes fusion of mouse alveolar macrophages both by a direct mechanism and by a spleen cell-mediated indirect mechanism. Proc Natl Acad Sci U S A 1983; 80:5583.
6. Bhalla AK, Amento EP, Serog B, et al. 1,25-Dihydroxyvitamin D3 inhibits antigen-induced T cell activation. J Immunol 1984;133:1748.

7. Bell NH, Stern PH, Pantzer E, et al. Evidence that increased circulating 1alpha, 25-dihydroxyvitamin D is the probable cause for abnormal calcium metabolism in sarcoidosis. J Clin Invest 1979;64:218.

8. Papapoulos SE, Clemens TL, Fraher LJ, et al. 1,25-Dihydroxycholecalciferol in the pathogenesis of the hypercalcaemia of sarcoidosis. Lancet 1979;1:627.

9. Adams JS, Gacad MA. Characterization of 1 alpha-hydroxylation of vitamin D3 sterols by cultured alveolar macrophages from patients with sarcoidosis. J Exp Med 1985;161:755.

10. Adams JS, Sharma OP, Gacad MA, et al. Metabolism of 25-hydroxyvitamin D3 by cultured pulmonary alveolar macrophages in sarcoidosis. J Clin Invest 1983;72:1856.

11. Barbour GL, Coburn JW, Slatopolsky E, et al. Hypercalcemia in an anephric patient with sarcoidosis: evidence for extrarenal generation of 1,25-dihydroxyvitamin D. N Engl J Med 1981;305:440.

12. Hewison M. Vitamin D and the immune system. J Endocrinol 1992;132:173.

13. Hewison M, Burke F, Evans KN, et al. Extra-renal 25-hydroxyvitamin D3-1alpha-hydroxylase in human health and disease. J Steroid Biochem Mol Biol 2007; 103:316.

14. Griffin MD, Xing N, Kumar R. Vitamin D and its analogs as regulators of immune activation and antigen presentation. Annu Rev Nutr 2003;23:117.

15. Van Etten E, Decallonne B, Verlinden L, et al. Analogs of 1alpha,25-dihydroxyvitamin D3 as pluripotent immunomodulators. J Cell Biochem 2003;88:223.

16. Koeffler HP, Amatruda T, Ikekawa N, et al. Induction of macrophage differentiation of human normal and leukemic myeloid stem cells by 1,25-dihydroxyvitamin D3 and its fluorinated analogues. Cancer Res 1984;44:5624.

17. Tanaka H, Abe E, Miyaura C, et al. 1 alpha,25-Dihydroxyvitamin D3 induces differentiation of human promyelocytic leukemia cells (HL-60) into monocyte-macrophages, but not into granulocytes. Biochem Biophys Res Commun 1983;117:86.

18. Kreutz M, Andreesen R, Krause SW, et al. 1,25-Sihydroxyvitamin D3 production and vitamin D3 receptor expression are developmentally regulated during differentiation of human monocytes into macrophages. Blood 1993;82:1300.

19. Koeffler HP, Reichel H, Bishop JE, et al. Gamma-interferon stimulates production of 1,25-dihydroxyvitamin D3 by normal human macrophages. Biochem Biophys Res Commun 1985;127:596.

20. Liu PT, Stenger S, Li H, et al. Toll-like receptor triggering of a vitamin D-mediated human antimicrobial response. Science 2006;311:1770.

21. Adams JS, Ren S, Liu PT, et al. Vitamin D-directed rheostatic regulation of monocyte antibacterial responses. J Immunol 2009;182:4289.

22. Gombart AF, Borregaard N, Koeffler HP. Human cathelicidin antimicrobial peptide (CAMP) gene is a direct target of the vitamin D receptor and is strongly up-regulated in myeloid cells by 1,25-dihydroxyvitamin D3. FASEB J 2005;19:1067.

23. Wang TT, Nestel FP, Bourdeau V, et al. Cutting edge: 1,25-dihydroxyvitamin D3 is a direct inducer of antimicrobial peptide gene expression. J Immunol 2004; 173:2909.

24. Stoffels K, Overbergh L, Giulietti A, et al. Immune regulation of 25-hydroxyvitamin-d(3)-1alpha-hydroxylase in human monocytes. J Bone Miner Res 2006; 21:37.

25. Krutzik SR, Hewison M, Liu PT, et al. IL-15 links TLR2/1-induced macrophage differentiation to the vitamin D-dependent antimicrobial pathway. J Immunol 2008;181:7115.

26. Peric M, Koglin S, Kim SM, et al. IL-17A enhances vitamin D3-induced expression of cathelicidin antimicrobial peptide in human keratinocytes. J Immunol 2008;181:8504.

27. Ren S, Nguyen L, Wu S, et al. Alternative splicing of vitamin D-24-hydroxylase: a novel mechanism for the regulation of extrarenal 1,25-dihydroxyvitamin D synthesis. J Biol Chem 2005;280:20604.

28. Schauber J, Dorschner RA, Coda AB, et al. Injury enhances TLR2 function and antimicrobial peptide expression through a vitamin D-dependent mechanism. J Clin Invest 2007;117:803.

29. Schauber J, Dorschner RA, Yamasaki K, et al. Control of the innate epithelial antimicrobial response is cell-type specific and dependent on relevant microenvironmental stimuli. Immunology 2006;118:509.

30. Yim S, Dhawan P, Ragunath C, et al. Induction of cathelicidin in normal and CF bronchial epithelial cells by 1,25-dihydroxyvitamin D(3). J Cyst Fibros 2007;6: 403.

31. Liu N, Kaplan AT, Low J, et al. Vitamin D induces innate antibacterial responses in human trophoblasts via an intracrine pathway. Biol Reprod 2009;80:398.

32. Evans KN, Bulmer JN, Kilby MD, et al. Vitamin D and placental-decidual function. J Soc Gynecol Investig 2004;11:263.

33. Makishima M, Lu TT, Xie W, et al. Vitamin D receptor as an intestinal bile acid sensor. Science 2002;296:1313.

34. D'Aldebert E, Biyeyeme Bi Mve MJ, Mergey M, et al. Bile salts control the antimicrobial peptide cathelicidin through nuclear receptors in the human biliary epithelium. Gastroenterology 2009;136:1435.

35. Matsunawa M, Amano Y, Endo K, et al. The aryl hydrocarbon receptor activator benzo[a]pyrene enhances vitamin D3 catabolism in macrophages. Toxicol Sci 2009;109:50–8.

36. Sadeghi K, Wessner B, Laggner U, et al. Vitamin D3 down-regulates monocyte TLR expression and triggers hyporesponsiveness to pathogen-associated molecular patterns. Eur J Immunol 2006;36:361.

37. Brennan A, Katz DR, Nunn JD, et al. Dendritic cells from human tissues express receptors for the immunoregulatory vitamin D3 metabolite, dihydroxycholecalciferol. Immunology 1987;61:457.

38. Dam TN, Moller B, Hindkjaer J, et al. The vitamin D3 analog calcipotriol suppresses the number and antigen-presenting function of Langerhans cells in normal human skin. J Investig Dermatol Symp Proc 1996;1:72.

39. Penna G, Adorini L. 1 Alpha,25-dihydroxyvitamin D3 inhibits differentiation, maturation, activation, and survival of dendritic cells leading to impaired alloreactive T cell activation. J Immunol 2000;164:2405.

40. Griffin MD, Lutz WH, Phan VA, et al. Potent inhibition of dendritic cell differentiation and maturation by vitamin D analogs. Biochem Biophys Res Commun 2000;270:701.

41. Gregori S, Casorati M, Amuchastegui S, et al. Regulatory T cells induced by 1 alpha,25-dihydroxyvitamin D3 and mycophenolate mofetil treatment mediate transplantation tolerance. J Immunol 1945;167:2001.

42. O'Garra A, Barrat FJ. In vitro generation of IL-10-producing regulatory CD4+ T cells is induced by immunosuppressive drugs and inhibited by Th1- and Th2-inducing cytokines. Immunol Lett 2003;85:135.

43. Fritsche J, Mondal K, Ehrnsperger A, et al. Regulation of 25-hydroxyvitamin D3-1 alpha-hydroxylase and production of 1 alpha,25-dihydroxyvitamin D3 by human dendritic cells. Blood 2003;102:3314.

44. Hewison M, Freeman L, Hughes SV, et al. Differential regulation of vitamin D receptor and its ligand in human monocyte-derived dendritic cells. J Immunol 2003;170:5382.

45. Hewison M, Zehnder D, Chakraverty R, et al. Vitamin D and barrier function: a novel role for extra-renal 1 alpha-hydroxylase. Mol Cell Endocrinol 2004;215:31.

46. Liu YJ. IPC: professional type 1 interferon-producing cells and plasmacytoid dendritic cell precursors. Annu Rev Immunol 2005;23:275.

47. Steinman RM, Hawiger D, Nussenzweig MC. Tolerogenic dendritic cells. Annu Rev Immunol 2003;21:685.

48. Karmali R, Hewison M, Rayment N, et al. 1,25(OH)2D3 regulates c-myc mRNA levels in tonsillar T lymphocytes. Immunology 1991;74:589.

49. Nunn JD, Katz DR, Barker S, et al. Regulation of human tonsillar T-cell proliferation by the active metabolite of vitamin D3. Immunology 1986;59:479.

50. Provvedini DM, Manolagas SC. 1 alpha,25-dihydroxyvitamin D3 receptor distribution and effects in subpopulations of normal human T lymphocytes. J Clin Endocrinol Metab 1989;68:774.

51. Lemire JM, Archer DC, Beck L, et al. Immunosuppressive actions of 1,25-dihydroxyvitamin D3: preferential inhibition of Th1 functions. J Nutr 1995;125:1704S.

52. Boonstra A, Barrat FJ, Crain C, et al. 1alpha,25-Dihydroxyvitamin d3 has a direct effect on naive CD4(+) T cells to enhance the development of Th2 cells. J Immunol 2001;167:4974.

53. Overbergh L, Decallonne B, Waer M, et al. 1alpha,25-dihydroxyvitamin D3 induces an autoantigen-specific T-helper 1/T-helper 2 immune shift in NOD mice immunized with GAD65 (p524-543). Diabetes 2000;49:1301.

54. O'Kelly J, Hisatake J, Hisatake Y, et al. Normal myelopoiesis but abnormal T lymphocyte responses in vitamin D receptor knockout mice. J Clin Invest 2002;109:1091.

55. Harrington LE, Mangan PR, Weaver CT. Expanding the effector CD4 T-cell repertoire: the Th17 lineage. Curr Opin Immunol 2006;18:349.

56. Weaver CT, Hatton RD, Mangan PR, et al. IL-17 family cytokines and the expanding diversity of effector T cell lineages. Annu Rev Immunol 2007;25:821.

57. Bettelli E, Korn T, Kuchroo VK. Th17: the third member of the effector T cell trilogy. Curr Opin Immunol 2007;19:652.

58. Korn T, Oukka M, Kuchroo V, et al. Th17 cells: effector T cells with inflammatory properties. Semin Immunol 2007;19:362.

59. Daniel C, Sartory NA, Zahn N, et al. Immune modulatory treatment of TNBS colitis with calcitriol is associated with a change of a Th1/Th17 to a Th2 and regulatory T cell profile. J Pharmacol Exp Ther 2007;323:23–33.

60. Liu N, Nguyen L, Chun RF, et al. Altered endocrine and autocrine metabolism of vitamin D in a mouse model of gastrointestinal inflammation. Endocrinology 2008;149:4799.

61. Barrat FJ, Cua DJ, Boonstra A, et al. In vitro generation of interleukin 10-producing regulatory CD4(+) T cells is induced by immunosuppressive drugs and inhibited by T helper type 1 (Th1)- and Th2-inducing cytokines. J Exp Med 2002;195:603.

62. Gorman S, Kuritzky LA, Judge MA, et al. Topically applied 1,25-dihydroxyvitamin D3 enhances the suppressive activity of CD4+CD25+ cells in the draining lymph nodes. J Immunol 2007;179:6273.

63. Gregori S, Giarratana N, Smiroldo S, et al. A 1alpha,25-dihydroxyvitamin D(3) analog enhances regulatory T-cells and arrests autoimmune diabetes in NOD mice. Diabetes 2002;51:1367.

64. Mathieu C, Badenhoop K. Vitamin D and type 1 diabetes mellitus: state of the art. Trends Endocrinol Metab 2005;16:261.
65. Spach KM, Nashold FE, Dittel BN, et al. IL-10 signaling is essential for 1,25-di-hydroxyvitamin D3-mediated inhibition of experimental autoimmune encephalo-myelitis. J Immunol 2006;177:6030.
66. Adorini L, Penna G, Giarratana N, et al. Dendritic cells as key targets for immu-nomodulation by vitamin D receptor ligands. J Steroid Biochem Mol Biol 2004; 89-90:437.
67. Dong X, Bachman LA, Kumar R, et al. Generation of antigen-specific, inter-leukin-10-producing T-cells using dendritic cell stimulation and steroid hormone conditioning. Transpl Immunol 2003;11:323.
68. Urry Z, Xystrakis E, Richards DF, et al. Ligation of TLR9 induced on human IL-10-secreting Tregs by 1alpha,25-dihydroxyvitamin D3 abrogates regulatory function. J Clin Invest 2009;119:387.
69. Vanham G, Ceuppens JL, Bouillon R. T lymphocytes and their CD4 subset are direct targets for the inhibitory effect of calcitriol. Cell Immunol 1989; 124:320.
70. Veldman CM, Cantorna MT, DeLuca HF. Expression of 1,25-dihydroxyvitamin D(3) receptor in the immune system. Arch Biochem Biophys 2000;374:334.
71. Willheim M, Thien R, Schrattbauer K, et al. Regulatory effects of 1alpha,25-dihy-droxyvitamin D3 on the cytokine production of human peripheral blood lympho-cytes. J Clin Endocrinol Metab 1999;84:3739.
72. Iho S, Iwamoto K, Kura F, et al. Mechanism in 1,25(OH)2D3-induced suppres-sion of helper/suppressor function of CD4/CD8 cells to immunoglobulin produc-tion in B cells. Cell Immunol 1990;127:12.
73. Meehan TF, DeLuca HF. CD8(+) T cells are not necessary for 1 alpha,25-dihy-droxyvitamin D(3) to suppress experimental autoimmune encephalomyelitis in mice. Proc Natl Acad Sci U S A 2002;99:5557.
74. Topilski I, Flaishon L, Naveh Y, et al. The anti-inflammatory effects of 1,25-dihy-droxyvitamin D3 on Th2 cells in vivo are due in part to the control of integrin-mediated T lymphocyte homing. Eur J Immunol 2004;34:1068.
75. Sigmundsdottir H, Pan J, Debes GF, et al. DCs metabolize sunlight-induced vitamin D3 to 'program' T cell attraction to the epidermal chemokine CCL27. Nat Immunol 2007;8:285.
76. Yu S, Bruce D, Froicu M, et al. Failure of T cell homing, reduced CD4/CD8al-phaalpha intraepithelial lymphocytes, and inflammation in the gut of vitamin D receptor KO mice. Proc Natl Acad Sci U S A 2008;105:20834.
77. Provvedini DM, Tsoukas CD, Deftos LJ, et al. 1 alpha,25-Dihydroxyvitamin D3-binding macromolecules in human B lymphocytes: effects on immunoglobulin production. J Immunol 1986;136:2734.
78. Shiozawa K, Shiozawa S, Shimizu S, et al. 1 alpha,25-dihydroxyvitamin D3 inhibits pokeweed mitogen-stimulated human B-cell activation: an analysis using serum-free culture conditions. Immunology 1985;56:161.
79. Lemire JM, Adams JS, Sakai R, et al. 1 alpha,25-dihydroxyvitamin D3 suppresses proliferation and immunoglobulin production by normal human peripheral blood mononuclear cells. J Clin Invest 1984;74:657.
80. Chen S, Sims GP, Chen XX, et al. Modulatory effects of 1,25-dihydroxyvitamin d3 on human B cell differentiation. J Immunol 2007;179:1634.
81. Chapuy MC, Preziosi P, Maamer M, et al. Prevalence of vitamin D insufficiency in an adult normal population. Osteoporos Int 1997;7:439.
82. Holick MF. Vitamin D deficiency. N Engl J Med 2007;357:266.

83. Ginde AA, Liu MC, Camargo CA Jr. Demographic differences and trends of vitamin D insufficiency in the US population, 1988–2004. Arch Intern Med 2009;169:626.

84. Martineau AR, Honecker FU, Wilkinson RJ, et al. Vitamin D in the treatment of pulmonary tuberculosis. J Steroid Biochem Mol Biol 2007;103:793.

85. Martineau AR, Wilkinson RJ, Wilkinson KA, et al. A single dose of vitamin D enhances immunity to mycobacteria. Am J Respir Crit Care Med 2007;176:208.

86. Nursyam EW, Amin Z, Rumende CM. The effect of vitamin D as supplementary treatment in patients with moderately advanced pulmonary tuberculous lesion. Acta Med Indones 2006;38:3.

87. Wejse C, Gomes VF, Rabna P, et al. Vitamin D as supplementary treatment for tuberculosis: a double-blind, randomized, placebo-controlled trial. Am J Respir Crit Care Med 2009;179:843.

88. Raghuwanshi A, Joshi SS, Christakos S. Vitamin D and multiple sclerosis. J Cell Biochem 2008;105:338.

89. Spach KM, Hayes CE. Vitamin D3 confers protection from autoimmune encephalomyelitis only in female mice. J Immunol 2005;175:4119.

90. Pedersen LB, Nashold FE, Spach KM, et al. 1,25-Dihydroxyvitamin D3 reverses experimental autoimmune encephalomyelitis by inhibiting chemokine synthesis and monocyte trafficking. J Neurosci Res 2007;85:2480.

91. Spach KM, Pedersen LB, Nashold FE, et al. Gene expression analysis suggests that 1,25-dihydroxyvitamin D3 reverses experimental autoimmune encephalomyelitis by stimulating inflammatory cell apoptosis. Physiol Genomics 2004; 18:141.

92. Mathieu C, Gysemans C, Giulietti A, et al. Vitamin D and diabetes. Diabetologia 2005;48:1247.

93. Littorin B, Blom P, Scholin A, et al. Lower levels of plasma 25-hydroxyvitamin D among young adults at diagnosis of autoimmune type 1 diabetes compared with control subjects: results from the nationwide Diabetes Incidence Study in Sweden (DISS). Diabetologia 2006;49:2847.

94. Harris SS. Vitamin D in type 1 diabetes prevention. J Nutr 2005;135:323.

95. Ramos-Lopez E, Jansen T, Ivaskevicius V, et al. Protection from type 1 diabetes by vitamin D receptor haplotypes. Ann N Y Acad Sci 2006;1079:327.

96. Bailey R, Cooper JD, Zeitels L, et al. Association of the vitamin D metabolism gene CYP27B1 with type 1 diabetes. Diabetes 2007;56(10):2616.

97. Giulietti A, Gysemans C, Stoffels K, et al. Vitamin D deficiency in early life accelerates type 1 diabetes in non-obese diabetic mice. Diabetologia 2004;47:451.

98. Pappa HM, Gordon CM, Saslowsky TM, et al. Vitamin D status in children and young adults with inflammatory bowel disease. Pediatrics 1950;118:2006.

99. Pappa HM, Grand RJ, Gordon CM. Report on the vitamin D status of adult and pediatric patients with inflammatory bowel disease and its significance for bone health and disease. Inflamm Bowel Dis 2006;12:1162.

100. Vagianos K, Bector S, McConnell J, et al. Nutrition assessment of patients with inflammatory bowel disease. JPEN J Parenter Enteral Nutr 2007;31:311.

101. Froicu M, Cantorna MT. Vitamin D and the vitamin D receptor are critical for control of the innate immune response to colonic injury. BMC Immunol 2007;8:5.

102. Froicu M, Weaver V, Wynn TA, et al. A crucial role for the vitamin D receptor in experimental inflammatory bowel diseases. Mol Endocrinol 2003;17:2386.

103. Kong J, Zhang Z, Musch MW, et al. Novel role of the vitamin D receptor in maintaining the integrity of the intestinal mucosal barrier. Am J Physiol Gastrointest Liver Physiol 2007;294:G208–16.

104. Zehnder D, Bland R, Williams MC, et al. Extrarenal expression of 25-hydroxyvitamin d(3)-1 alpha-hydroxylase. J Clin Endocrinol Metab 2001;86:888.
105. Abreu MT, Kantorovich V, Vasiliauskas EA, et al. Measurement of vitamin D levels in inflammatory bowel disease patients reveals a subset of Crohn's disease patients with elevated 1,25-dihydroxyvitamin D and low bone mineral density. Gut 2004;53:1129.
106. Packey CD, Sartor RB. Commensal bacteria, traditional and opportunistic pathogens, dysbiosis and bacterial killing in inflammatory bowel diseases. Curr Opin Infect Dis 2009;22:292.

Vitamin D: Extraskeletal Health

Michael F. Holick, MD, PhD

KEYWORDS

- Vitamin D • Extraskeletal effects • Psoriasis • Cancer
- Diabetes • Autoimmune diseases • Cardiovascular

Vitamin D is one of the oldest hormones.[1] Early in evolution as unicellular organisms evolved and took advantage of the sun's energy for photosynthesis of sugars, they also began to photosynthesize vitamin D.[1] A phytoplankton species that has existed in the Sargasso sea (Atlantic Ocean) for more than 500 million years unchanged was found to have more than 1% of its total dry weight as provitamin D_2 (ergosterol). When this organism was cultured and exposed to simulated sunlight it produced vitamin D_2.[2] As life forms evolved in the ocean, which has a high calcium content, and ventured onto land where calcium was stored in the soil, they needed to develop a method to efficiently absorb calcium from the plants and roots that they ate. It is likely that these organisms when exposed to sunlight produced vitamin D in their skin, which was critical for them to be able to absorb their dietary calcium efficiently. Vitamin D has evolved over millions of years to play and essential role in vertebrate evolution not only for bone health but for their overall health and well being.

SOURCES OF VITAMIN D

Humans have always depended on the sun for their vitamin D requirement.[1,3] Thus the major source of vitamin D for children and adults is exposure of the skin to sunlight.[3] Adults in a bathing suit exposed to an amount of sunlight that causes a slight pinkness to the skin 24 hours later (1MED) is equivalent to ingesting about 20,000 IU of vitamin D.[3] There are few foods that naturally contain vitamin D. Because vitamin D is fat-soluble it is found in oily fish, including salmon, mackerel, and herring. Fish that have little fat in their flesh concentrate their fat in their liver, which is why cod liver oil and oil from other nonoily fish are good sources of vitamin D. Yeast and mushrooms make huge quantities of ergosterol and when exposed to sunlight or ultraviolet irradiation are excellent sources of vitamin D. In the United States and Canada, milk and

This work was supported in part by the UV Foundation.
Section of Endocrinology, Nutrition, and Diabetes, Department of Medicine, Vitamin D, Skin and Bone Research Laboratory, Boston University School of Medicine, Boston University Medical Center, 85 East Newton Street, M-1013, Boston, MA 02118, USA
E-mail address: mfholick@bu.edu

Endocrinol Metab Clin N Am 39 (2010) 381–400
doi:10.1016/j.ecl.2010.02.016
0889-8529/10/$ – see front matter © 2010 Elsevier Inc. All rights reserved.

several other dairy products are fortified with vitamin D. Some orange juices are also fortified with calcium and vitamin D.[4]

HISTORICAL PERSPECTIVE ON EXTRASKELETAL EFFECTS OF VITAMIN D

At the turn of the twentieth century it was estimated that more than 90% of children in the industrialized cities of northern Europe and 80% of children living in the northeastern United States had skeletal evidence of rickets.[5,6] Besides the obvious deformities associated with rickets, it was noted that these children had severe muscle weakness, poor tooth eruption with dental caries, and were plagued by upper respiratory tract infections.[5,7] In the early 1900s Finsen observed that exposure to sunlight was effective in treating several skin disorders, including lupus vulgaris, which is caused by a tuberculosis infection of the skin. His remarkable observations resulted in him receiving the Nobel prize in 1903. In 1915 Hoffman compared cancer mortality in cities according to latitude, and demonstrated that cancer mortality increased with increasing distance from the equator (**Table 1**).[8] In 1941 Apperly[9] reported that people who lived in the Northeast were more likely to die of cancer than people who lived in the South. In the 1980s it was reported that there was a latitudinal association with colorectal cancer risk.[10]

In the 1970s it was appreciated that vitamin D (D represents D_2 or D_3) that came from the diet or was synthesized in the skin required a hydroxylation in the liver to form the major circulating form of vitamin D, 25-hydroxyvitamin D (25(OH)D).[11] 25(OH)D is metabolized in the kidneys to its active form 1,25-dihydroxyvitamin D $(1,25(OH)_2D)$.[3] Because $1,25(OH)_2D$ is fat-soluble it was assumed that it functioned by interacting with a nuclear vitamin D receptor (VDR) to up- and down-regulate genes responsible for calcium and bone metabolism.[3,11–13] It was quickly demonstrated that kidneys, small intestine, and osteoblasts had a VDR and that several genes, including calbindin9k, epithelial calcium channel, and receptor activator of nuclear factor-κB (RANKL) were up-regulated to control calcium and phosphorus absorption in the small intestine as well as calcium and phosphorus metabolism in the kidneys, and to enhance bone calcium mobilization from the skeleton.[3,12,13]

When radiolabeled $1,25(OH)_2D_3$ was given to vitamin D–deficient rats it had been assumed that it would concentrate only in the organs that were responsible for calcium and bone metabolism that had a VDR. However, when other tissues in the body were recovered to serve as a negative control it was found that nuclei in essentially every tissue and organ in the body were able to concentrate and localize

Table 1
Mortality from cancer in cities according to latitude measured between 1908 and 1912

Number of Cities	Latitude	Deaths from Cancer	Rate (per 100,000)
35	60N–50N	119374	105.7
48	50N–40N	121216	92.4
24	40N–30N	37451	78.1
7	30N–10N	5696	42.3
4	10N–10S	1056	40.9
7	10S–30S	3040	37.7
5	30S–40S	11048	89.8

Modified from Hoffman FL. The mortality of cancer throughout the world. Appendix E. Prudential Press; 1915.

^{3}H-1,25(OH)$_2$D$_3$, including the skin, colon, brain, and pancreas, among many other organs.[14] Within a decade a multitude of laboratories demonstrated the presence of a VDR in essentially every tissue and cell in the body including skin, colon, brain, pancreas, and breast as well as activated T and B lymphocytes, monocytes, and macrophages.[2,13]

The first insight into the noncalcium, nonskeletal effects of vitamin D was reported in the early 1980s, when it was observed that mouse and human leukemia cells had a VDR and when they were exposed to 1,25(OH)$_2$D$_3$ their proliferative activity was reduced, and the leukemic cells differentiated into normal-appearing macrophages.[15] This observation was quickly followed by reports that a variety of cancer cell lines developed from melanoma, colon cancer and prostate cancer had a VDR, and when these cell lines were incubated with 1,25(OH)$_2$D$_3$ their cellular proliferation was reduced and they showed signs of differentiation.[16–19]

In the 1980s the first reports for extrarenal synthesis of 1,25(OH)$_2$D came from observations that patients with sarcoidosis or tuberculosis who had hypercalcemia had inappropriately normal or elevated levels of 1,25(OH)$_2$D$_3$. Initially it was believed that this was due to a unregulated synthesis of 1,25(OH)$_2$D by the kidneys.[3,20] When it was reported that a sarcoid patient who developed nephritis and lost all kidney function remained hypercalcemic with an elevated blood level of 1,25(OH)$_2$D, it was suggested that there was a nonrenal source for this metabolite.[20] This result was quickly followed by the observation that macrophages converted 25(OH)D$_3$ to 1,25(OH)$_2$D$_3$.[21] Within a decade several investigators began reporting that cultured cells from the skin, colon, prostate, breast, lung, and brain all had the enzymatic machinery to produce 1,25(OH)$_2$D$_3$.[3,13,16–18,22–25]

CANCER PREVENTION

Epidemiologic studies over the past decade have confirmed the observations of Garland and colleagues[25] Hanchette and Schwartz,[26] who reported that adults who lived at higher latitudes were more likely to develop and die of colorectal and prostate cancer. Other observations revealed that living at higher latitudes increased the risk of dying of ovarian,[27] breast,[28] lung,[29] and esophageal cancer[30] among many others. Compelling retrospective and prospective epidemiologic studies have demonstrated that when 25(OH)D levels are less than 20 ng/mL there is a 30% to 50% increased risk of developing and dying of colorectal, prostate, breast, pancreatic, and esophageal cancer, among others (**Fig. 1**).[10,29,31–33] Men who had the most exposure to sunlight had a 3- to 5-year reprieve from developing prostate cancer compared with men who worked indoors.[34] When 972 women in Canada who had a history of breast cancer were asked about their sun exposure history as teenagers and young adults and compared their sun exposure to 1135 women matched for age and location who did not have breast cancer, it was revealed that the women with breast cancer had much less sun exposure as teenagers and young adults compared with women with no history of breast cancer. It was estimated that women who had had the most sun exposure during their teens and 20s reduced their risk of developing breast cancer by 69%, and young and middle-aged women who had the most sun exposure reduced their risk by 51%.[35] Women older than 45 years received no benefit in reducing their risk for breast cancer by being exposed to more sunlight.

The Women's Health Initiative reported that 1000 mg calcium and 400 IU vitamin D/d did not decrease the risk of developing colorectal cancer, raising questions about the benefits of vitamin D in reducing the risk of this deadly cancer.[36] The study results, however, came into question because most of the women admitted that they were not

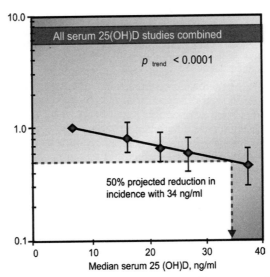

Fig. 1. Dose-response gradient for colorectal cancer according to serum 25(OH)D concentration, of 5 studies combined. The 5 points are the odds ratios for each quintile of 25(OH)D based on the combined data from the 5 studies. (*From* Gorham ED, Garland CF, Garland FC, et al. Optimal Vitamin D Status for Colorectal Cancer Prevention: A Quantitative Meta Analysis. Am J Prev Med 2007;32(3):210–6; with permission.)

taking their calcium and vitamin D more than 40% of the time during the study. More importantly, a review of the data revealed that women who had a blood level of 25(OH)D less than 12 ng/mL at the start of the study and followed for 8 years on suboptimal doses of vitamin D compared with women who had an initial blood level of 25(OH)D of 24 ng/mL had a 253% increased risk of developing colorectal cancer.[37] Pooled data of 1761 women found the highest vitamin D consumption correlated with a 50% lower risk of breast cancer (they had on average a blood level of 48 ng/mL).[31]

Lappe and colleagues[38] reported that 1179 postmenopausal women who received 1500 mg of calcium a day with 1100 IU of vitamin D_3 a day and followed for 4 years reduced their risk of developing all cancers by more than 60%. When women during the first year were removed from the analysis because of the likelihood that these women had a small undetectable cancer at the initiation of the trial, there was a dramatic 77% reduced risk of developing cancer when taking 1100 IU of vitamin D_3 a day along with calcium supplementation compared with the group that received either calcium or placebo (**Fig. 2**). In the Physician Health Study, men who had the highest levels of 25(OH)D had a lower risk of developing several cancers, including colorectal, esophageal, pancreatic, and leukemia.[33] It has also been suggested that one possible cause for the health disparity in blacks who are at a higher risk for developing and dying of cancer is due to their high incidence of vitamin D deficiency, which not only could increase their risk of developing deadly cancers but also might make the cancers more aggressive and more difficult to treat.[39,40]

Nagpal and colleagues[41] reported that 1,25(OH)$_2$D$_3$ through its transcriptional activity was capable of regulating directly or indirectly at least 200 genes. Among these genes are those that control proliferation, differentiation, apoptosis, and angiogenesis (**Fig. 3**).[3,41] 1,25(OH)$_2$D$_3$ increased the expression of cell cycle inhibitors and decreased activators of cyclin-cyclin dependent kinase complexes, in addition to

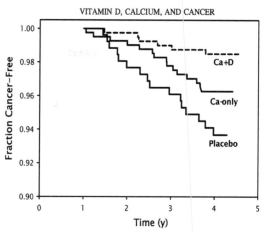

Fig. 2. Kaplan-Meier survival curves (ie, free of cancer) for the 3 treatment groups randomly assigned in the cohort of women who were free of cancer at 1 year after intervention (n = 1085). Sample sizes are 266 for the placebo group, 416 for the calcium-only (Ca-only) group, and 403 for the calcium plus vitamin D (Ca+D) group. The survival at the end of study for the Ca + D group is significantly higher than that for the placebo group, by logistic regression. (Copyright Robert P. Heaney, 2006. Used with permission.)

increasing levels of cyclin-dependent kinase inhibitors Cip/Kip proteins P21 and P27, which are known to keep the cell cycle in the G1/S phase, thus preventing DNA synthesis and cellular growth (**Fig. 4**). In addition, $1,25(OH)_2D_3$ increased the expression of the cell adhesion molecule E-cadherin and inhibited the expression of β-catenin.[42,43]

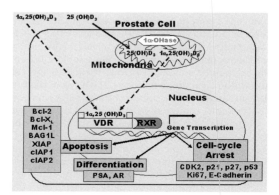

Fig. 3. Vitamin D maintains cellular growth by controlling several genes that control cellular proliferation and differentiation. 25-hydroxyvitamin D (25(OH)D) is converted to 1,25-dihydroxyvitamin D ($1,25(OH)_2D$) in a wide variety of nonrenal cells, including cells in the colon and prostate. $1,25(OH)_2D$ interacts with the vitamin D receptor (VDR) and regulates a variety of genes that control apoptosis, proliferation, and differentiation. (*Courtesy of* Michael F. Holick, PhD, MD; Copyright © 2009.)

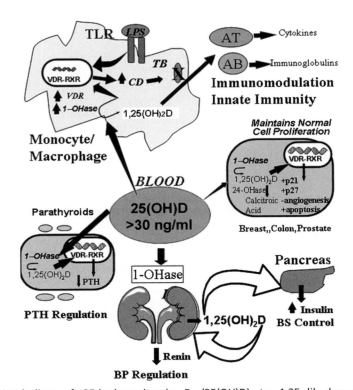

Fig. 4. Metabolism of 25-hydroxyvitamin D (25(OH)D) to 1,25-dihydroxyvitamin D (1,25(OH)$_2$D) for nonskeletal functions. When a monocyte/macrophage is stimulated through its toll-like receptor 2/1 (TLR2/1) by an infective agent such as *Mycobacterium tuberculosis* (TB), or its lipopolysaccharide (LPS), the signal up-regulates the expression of vitamin D receptor (VDR) and the 25-hydroxyvitamin D1-hydroxylase (1-OHase). A 25(OH)D level greater than 30 ng/mL provides adequate substrate for the 1-OHase to convert it to 1,25(OH)$_2$D. 1,25(OH)$_2$D returns to the nucleus where it increases the expression of cathelicidin (CD), which is a peptide capable of promoting innate immunity and inducing the destruction of infective agents such as TB. It is also likely that the 1,25(OH)$_2$D produced in the monocytes/macrophage is released to act locally on activated T (AT) and activated B (AB) lymphocytes, which regulate cytokine and immunoglobulin synthesis, respectively. When 25(OH)D levels are approximately 30 ng/mL, it reduces the risk of many common cancers. It is believed that the local production of 1,25(OH)$_2$D in the breast, colon, prostate, and other cells regulates a variety of genes that control proliferation, including p21 and p27 as well as genes that inhibit angiogenesis and induced apoptosis. Once 1,25(OH)$_2$D completes the task of maintaining normal cellular proliferation and differentiation, it induces the 25-hydroxyvitamin D24-hydroxylase (24-OHase). The 24-OHase enhances the metabolism of 1,25(OH)$_2$D to calcitroic acid, which is biologically inert. Thus, the local production of 1,25(OH)$_2$D does not enter the circulation and has no influence on calcium metabolism. The parathyroid glands have 1-OHase activity and the local production of 1,25(OH)$_2$D inhibits the expression and synthesis of parathyroid hormone (PTH). The production of 1,25(OH)2D in the kidney enters the circulation, and is able to down-regulate renin production in the kidney and to stimulate insulin secretion in the β-islet cells of the pancreas. (*Courtesy of* Michael F. Holick, PhD, MD; Copyright © 2007.)

The recognition that many human cancer cell lines had a VDR prompted an investigation to determine whether $1,25(OH)_2D_3$ could be used as a treatment for preleukemia. In a double-blind placebo-controlled trial, patients with preleukemia who received $1,25(OH)_2D_3$ initially responded well.[44] However, the trial proved to be unsuccessful due to the observation that patients on $1,25(OH)_2D_3$ not only developed hypercalcemia but ultimately went into blastic crisis.

There have been several thousand analogues of $1,25(OH)_2D_3$ that have been made and evaluated for their antiproliferative and calcemic activities.[45,46] Many of these analogues appeared to have great clinical promise in that they demonstrated 100 to 1000 times higher antiproliferative activity while having minimum calcemic activity. In animal models, some of these analogues including those with 2 side arms known as Gemini compounds, were shown to be effective in inhibiting MC-26 tumor cell growth progression in mice, with minimum calcemic activity.[47]

It was observed that men with metastatic prostate cancer who received 2000 IU of vitamin D_3 a day for up to 21 months showed a more than 50% reduction in rise in their prostate-specific antigen (PSA) levels compared with before receiving the vitamin D_3.[48] Men with prostate cancer who received daily $1,25(OH)_2D_3$ had a significant decrease in the rise of their PSA levels compared with men who were on placebo.[49] This prompted a phase 2 clinical trial in which a single oral dose of 45 μg of $1,25(OH)_2D_3$ was given once a week. The study was halted as a result of hypercalcemia and increased death rate in men who were taking $1,25(OH)_2D_3$.[50]

Cancer cells have developed several strategies to decrease the effectiveness of $1,25(OH)_2D_3$ from keeping cell growth in check. A human prostate cancer cell line, DU-145, is able to resist the antiproliferative activity of $1,25(OH)_2D_3$ by increasing the expression of the 25-hydroxyvitamin D24-hydroxylase (24-OHase).[51,52] This enzyme hydroxylates the side arm on carbons 24 and 23, causing a cleavage of the carbon bond at carbon 23 that results in the formation of a water-soluble carboxylic acid metabolite, calcitroic acid.[53]

Another clever strategy that malignant cells have developed to mitigate the antiproliferative activity of $1,25(OH)_2D_3$ is to increase the expression of the transcriptional factor Snail.[42] Snail is a zinc finger transcription factor that is involved in cell movement, and exists in both invertebrates and vertebrates. Snail-1 induces epithelial-to-mesenchymal transition and was found to not only inhibit the expression of VDR but also E-cadherin. Palmer and colleagues[42] observed that a human colon cancer cell line, SW-480–ADH, transfected with the Snail gene prevented the antiproliferative and prodifferentiating activity of $1,25(OH)_2D_3$ (**Fig. 5**).

PSORIASIS

In the 1980s it was appreciated that keratinocytes in the skin was not only the major source for 7-dehydrocholesterol, which could be converted to vitamin D_3 when exposed to sunlight, but also that this cell had a VDR and was able to convert $25(OH)D$ to $1,25(OH)_2D_3$.[2,43,53] Studies revealed that incubating keratinocytes with $1,25(OH)_2D_3$ resulted in marked decrease in DNA synthesis and proliferation, and a marked increase in markers of differentiation, including transglutaminase activity.[43,54]

It was reasoned that because $1,25(OH)_2D_3$ was such a potent inhibitor of keratinocyte proliferation in vitro, it could be used for the treatment of the nonmalignant hyperproliferative disease psoriasis (**Fig. 6**). Topically applied $1,25(OH)_2D_3$ was found to be both safe and effective for treating psoriasis.[55] Topically applied $1,25(OH)_2D_3$ resulted in marked reduction in the thickness of plaques, scaling, and erythema. Several

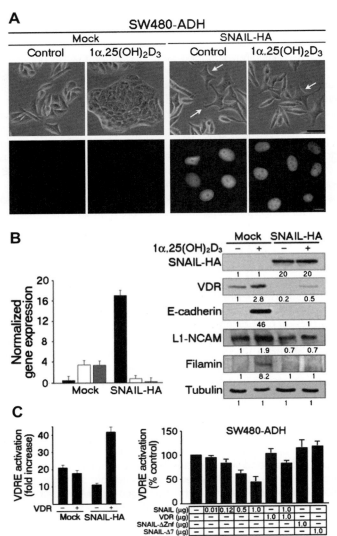

Fig. 5. (*A, top*) Micrographs of SNAIL-HA and mock-infected cells. Arrows indicate the phenotypic change induced by SNAIL. Bar, 50 μm. (*A, bottom*) Immunostaining of ectopic SNAIL expression using an antibody to HA. Bar, 10 μm. (*B, left*) normalized SNAIL. VDR and E-cadherin mRNA levels were measured by real-time reverse transcription-polymerase chain reaction. (*B, right*) Protein expression was estimated by Western blot. Numbers refer to fold increase over untreated mock-infected cells. (*C*) SNAIL inhibits the induction of L1-NCAM and filamin by 1,25(OH)$_2$D$_3$. Wild-type (*left*) but not mutant (*right*) SNAIL proteins inhibit VDR transcriptional activity (4XVDRE-tk-luciferase). (*From* Palmer HG, Larriba MJ, Garcia JM, et al. The transcription factor SNAIL represses vitamin D receptor expression and responsiveness in human colon cancer. Nat Med 2004;10:917–9; with permission.)

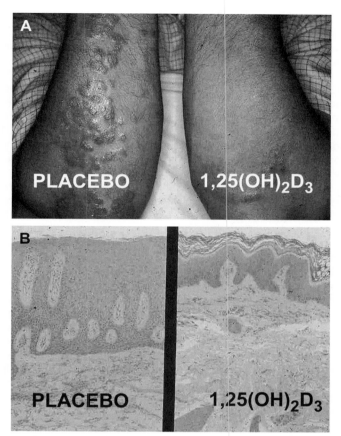

Fig. 6. (Top panel) A 28-year-old man with a more than 20-year history of psoriasis. The psoriatic lesions on the patient's right forearm were treated with placebo Vaseline and the psoriatic lesions on the left forearm were treated with Vaseline containing 1,25-dihydroxyvitamin D_3 (1,25(OH)$_2$D$_3$). (*Bottom panel*) Photomicrographs of biopsies from the right forearm and left forearm. (*Courtesy of* Michael F. Holick, PhD, MD; Copyright © 2009.)

analogues of 1,25(OH)$_2$D$_3$, including calcipotriene, 1,24-dihydroxyvitamin D_3, and 22-oxo-1,25(OH)$_2$D$_3$, were also evaluated for their antiproliferative activity in cultured keratinocytes.[56,57] These substances were all found to inhibit keratinocyte proliferation and induced maturation; along with 1,25(OH)$_2$D$_3$, they were consequently developed as a first-line therapy for the treatment of psoriasis.

VITAMIN D AND AUTOIMMUNE DISEASES

Living at a latitude above 35° for the first 10 years increases the risk of developing multiple sclerosis (MS) by 100% no matter where one lives thereafter.[58,59] A similar observation has been made for type I diabetes. There was a 10- to 15-fold increased risk of developing type 1 diabetes if living in far northern or southern regions of the globe compared with living near the equator.[60]

Epidemiologic evidence suggests that both men and women who have the highest blood levels of 25(OH)D had the lowest risk for developing MS.[61] In the Nurses' Health

Study it was observed that women who had the highest intake of vitamin D had a 42% reduced risk of developing MS.[62] A similar observation was made in that the women who had the highest intake of vitamin D and had a reduced risk of developing rheumatoid arthritis by 41%.[63]

In the 1960s children in Finland during their first year of life were recommended to take 2000 IU of vitamin D a day. A follow-up study 31 years later revealed that those children who took 2000 IU of vitamin D a day during their first year of life reduced their risk of developing type 1 diabetes by 88%.[64] Those children who had evidence of vitamin D deficiency had a 2.4-fold increased risk of developing type 1 diabetes. Wheezing disorders and asthma have been linked to vitamin D deficiency in utero. Children born from mothers who were vitamin D deficient had a 60% increased risk of having wheezing disorders during their first few years of life.[65,66]

Although the mechanism by which enhancing vitamin D status reduces risk of developing autoimmune diseases is not fully understood, it is known that when resting T and B lymphocytes are stimulated, one of the first genes that is turned on is the gene for the VDR. Activated T and B lymphocytes have a VDR and $1,25(OH)_2D_3$ is a potent regulator of both T- and B-cell activity. $1,25(OH)_2D_3$ suppresses proliferation and immunoglobulin synthesis,[43,67] and has a multitude of effects on T-lymphocyte function and activity. $1,25(OH)_2D_3$ inhibits T-cell proliferation, in particular T-helper (Th1) cells capable of producing interferon (IFN)-γ and interleukin (IL)-2. These actions in turn prevent further antigen presentation to and recruitment of T lymphocytes. In addition, $1,25(OH)_2D_3$ enhances the production of IL-4, IL-5, and IL-10, shifting the balance from Th1 to Th2 cell phenotype.[43,68] In addition to its effects on activated T lymphocytes, $1,25(OH)_2D_3$ regulates dendritic cell activity, which plays a key role in antigen presentation. These cells have a VDR, and respond to the antiproliferative and immunomodulatory activities of $1,25(OH)_2D_3$. It is also recognized that $1,25(OH)_2D_3$ inhibits the formation of Th17 cells, which are now considered to play an important role in autoimmunity.[43,69]

It is curious that whereas most tissues and cells in the body are capable of producing $1,25(OH)_2D_3$, lymphocytes do not express the 1-OHase. Instead, activated macrophages produce $1,25(OH)_2D_3$ not only for the regulation of cathelicidin production[70,71] but also to act in a paracrine fashion to interact with the VDR in activated T and B lymphocytes, in order to modulate their immune functions (see **Fig. 4**).[3]

It has been suggested that the potent immunomodulatory activity of $1,25(OH)_2D_3$ will lead to an increased risk of autoimmune diseases.[72] However, what these investigators do not appreciate is that vitamin D is a modulator, not an inhibitor, of the immune system and that it plays a central role in maintaining a healthy immune system. Several animal models have been used to demonstrate that $1,25(OH)_2D_3$ is very effective in either preventing or significantly reducing the progression of autoimmune encephalitis in models of MS, type 1 diabetes, and Crohn disease,[73,74] all of which support the epidemiologic evidence that vitamin D is important for immune health.

INNATE IMMUNITY

In the mid-1800s it was recognized that cod liver oil was effective in treating tuberculosis (TB). In the early 1900s solariums were developed, in part to treat patients with TB, and Finsen demonstrated that exposure of the skin to sunlight was an effective therapy for treating *Mycobacterium* infections of the skin. More recent studies have associated vitamin D deficiency with increased risk of not only developing TB but also other infectious diseases, including otitis media,[75] upper respiratory tract

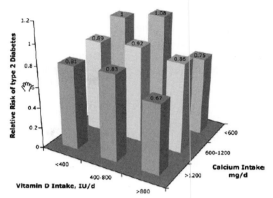

Fig. 7. Adjusted relative risk of incident type 2 DM in the Nurses' Health Study by calcium and vitamin D intake. (*From* Holick, MF. Diabetes and the Vitamin D Connection. Current Diabetes Reports 2008;8:393–8; with permission.)

infections,[76] and influenza infection.[77] It has been hypothesized that there is a seasonal stimulus for influenza infection; it usually appears in mid to end of winter, a time when the 25(OH)D levels are at the nadir.[77] Postmenopausal women who took 2000 IU of vitamin D a day for 1 year reduced their risk of upper respiratory tract infections by 90%.[78] Children and adults who had the highest blood levels of 25(OH)D had the lowest risk of developing upper respiratory tract infections throughout the year.[76]

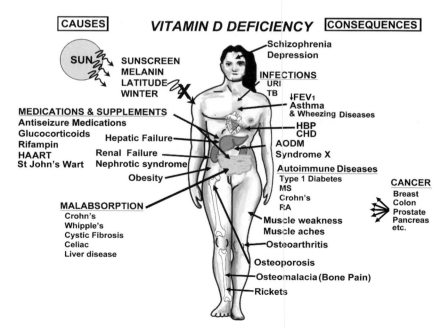

Fig. 8. Major Causes of vitamin D deficiency and potential health consequences. (*Courtesy of* Michael F. Holick, PhD, MD; Copyright © 2007.)

Although it was well known that activated T and B lymphocytes had a VDR and that $1,25(OH)_2D_3$ was a potent modulator of the immune response, it was unclear how this activity could reduce risk of infectious diseases. It was also known that circulating monocytes and macrophages have a VDR and also can produce $1,25(OH)_2D_3$.[3,43,79] Innate immunity is associated with the activation of toll-like receptors (TLRs), not

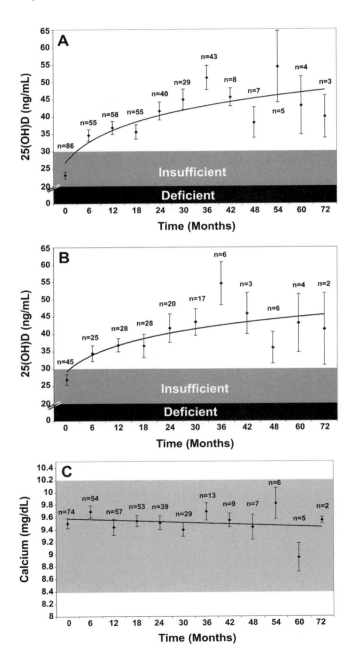

only on monocytes and macrophages but also in other barrier cells of the intestine, gingiva, bladder, lungs, and epidermis.[43] Activation of TLRs results in the production of antimicrobial peptides and reactive oxygen species, which in turn kill infective agents. When a macrophage ingests a mycobacterium the lipopolysaccharide on its cell wall interacts with the TLR2/1 receptor, resulting in the expression of VDR and 1-OHase.[70] The macrophage now has the capability of producing $1,25(OH)_2D_3$, which can in turn interact with its VDR to stimulate the production of the antimicrobial peptide cathelicidin. It has been demonstrated that monocytes infected with *Mycobacterium* and incubated in blood from an African American who had a 25(OH)D level of 8 ng/mL resulted in the death of the monocyte. When monocytes were exposed to the same mycobacterium but now incubated in blood that had added to it 25(OH)D to raise the level to 28 ng/mL, the monocyte was able to mount an effective response by enhancing cathelicidin production, resulting in the death of the mycobacterium. These results provide a mechanism by which vitamin D plays a crucial role in reducing the risk of infectious diseases.

CARDIOVASCULAR HEALTH

Adults who are vitamin D deficient have a 50% higher risk of developing a myocardial infarction.[80] Furthermore, patients who had a myocardial infarction and were vitamin D deficient were more likely to die from the event.[81] In 1979 Rostand[82] reported that living at higher latitudes increased the risk of hypertension. Studies have suggested that increasing vitamin D intake reduces the risk of hypertension. Exposure of patients to vitamin D producing simulated sunlight 3 times a week for 3 months on a tanning bed increased circulating levels of 25(OH)D by 180% and reduced systolic and diastolic blood pressure by 6 mm Hg, whereas hypertensive patients exposed to a tanning bed that only emitted ultraviolet A radiation and did not experience any increase in the blood level of 25(OH)D and had no change in their blood pressure.[83]

Fig. 9. (*A*) Mean serum 25-hydroxyvitamin D (25(OH)D) levels in all patients: includes patients treated with 50,000 IU vitamin D_2 every 2 weeks (maintenance therapy, N = 81), including those patients with vitamin D insufficiency who were initially treated with 8 weeks of 50,000 IU vitamin D_2 weekly before maintenance therapy (N = 39). Error bars represent standard error of the mean; mean result over 5 years is shown. Time 0 is initiation of treatment, results shown as mean values averaged for 6-month intervals. When mean 25(OH)D in each 6-month group was compared with mean initial 25(OH)D, $P<.001$ up until month 43; $P<.001$ when all remaining values after month 43 were compared with mean initial 25(OH)D. (*B*) Mean serum 25(OH)D levels in patients receiving maintenance therapy only: levels for 37 patients who were vitamin D insufficient (25(OH)D levels <30 ng/mL) and 5 patients who were vitamin D sufficient (25(OH)D levels ≥30 ng/mL) who were treated with maintenance therapy of 50,000 IU vitamin D_2 every 2 weeks. Error bars represent standard error of the mean; mean result over 5 years is shown. Time 0 is initiation of treatment, results shown as mean values averaged for 6-month intervals. When mean 25(OH)D in each 6-month group were compared with mean initial 25(OH)D, $P<.001$ up until month 37; $P<.001$ when all remaining values after month 43 were compared with mean initial 25(OH)D. (*C*) Serum calcium levels: results for all 81 patients who were treated with 50,000 IU of vitamin D_2. Error bars represent standard error of the mean. Time 0 is initiation of treatment, results shown as mean values averaged for 6-month intervals. Normal serum calcium: 8.5 to 10.2 mg/dL. (*From* Pietras SM, Obayan BK, Cai MH, et al. Vitamin D2 treatment for vitamin D deficiency and insufficiency for up to 6 years. Arch Intern Med 2009;169:1806–8; with permission. Copyright © 2009 American Medical Association. All rights reserved.)

1,25(OH)$_2$D$_3$ is a potent down-regulator of renin production, a hormone that is responsible for regulating blood pressure.[84] Vascular smooth muscle and cardio-myocytes have a VDR, and it has been estimated that 200 genes that regulate cardiovascular health may be influenced by 1,25(OH)$_2$D$_3$.[85,86] In addition to these cardioprotective effects 1,25(OH)$_2$D$_3$ has anti-inflammatory activity, and reduces C-reactive protein (CRP) and IL-10 production.[85,86] In addition, 1,25(OH)$_2$D$_3$ suppressed foam cell formation by reducing acetylated or oxidized low-density lipoprotein cholesterol uptake in macrophages obtained from diabetes patients.[87]

This finding may help explain the observation of an 80% reduction in development of peripheral vascular disease when the 25(OH)D was above 25 ng/mL.[88]

TYPE 2 DIABETES

β-Islet cells in the pancreas have a VDR, and 1,25(OH)$_2$D$_3$ stimulates insulin production.[60,89] In addition, it has been reported that improvement in vitamin D status in type 2 diabetic patients improves insulin resistance.[60,89] Men and women who had an intake of calcium of greater than 1000 mg a day and more than 800 IU of vitamin D a day had a relative risk of reduction in developing type 2 diabetes of 33% (**Fig. 7**).[90] It has also been observed that there is an inverse relationship between blood levels of 25(OH)D and risk of type 2 diabetes, with a 75% reduction in whites and 83% reduction in Mexican Americans.[91]

SUMMARY

Vitamin D deficiency is the most common nutritional deficiency and likely the most common medical condition in the world.[3] There is a multitude of causes of vitamin D deficiency (**Fig. 8**), but the major cause has been the lack of appreciation that the body requires 5- to 10-fold higher intakes than is currently recommended by the Institute of Medicine and other health agencies.[92] It is likely that our hunter gatherer forefathers being exposed to sunlight on a daily basis were making several thousand IU of vitamin D a day. The fact that 100 IU of vitamin D prevented overt signs of rickets led to the false security that ingesting twice this amount was more than adequate to satisfy the body's vitamin D requirement.[93] Although this may be true for preventing overt skeletal deformities associated with rickets, there is now overwhelming and compelling scientific and epidemiologic data suggesting that the human body requires a blood level of 25(OH)D above 30 ng/mL for maximum health.[94] The likely reason is that essentially every tissue and cell in the body has a VDR and thus, to have enough vitamin D to satisfy all of these cellular requirements, the blood level of 25(OH)D needs to be above 30 ng/mL. It has been estimated that for every 100 IU of vitamin D ingested that the blood level of 25(OH)D increases by 1 ng/mL.[95,96] Thus to theoretically achieve a blood level above 30 ng/mL requires the ingestion of 3000 IU of vitamin D a day. There is evidence, however, that when the blood levels of 25(OH)D are less than 15 ng/mL, the body is able to more efficiently use vitamin D to raise the blood level to about 20 ng/mL.[97] To raise the blood level of 25(OH)D above 20 ng/mL requires the ingestion of 100 IU of vitamin D for every 1-ng increase; therefore to increase the blood level to the minimum 30 ng/mL requires the ingestion of at least 1000 IU of vitamin D a day for adults.

There is a great need to significantly increase the recommended adequate intakes of vitamin D. All neonates during the first year of life should take at least 400 IU/d of vitamin D, and increasing it to 1000 IU/d may provide additional health benefits. Children 1 year and older should take at least 400 IU/d of vitamin D as recently recommended by the American Academy of Pediatrics,[98] but they should consider increasing intake up to 2000 IU/d derive maximum health benefits from vitamin D. Prepubertal and teenage girls who received 2000 IU of vitamin D per day for a year showed improvement in their musculoskeletal health with no untoward toxicity.[99] All adults should be taking 2000 IU of vitamin D per day. A recent study reported that adults who took 50,000 IU of vitamin D once every 2 weeks, which is equivalent to taking 3000 IU of vitamin D a day, for up to 6 years was effective in maintaining blood levels of 25(OH)D of between 40 and 60 ng/mL without any toxicity (**Fig. 9**).[100]

There is no downside to increasing either a child's or adult's vitamin D intake, with the exception of acquired disorders such as granulomatous diseases including sarcoidosis and tuberculosis, as well as some lymphomas with activated macrophages that produce $1,25(OH)_2D_3$ in an unregulated fashion.[3,79]

REFERENCES

1. Holick MF. Phylogenetic and evolutionary aspects of vitamin D from phytoplankton to humans. In: Pang PK, Schreibman MP, editors, Vertebrate endocrinology: fundamentals and biomedical implications, vol. 3. Orlando (FL): Academic Press, Inc. (Harcourt Brace Jovanovich); 1989. p. 7–43.
2. Holick MF. Vitamin D: a millennium perspective. J Cell Biochem 2003;88: 296–307.
3. Holick MF. Vitamin D deficiency. N Engl J Med 2007;357:266–81.
4. Tangpricha V, Koutkia P, Rieke SM, et al. Fortification of orange juice with vitamin D: a novel approach to enhance vitamin D nutritional health. Am J Clin Nutr 2003;77:1478–83.
5. Holick MF. Resurrection of vitamin D deficiency and rickets. J Clin Invest 2006; 116(8):2062–72.
6. Rajakumar, K, Greenspan, SL, Thomas, SB and et al. Solar ultraviolet radiation and vitamin D. A historical perspective. 2007. Am J Public Health. 97(10):1746–8.
7. Hess AF. Collected writings, volume I. Springfield (IL): Charles C. Thomas; 1936. 669–719.
8. Hoffman FL. The mortality of cancer throughout the world. Appendix E. Newark (NJ): Prudential Press; 1915.
9. Apperly FL. The relation of solar radiation to cancer mortality in North America. Cancer Res 1941;1:191–5.
10. Gorham ED, Garland CF, Garland FC, et al. Optimal vitamin D status for colorectal cancer prevention: a quantitative meta analysis. Am J Prev Med 2007; 32(3):210–6; with permission.
11. Jones G. Expanding role for Vitamin D in chronic kidney disease: importance of blood 25-OH-D levels and extra-renal 1α-hydroxylase in the classical and nonclassical actions of 1α,25-dihydroxyvitamin D3. Semin Dial 2007;20(4):316–24.
12. Christakos S, Dhawan P, Liu Y, et al. New insights into the mechanisms of vitamin D action. J Cell Biochem 2003;88:695–705.
13. Dusso AS, Brown AJ. Slatopolsky. Vitamin D. Am J Physiol Renal Physiol 2005; 289:F8–28.
14. Stumpf WE, Sar M, Reid FA, et al. Target cells for 1,25-dihydroxyvitamin D3 in intestinal tract, stomach, kidney, skin, pituitary, and parathyroid. Science 1979;206:1188–90.
15. Tanaka H, Abe E, Miyaura C, et al. 1,25-Dihydroxycholeciferol and human myeloid leukemia cell line (HL-60): The presence of cytosol receptor and induction of differentiation. Biochem J 1982;204(3):713–9.

16. Colston K, Colston MJ, Feldman D. 1,25-Dihydroxyvitamin D_3 and malignant melanoma: the presence of receptors and inhibition of cell growth in culture. Endocrinology 1981;108:1083–6.
17. Cross HS, Bareis P, Hofer H, et al. 25- Hydroxyvitamin D_3-1-hydroxylase and vitamin D receptor gene expression in human colonic mucosa is elevated during early cancerogenesis. Steroids 2001;66:287–92.
18. Schwartz GG, Whitlatch LW, Chen TC, et al. Human prostate cells synthesize 1,25-dihydroxyvitamin D_3 from 25-hydroxyvitamin D_3. Cancer Epidemiol Biomarkers Prev 1998;7:391–5.
19. Feldman D, Zhao XY, Krishnan AV. Editorial/mini-review: vitamin D and prostate cancer. Endocrinology 2000;141:5–9.
20. Gkonos PJ, London R, Hendler ED. Hypercalcemia and elevated 1,25-dihydroxyvitamin D levels in a patient with end-stage renal disease and active tuberculosis. N Engl J Med 1984;311:1683–5.
21. Adams JS, Singer FR, Gacad MA, et al. Isolation and structural identification of 1,25-dihydroxyvitamin D_3 produced by cultured alveolar macrophages in sarcoidosis. J Clin Endocrinol Metab 1985;60:960–6.
22. Tangpricha V, Flanagan JN, Whitlatch LW, et al. 25-hydroxyvitamin D-1α-hydroxylase in normal and malignant colon tissue. Lancet 2001; 357(9269):1673–4.
23. Mawer EB, Hayes ME, Heys SE, et al. Constitutive synthesis of 1,25-dihydroxyvitamin D_3 by a human small cell lung cell line. J Clin Endocrinol Metab 1994; 79(2):554–60.
24. Radermacher J, Diesel B, Seifert M, et al. Expression analysis of CYP27B1 in tumor biopsies and cell cultures. Anticancer Res 2006;26:2683–6.
25. Garland CF, Garland FC, Gorham ED. Can colon cancer incidence and death rates be reduced with calcium and vitamin D? Am J Clin Nutr 1991;54: 93S–201S.
26. Hanchette CL, Schwartz GG. Geographic patterns of prostate cancer mortality. Cancer 1992;70:2861–9.
27. Bischoff-Ferrari HA, Giovannucci E, Willett WC, et al. Estimation of optimal serum concentrations of 25-hydroxyvitamin D for multiple health outcomes. Am J Clin Nutr 2006;84:18–28.
28. Bertone-Johnson ER, Chen WY, Holick MF, et al. Plasma 25-hydroxyvitamin D and 1,25-dihydroxyvitamin D and risk of breast cancer. Cancer Epidemiol Biomarkers Prev 2005;14:1991–7.
29. Moan J, Porojnicu AC, Dahlback A, et al. Addressing the health benefits and risks, involving vitamin D or skin cancer, of increased sun exposure. Proc Natl Acad Sci USA 2008;105(2):668–73.
30. Grant WB. Lower vitamin-D production from solar ultraviolet-B Irradiance may explain some differences in cancer survival rates. J Natl Med Assoc 2006; 98(3):357–64.
31. Garland CF, Gorham ED, Mohr SB, et al. Vitamin D and prevention of breast cancer: Pooled analysis. J Steroid Biochem Mol Biol 2007; 103(3–5):708–11.
32. Ahonen MH, Tenkanen L, Teppo L, et al. Prostate cancer risk and prediagnostic serum 25-hydroxyvitamin D levels (Finland). Cancer Causes Control 2000;11: 847–52.
33. Giovannucci E, Liu Y, Rimm EB, et al. Prospective study of predictors of vitamin D status and cancer incidence and mortality in men. J Natl Cancer Inst 2006; 98(7):451–9.

34. Luscombe CJ, Fryer AA, French ME, et al. Exposure to ultraviolet radiation: association with susceptibility and age at presentation with prostate cancer. Lancet 2001;358:641–2.
35. Knight JA, Lesosky M, Barnett H, et al. Vitamin D and reduced risk of breast cancer: a population-based case-control study. Cancer Epidemiol Biomarkers Prev 2007;16(3):422–99.
36. Wactawski-Wende J, Kotchen JM, Anderson GL, et al. Calcium plus vitamin D supplementation and the risk of colorectal cancer. N Engl J Med 2006;354: 684–96.
37. Holick MF. Calcium plus vitamin D and the risk of colorectal cancer. N Engl J Med 2006;354(21):2287.
38. Lappe JM, Travers-Gustafson D, Davies KM, et al. Vitamin D and calcium supplementation reduces cancer risk: results of a randomized trial. Am J Clin Nutr 2007;85(6):1586–91.
39. Giovannucci E, Liu Y, Willett WC. Cancer incidence and mortality and vitamin D in black ad white male health professionals. Cancer Epidemiol Biomarkers Prev 2006;15(12):2467–72.
40. Bibuld D. Health disparities and vitamin D. Humana Press Inc. 2009;7(1): 63–76.
41. Nagpal S, Na S, Rathnachalam R. Noncalcemic actions of vitamin D receptor ligands. Endocr Rev 2005;26:662–87.
42. Palmer HG, Larriba MJ, Garcia JM, et al. The transcription factor SNAIL represses vitamin D receptor expression and responsiveness in human colon cancer. Nat Med 2004;10:917–9.
43. Bikle DD. Nonclassic actions of vitamin D. J Clin Endocrinol Metab 2009;94(1): 26–34.
44. Koeffler HP, Hirjik J, Iti L, et al. 1,25-Dihydroxyvitamin D3: in vivo and in vitro effects on human preleukemic and leukemic cells. Cancer Treat Rep 1985;69: 1399–407.
45. Bouillon R, Okamura WH, Norman AW. Structure-function relationships in the vitamin D endocrine system. Endocr Rev 1995;16:200–57.
46. Spina C, Tangpricha V, Yao M, et al. Colon cancer and solar ultraviolet B radiation and prevention and treatment of colon cancer in mice with vitamin D and its Gemini analogs. J Steroid Biochem Mol Biol 2005;97:111–20.
47. Spina CS, Tangpricha V, Uskokovic M, et al. Vitamin D and cancer. Anticancer Res 2006;26(4a):2515–24.
48. Woo TCS, Choo R, Jamieson M, et al. Pilot study: potential role of vitamin D (cholecalciferol) in patients with PSA relapse after definitive therapy. Nutr Cancer 2005;51(1):32–6.
49. Gross C, Stamey T, Hancock S, et al. Treatment of early recurrent prostate cancer with 1,25-di-hydroxyvitamin D_3 (calcitriol). J Urol 1998;159:2035–40.
50. Beer TM, Javle MM, Ryan CW, et al. Phase I study of weekly DN-101, a new formulation of calcitriol, in patients with cancer. Cancer Chemother Pharmacol 2007;59:581–7.
51. Chen TC, Holick MF. Vitamin D and prostate cancer prevention and treatment. Trends Endocrinol Metab 2003;14:423–30.
52. Zhao XY, Feldman D. The role of vitamin D in prostate cancer. Steroids 2001;66: 293–300.
53. Holick MF. Vitamin D and sunlight: strategies for cancer prevention and other health benefits. Clin J Am Soc Nephrol 2008;3:1548–54. doi:10.2215/CJN. 0135038.

54. Holick MF, Chen TC, Sauter ER. Vitamin D and skin physiology: a D-lightful story. J Bone Miner Res 2007;22(S2):V28–33.

55. Perez A, Chen TC, Turner A, et al. Efficacy and safety of topical calcitriol (1,25-dihydroxyvitamin D_3) for the treatment of psoriasis. Br J Dermatol 1996;134:238–46.

56. Kragballe K. Treatment of psoriasis by the topical application of the novel vitamin D_3 analogue MC 903. Arch Dermatol 1989;125:1647–52.

57. Holick MF. Clinical efficacy of 1,25-dihydroxyvitamin D_3 and its analogues in the treatment of psoriasis. Retinoids 1998;14:7–12.

58. Embry AF, Snowdon LR, Vieth R. Vitamin D and seasonal fluctuations of gadolinium-enhancing magnetic resonance imaging lesions in multiple sclerosis. Ann Neurol 2000;48:271–2.

59. Hernán MA, Olek MJ, Ascherio A. Geographic variation of MS incidence in two prospective studies of US women. Neurology 1999;51:1711–8.

60. Mohr SB, Garland CF, Gorham ED, et al. The association between ultraviolet B irradiance, vitamin D status and incidence rates of type 1 diabetes in 51 regions worldwide. Diabetologia 2008;51(8):1391–8.

61. Munger KL, Levin LI, Hollis BW, et al. Serum 25-hydroxyvitamin D levels and risk of multiple sclerosis. JAMA 2006;296:2832–8.

62. Munger KL, Zhang SM, O'Reilly E, et al. Vitamin D intake and incidence of multiple sclerosis. Neurology 2004;62(1):60–5.

63. Merlino LA, Curtis J, Mikuls TR, et al. Iowa Women's Health Study. Vitamin D intake is inversely associated with rheumatoid arthritis. Arthritis Rheum 2004; 50(1):72–7.

64. Hypponen E, Laara E, Jarvelin M-R, et al. Intake of vitamin D and risk of type 1 diabetes: a birth-cohort study. Lancet 2001;358:1500–3.

65. Camargo CA Jr, Rifas-Shiman SL, Litonjua AA, et al. Maternal intake of vitamin D during pregnancy and risk of recurrent wheeze in children at 3 y of age. Am J Clin Nutr 2007;85(3):788–95.

66. Black PN, Scragg R. Relationship between serum 25-hydroxyvitamin D and pulmonary function in the third national health and nutrition examination survey. Clin Investig 2005;128:3792–8.

67. Cantorna MT, Zhu Y, Froicu M, et al. Vitamin D status, 1,25-dihydroxyvitamin D_3, and the immune system. Am J Clin Nutr 2004;80(Suppl):1717S–20S.

68. Adorini L, Giarratana N, Penna G. Pharmacological induction of tolerogenic dendritic cells and regulatory T cells. Semin Immunol 2004;16:127–34.

69. Daniel C, Satory NA, Zahn N, et al. Immune modulatory treatment of trinitrobenzene sulfonic acid colitis with calcitriol is associated with a change of a T helper (Th) 1/Th17 to a Th2 and regulatory T cell profile. J Pharmacol Exp Ther 2008; 324:23–33.

70. Liu PT, Stenger S, Li H, et al. Toll-like receptor triggering of a vitamin D-mediated human antimicrobial response. Science 2006;3:1770–3.

71. White JH. Vitamin D signaling, infectious diseases, and regulation of innate immunity. Infect Immun 2008;76(9):3837–43.

72. Albert PJ, Proal AD, Marshall TG. Vitamin D: the alternative hypothesis. Autoimmun Rev 2009;8:639–44.

73. Cantorna MT, Hayes CE, DeLuca HF. 1,25-Dihydroxyvitamin D_3 reversibly blocks the progression of relapsing encephalomyelitis, a model of multiple sclerosis. Proc Natl Acad Sci 1996;93:7861–4.

74. Cantorna MT, Munsick C, Bemiss C, et al. 1,25-dihydroxycholecalciferol prevents and ameliorates symptoms of experimental murine inflammatory bowel disease. J Nutr 2000;130:2648–52.

75. Linday LA, Shindledecker RD, Dolitsky JN, et al. Plasma 25-hydroxyvitamin D levels in young children undergoing placement of tympanostomy tubes. Ann Otol Rhinol Laryngol 2008;117:740–4.
76. Ginde AA, Mansbach JM, Camargo CA. Association between serum 25-hydroxyvitamin D level and upper respiratory tract infection in the third national health and nutrition examination survey. Arch Intern Med 2009;169(4):384–90.
77. Cannell JJ, Vieth R, Umhau JC, et al. Epidemic influenza and vitamin D. Epidemiol Infect 2006;134(6):1129–40.
78. Aloia JF, Talwar SA, Pollack S, et al. A Randomized controlled trial of vitamin D_3 supplementation in African American women. Arch Intern Med 2005;165: 1618–23.
79. Adams JS, Hewison M. Hypercalcemia caused by granuloma-forming disorders. In: Favus MJ, editor. Primer on the metabolic bone diseases and disorders of mineral metabolism. 6th edition. Washington, DC: American Society for Bone and Mineral Research; 2006. p. 200–2.
80. Wang TJ, Pencina MJ, Booth SL, et al. Vitamin D deficiency and risk of cardiovascular disease. Circulation 2008;117(4):503–11.
81. Autier P, Gandini S. Vitamin D supplementation and total mortality: a meta-analysis of randomized controlled trials. Arch Intern Med 2007;167(16):1730–7.
82. Rostand SG. Ultraviolet light may contribute to geographic and racial blood pressure differences. Hypertension 1997;30(2 pt 1):150–6.
83. Krause R, Buhring M, Hopfenmuller W, et al. Ultraviolet B and blood pressure. Lancet 1998;352(9129):709–10.
84. Li Y, Kong J, Wei M, et al. 1,25-dihydroxyvitamin D_3 is a negative endocrine regulator of the renin-angiotensin system. J Clin Invest 2002;110(2):229–38.
85. Lee JH, O'Keefe JH, Bell D, et al. Vitamin D Deficiency: an important, common, and easily treatable cardiovascular risk factor. J Am Coll Cardiol 2008;52: 1949–56.
86. Zittermann A, Schleithoff SS, Tenderich G, et al. Low vitamin D status: a contributing factor in the pathogenesis of congestive heart failure? J Am Coll Cardiol 2003;41:105–12.
87. Oh J, Weng S, Felton SK, et al. 1,25$(OH)_2$ vitamin D inhibits foam cell formation and suppresses macrophage cholesterol uptake in patients with type 2 diabetes mellitus. Circulation 2009;120(8):687–712.
88. Holick MF. Vitamin D. The underappreciated D-lightful hormone that is important for skeletal and cellular health. Curr Opin Endocrinol Diabetes 2002;9: 87–98.
89. Chiu KC, Chu A, Go VLW, et al. Hypovitaminosis D is associated with insulin resistance and β cell dysfunction. Am J Clin Nutr 2004;79:820–5.
90. Pittas AG, Dawson-Hughes B, Li T, et al. Vitamin D and calcium intake in relation to type 2 diabetes in women. Diabetes Care 2006;29(3):650–6.
91. Scragg R, Sowers M, Bell C. Serum 25-hydroxyvitamin D, diabetes, and ethnicity in the third national health and nutrition examination survey. Diabetes Care 2004;27:2813–8.
92. Standing Committee on the Scientific Evaluation of Dietary Reference Intakes Food and Nutrition Board, Institute of medicine. Dietary reference intakes for calcium, phosphorus, magnesium, vitamin D and fluoride. Washington, DC: National Academy Press; 1999.
93. Jeans PC. Vitamin D. JAMA 1950;1243:177–81.
94. Grant WB, Holick MF. Benefits and requirements of vitamin D for optimal health: a review. Altern Med Rev 2005;10:94–111.

95. Holick MF, Biancuzzo RM, Chen TC, et al. Vitamin D_2 is as effective as vitamin D_3 in maintaining circulating concentrations of 25-hydroxyvitamin D. J Clin Endocrinol Metab 2008;93(3):677–81.

96. Heaney RP, Davies KM, Chen TC, et al. Human serum 25-hydroxycholecalciferol response to extended oral dosing with cholecalciferol. Am J Clin Nutr 2003;77: 204–10.

97. Holick MF, Chen TC. Vitamin D deficiency: a worldwide problem with health consequences. Am J Clin Nutr 2008;87(4):1080S–6S.

98. Wagner CL, Greeer FR, Section on Breastfeeeding and Committee on Nutrition. Prevention of rickets and vitamin D deficiency in infants, children, and adolescents. Pediatrics 2008;122:1142–52.

99. El-Hajj Fuleihan G, Nabulsi M, Tamim H, et al. Effect of vitamin D replacement on musculoskeletal parameters in school children: a randomized controlled trial. J Clin Endocrinol Metab 2006;91:405–12.

100. Pietras SM, Obayan BK, Cai MH, et al. Vitamin D_2 treatment for vitamin D deficiency and insufficiency for up to 6 years. Arch Intern Med 2009;169:1806–8.

The Role of Vitamin D in Cancer Prevention and Treatment

Aruna V. Krishnan, PhD[a], Donald L. Trump, MD[b],
Candace S. Johnson, PhD[c], David Feldman, MD[a],*

KEYWORDS

- Vitamin D • Gene regulation • Antiproliferation
- Antiinflammation • Cancer • Prevention • Treatment

Calcitriol (1,25-dihydroxyvitamin D_3), the biologically most active form of vitamin D, maintains calcium homeostasis through its actions in intestine, bone, kidneys, and the parathyroid glands.[1] The hormone exerts its effects through the vitamin D receptor (VDR), a member of the nuclear receptor superfamily.[1] VDR is present not only in cells and tissues involved in calcium regulation but also a wide variety of other cells including malignant cells. In recent years it has been recognized that calcitriol exerts antiproliferative and prodifferentiating effects in many malignant cells, and retards the development and growth of tumors in animal models raising the possibility of its use as an anticancer agent.[2]

EPIDEMIOLOGY

Epidemiologic studies have noted lower incidence and mortality rates from several cancers in regions with greater solar ultraviolet (UV)-B exposure.[3–5] The potential benefit from sunlight is attributed to vitamin D, because UV light is essential for the cutaneous synthesis of vitamin D.[1] The sunlight hypothesis (assuming that sunlight is a surrogate for vitamin D levels in circulation) has been proposed to determine the risk for several cancers[6,7] including colorectal cancer (CRC)[3] prostate cancer (PCa),[4,5] and breast cancer (BCa).[8] An inverse association between cancer risk and

This work was supported by NCI grant CA130991 and Komen Grant KG080101 (Feldman) and NCI grants CA067267, CA085142, CA095045, and P30 CA016056-32, as well as DOD grant PC040238 (Trump and Johnson).

[a] Department of Medicine, Division of Endocrinology, Stanford University School of Medicine, 300 Pasteur Drive, Room S-025, Stanford, CA 94305-5103, USA
[b] Department of Medicine, Roswell Park Cancer Institute, Elm and Carlton Streets, Buffalo, NY 14263, USA
[c] Department of Pharmacology & Therapeutics, Roswell Park Cancer Institute, Elm and Carlton Streets, Buffalo, NY 14263, USA
* Corresponding author.
E-mail address: dfeldman@stanford.edu

circulating levels of 25-hydroxyvitamin D (25(OH)D, the circulating precursor to calcitriol), which reflect sun exposure and dietary vitamin D intake, has also been reported.[7] The evidence is strongest for CRC; circulating 25(OH)D levels and vitamin D intake are inversely associated with colorectal adenoma incidence and recurrence.[9,10] In addition, higher prediagnosis plasma 25(OH)D levels were associated with a significant improvement in overall survival in CRC patients.[11] A recent reanalysis of data from the Women's Health Initiative (WHI) randomized trial concluded that concurrent estrogen therapy modified the effect of calcium and vitamin D supplementation on CRC risk and in the women assigned to placebo arms of the estrogen trials, the supplementation was beneficial.[12] The evidence is somewhat weaker for PCa, with some studies suggesting an inverse correlation between serum 25(OH)D levels and PCa risk[13,14] although others do not support such a correlation.[15,16] In general, a serum 25(OH)D level exceeding 20 ng/mL was associated with a 30% to 50% reduction in the risk of developing CRC and PCa,[17,18] and a level of approximately 52 ng/mL was associated with a reduction by 50% in the incidence of BCa.[8] Higher dietary intake of vitamin D has been associated with a lower incidence of pancreatic cancer.[19]

MECHANISMS OF THE ANTICANCER EFFECTS OF CALCITRIOL

In addition to the epidemiologic evidence described earlier, data from in vitro studies in cultured malignant cells reveal that calcitriol exerts antiproliferative and prodifferentiating effects; in vivo studies in animal models of cancer demonstrate that calcitriol retards tumor growth.[2,20–31] Several important mechanisms have been implicated in the anticancer effects of calcitriol. The molecular mediators of these calcitriol actions are currently being intensively investigated and characterized.[2]

Growth Arrest and Differentiation

Calcitriol inhibits the proliferation of many malignant cells by inducing cell cycle arrest and the accumulation of cells in the G_0/G_1 phase of the cell cycle.[20,31,32] In PCa cells calcitriol causes G_1/G_0 arrest[26,30,33] in a p53-dependent manner[30] by increasing the expression of the cyclin-dependent kinase inhibitors p21[Waf/Cip1] and p27[Kip1],[32–34] decreasing cyclin-dependent kinase 2 (CDK2) activity,[33] and causing the hypophosphorylation of the retinoblastoma protein (pRb).[35] Calcitriol also enhances the expression of p73, a p53 homolog, which has been shown to be associated with apoptosis induction in several human and murine tumor systems. Suppression of p73 abrogates calcitriol-induced apoptosis and reduces the ability of calcitriol to augment the cytotoxic effects of agents such as gemcitabine and cisplatin in a squamous cell carcinoma (SCC) model.[36] Calcitriol also increases the expression of CDK inhibitors in other cancer cells.[2,20,31] It has been shown that calcitriol controls cell growth in part by modulating the expression and activity of key growth factors in cancer cells.[2,20,26,27,30,31] For example, in PCa cells calcitriol up-regulates the expression of insulinlike growth factor binding protein-3 (IGFBP-3),[37,38] which functions to inhibit cell proliferation in part by increasing the expression of p21[Waf/Cip1].[37]

In many neoplastic cells, calcitriol also induces differentiation resulting in the generation of cells that acquire a more mature and less malignant phenotype. The mechanisms of the prodifferentiation effects of calcitriol in various cancer cells are specific to the cell type and cell context and include, for example, the regulation of signaling pathways involving β-catenin, Jun-N-terminal kinase (JNK), phosphatidyl inositol 3-kinase, nuclear factor κB (NFκB) as well as the regulation of the activity of several transcription factors such as the activator protein-1 (AP-1) complex and CCAAT/enhancer-binding protein (C/EBP).[2,39]

Apoptosis

Calcitriol induces apoptosis in several cancer cells, although this effect is not uniformly seen in all malignant cells. In PCa and BCa cells, calcitriol activates the intrinsic pathway of apoptosis causing the disruption of mitochondrial function, cytochrome release and production of reactive oxygen species.[31,40–42] These effects are related to the repression of the expression of antiapoptotic proteins such as Bcl$_2$[31,40] and enhancement of the expression of proapoptotic proteins such as Bax and Bad.[42] In some cells calcitriol also directly activates caspases to induce apoptosis.[42,43] In addition, calcitriol analogues have been shown to enhance cancer cell death in response to radiation and chemotherapeutic drugs.[44,45]

Inhibition of Invasion and Metastasis

Calcitriol reduces the invasive and metastatic potential of many malignant cells as demonstrated in murine models of prostate and lung cancer.[46,47] The mechanisms underlying this effect include the inhibition of angiogenesis (as discussed later) and the regulation of the expression of key molecules involved in invasion and metastasis such as the components of the plasminogen activator (PA) system and matrix metalloproteinases (MMPs),[48] decreasing the expression of tenascin-C, an extracellular matrix protein that promotes growth, invasion, and angiogenesis,[49] down-regulation of the expression of α6 and β4 integrins,[50] and increase in the expression of E-cadherin, a tumor suppressor gene whose expression is inversely correlated to metastatic potential.[32] Calcitriol-mediated suppression of MMP-9 activity and increase in tissue inhibitor of metalloproteinase-1 (TIMP-1) also decrease the invasive potential of PCa cells.[51]

Antiinflammatory Effects

Chronic inflammation, triggered by a variety of stimuli such as injury, infection, carcinogens, autoimmune disease, the development of tumors, hormonal factors, and so forth, has been recognized as a risk factor for cancer development.[52–54] Cancer-related inflammation is characterized by the presence of inflammatory cells at the tumor sites and over-expression of inflammatory mediators such as cytokines, chemokines, prostaglandins (PGs) and reactive oxygen and nitrogen species in tumor tissue.[52–56] Many of these proinflammatory mediators activate angiogenic switches usually under the control of vascular endothelial growth factor (VEGF) and thereby promote tumor progression, metastasis, and invasion.[57,58] Epidemiologic studies show a decrease in the risk of developing several cancers associated with the intake of antioxidants and nonsteroidal antiinflammatory drugs (NSAIDs).[58–60] Recent research suggests that calcitriol exhibits antiinflammatory actions that may contribute to its beneficial effects in several cancers in addition to the other antiproliferative actions discussed earlier. We used cDNA microarrays to uncover the molecular pathways that mediate the anticancer effects of calcitriol in PCa cells.[61,62] The results show that calcitriol regulation of gene expression leads to the inhibition of the synthesis and biologic actions of prostaglandins (PGs), stress-activated kinase signaling, and production of proinflammatory cytokines. Calcitriol also suppresses the activation and signaling of NFκB, a transcription factor that regulates the expression of genes involved in inflammatory and immune responses and cellular proliferation[63] and believed to play a key role in the process leading from inflammation to carcinogenesis.[64]

Regulation of prostaglandin metabolism and signaling

In multiple PCa cell lines as well as primary prostatic epithelial cells established from prostatectomy samples, calcitriol decreases the mRNA and protein levels of cyclooxygenase-2 (COX-2), the enzyme responsible for PG synthesis, and increases the expression of 15-hyroxyprostaglandin dehydrogenase(15-PGDH), the enzyme that initiates PG catabolism.[65] As a result calcitriol decreases the levels of biologically active PGs in these cells. In addition, calcitriol decreases the expression of EP and FP PG receptors and thereby attenuates PG-mediated functional responses including stimulation of cell growth.[65] Thus, reduction in the levels of biologically active PGs and inhibition of PG signaling through their receptors by calcitriol results in suppression of the proliferative and angiogenic stimuli provided by PGs. Combinations of calcitriol with NSAIDs cause a synergistic enhancement of the inhibition of PCa cell proliferation, suggesting that this drug combination might have clinical usefulness in PCa therapy.[65,66]

Induction of mitogen-activated protein kinase phosphatase-5 (MKP5) and inhibition of stress-activated kinase signaling

cDNA microarray analysis in normal human prostate epithelial cells[62] revealed a novel calcitriol-responsive gene, MKP5, also known as DUSP10, a member of the dual specificity MKP family of enzymes that dephosphorylate, and thereby inactivate, mitogen-activated protein kinases (MAPKs). MKP5 specifically dephosphorylates p38 MAPK and the stress-activated protein kinase JNK, leading to their inactivation. Calcitriol increases MKP5 transcription by the activation of VDR and its binding to a vitamin D response element (VDRE) in the MKP5 promoter.[67] The calcitriol-mediated increase in MKP5 causes the dephosphorylation and inactivation of the p38 stress-induced kinase, resulting in a decrease in the production of proinflammatory cytokines that sustain and amplify the inflammatory response, such as interleukin-6 (IL-6). IL-6 stimulates PCa growth and progression[68] and IL-6 synthesized in periprostatic adipose tissue has recently been shown to modulate PCa aggressiveness.[69] Calcitriol up-regulation of MKP5 is seen in primary cells derived from normal prostate epithelium and primary localized adenocarcinoma but not in the established cell lines derived from metastatic PCa,[67] suggesting that the loss of MKP5 might occur during PCa progression, as a result of a selective pressure to eliminate the tumor suppressor activity of MKP5 and/or calcitriol.

Inhibition of NFκB activation and signaling

NFκB comprises a family of inducible transcription factors ubiquitously present in cells that are important regulators of innate immune responses and inflammation.[70] In the basal state, most NFκB dimers are bound to specific inhibitory proteins called IκB and proinflammatory signals activate NFκB mainly through IκB kinase (IKK)-dependent phosphorylation and degradation of the inhibitory IκB proteins.[64] Free NFκB then translocates to the nucleus and activates the transcription of proinflammatory cytokines, chemokines, and antiapoptotic factors.[71] In contrast to normal cells, many malignant cells have increased levels of active NFκB.[72,73] Calcitriol directly modulates basal and cytokine-induced NFκB activity in many cells including human lymphocytes,[74] fibroblasts,[75] and peripheral blood monocytes.[76] A reduction in the levels of the NFκB inhibitory protein IκB has been reported in mice lacking the VDR.[77] Addition of a VDR antagonist to colon cancer cells up-regulates NFκB activity by decreasing the levels of IκB, suggesting that VDR ligands suppress NFκB activation.[78] Calcitriol decreases the production of the angiogenic and proinflammatory cytokine IL-8 in immortalized normal human prostate epithelial cell lines and established PCa cell lines by inhibiting the nuclear translocation of the NFκB subunit p65 and subsequent transcriptional stimulation of the NFκB downstream target IL-8.[79] Thus calcitriol could delay the progression of PCa by suppressing the expression of angiogenic and proinflammatory factors such as VEGF and IL-8. In addition, calcitriol indirectly inhibits NFκB signaling by up-regulating the expression of IGFBP-3, which has been shown to interfere with NFκB signaling in PCa cells.[80] NFκB also provides an adaptive response to PCa cells against cytotoxicity induced by redox active therapeutic agents and is implicated in radiation resistance of cancers.[81,82] Calcitriol significantly enhances the sensitivity of PCa cells to ionizing radiation by selectively suppressing radiation-mediated RelB activation.[83] Thus calcitriol may serve as an effective agent for sensitizing PCa cells to radiation therapy via suppression of the NFκB pathway. There is also considerable evidence that calcitriol potentiates the antitumor activity of a wide variety of cytotoxic chemotherapy agents (described later). As noted earlier, the induction of p73 by calcitriol seems to contribute to the synergistic activity of calcitriol and platinum analogues and some antimetabolites.[36]

The Role of Antiinflammatory Effects of Calcitriol in Cancer Prevention and Treatment

As discussed earlier current perspectives in cancer biology suggest that inflammation plays a role in the development of cancer.[52–54] De Marzo and colleagues[84] have proposed that precursor lesions called proliferative inflammatory atrophy (PIA) in the prostate, which are associated with acute or chronic inflammation, are the precursors of prostate intraepithelial neoplasia (PIN) and PCa. The epithelial cells in PIA lesions exhibit many molecular signs of stress including increased expression of COX-2.[85,86] Similarly, inflammatory bowel disease is associated with the development of CRC.[87–89] Based on the evidence demonstrating antiinflammatory effects of calcitriol, we postulate that calcitriol may play a role in delaying or preventing cancer development and/or progression. PCa generally progresses very slowly, likely over decades, before symptoms become obvious and the diagnosis is made.[90] The observed latency in PCa provides a long window of opportunity for intervention by chemopreventive agents. Dietary supplementation of COX-2 selective NSAIDs such as celecoxib has been shown to suppress prostate carcinogenesis in the Transgenic Adenocarcinoma of the Mouse Prostate (TRAMP) model of PCa.[91] The inhibitory effects of calcitriol on COX-2 expression and the PG pathway, production of proinflammatory cytokines, NFκB signaling, and tumor angiogenesis suggest that calcitriol has the potential to be useful as a chemopreventive agent in malignancies such as PCa. Foster and colleagues have shown that administration of high-dose calcitriol (20 μg/kg), intermittently 3 days per week for up to 14 to 30 weeks, suppresses prostate tumor development in TRAMP mice.[92,93] The efficacy of calcitriol as a chemopreventive agent has also been examined in Nkx3.1;Pten mutant mice, which recapitulate stages of prostate carcinogenesis from PIN lesions to adenocarcinoma.[94] The data reveal that calcitriol significantly reduces the progression of PIN from a lower to a higher grade. Calcitriol is more effective when administered before, rather than after, the initial occurrence of PIN. These animal studies as well as in vitro observations suggest that clinical trials in PCa patients with PIN or early disease evaluating calcitriol and its analogues as agents that prevent and/or delay progression, are warranted.

Inhibition of Angiogenesis

Angiogenesis is the process of formation of new blood vessels from existing vasculature and is a crucial step in the continued growth, progression, and metastasis of tumors.[95] VEGF is the most potent stimulator of angiogenesis. PGs are also important proangiogenic factors. The initiation of angiogenesis is controlled by local hypoxia, which induces the synthesis of proangiogenic factors that activate signaling pathways leading to the structural reorganization of endothelial cells favoring new capillary formation.[96] Stimulation of angiogenesis in response to hypoxia is mediated by hypoxia-inducible factor 1 (HIF-1), which directly increases the expression of several proangiogenic factors including VEGF.[97,98] Early studies indicate that calcitriol is a potent inhibitor of tumor cell–induced angiogenesis in experimental models.[99] Calcitriol inhibits VEGF-induced endothelial cell tube formation in vitro and decreases tumor vascularization in vivo in mice bearing xenografts of BCa cells over-expressing VEGF.[100] Calcitriol and its analogues also directly inhibit the proliferation of endothelial cells[101–103] leading to the inhibition of angiogenesis.

At the molecular level, calcitriol may exert its antiangiogenic effects through a direct antiproliferative action on endothelial cells in the tumor microenvironment and/or by regulating the expression of key factors that control angiogenesis. Calcitriol reduces VEGF expression in PCa cells through transcriptional repression of HIF-1.[101] Calcitriol also suppresses the expression of the proangiogenic factor IL-8 in an NFκB-dependent manner.[79] Chung and colleagues[103] established TRAMP-2 tumors in wild-type mice and VDR knockout mice and found enlarged vessels and increased vessel volume in TRAMP tumors in the VDR knockout mice, suggesting an inhibitory role for VDR and calcitriol in tumor angiogenesis. Their study further showed increased expression of proangiogenic factors such as HIF-1α, VEGF, angiopoietin-1 and platelet-derived growth factor (PDGF) in the tumors in the VDR knockout mice.[103] Another important mechanism by which COX-2 promotes tumor progression is through the stimulation of angiogenesis. The proangiogenic effect of COX-2–generated PGE_2 might be a result of its action to increase HIF-1α protein synthesis in cancer cells.[104] Suppression of COX-2 expression by calcitriol therefore provides an important indirect mechanism by which calcitriol inhibits angiogenesis, in addition to its direct suppressive effects on proangiogenic factors such as HIF-1 and VEGF.

ANTICANCER EFFECTS OF CALCITRIOL IN ANIMAL MODELS

Considerable data indicate antitumor effects of vitamin D compounds in in vivo models and calcitriol and calcitriol analogues also potentiate the antitumor actions of many more traditional anticancer agents. In model systems of murine SCC[105] and human carcinomas arising in the prostate,[46] lung,[47] ovary,[106] breast,[107,108] bladder,[109] pancreas,[110] as well as neuroblastoma,[111] calcitriol or calcitriol analogues have substantial anticancer effects. Significant inhibition of metastasis is observed in murine models of prostate and lung cancer treated with calcitriol; these effects may be based, at least in part, on antiangiogenic effects.[46,47] In tumor-derived endothelial cells (TDECs), calcitriol induces apoptosis and cell cycle arrest; however, these effects are not seen in endothelial cells isolated from normal tissues or from Matrigel.[103,112] Recently, Chung and colleagues[113] reported that tumor-derived endothelial cells may be more sensitive to calcitriol as a result of novel epigenetic silencing of CYP24A1. Because Cyp24 (24-hydroxylase) initiates the degradation of calcitriol,[1] inhibition of this enzyme has been shown to enhance calcitriol actions and tumors expressing high levels of the enzyme are resistant to calcitriol action.[114–116] Direct effects of calcitriol on endothelial cells may play a primary role in the calcitriol-mediated antitumor activity that is observed in animal tumor models. There are no in vitro data to suggest that particular histotypes of cancer are more, or less, responsive to calcitriol-mediated antitumor effects except in the case of cells that have lost their VDR[31] or over-express CYP24.[114–116]

In Vivo Animal Studies of Calcitriol in Combination Regimens

In vivo analyses in mouse tumor models indicate that calcitriol acts synergistically with a wide range of chemotherapeutic agents. Calcitriol potentiates the anticancer activity of platinum analogues,[117,118] taxanes,[119] and DNA-intercalating agents.[36] Optimal potentiation is seen when calcitriol is administered before or simultaneously with chemotherapy treatment; administration of calcitriol after the cytotoxic agent does not provide potentiation.[119] In SCC and PC-3 (PCa) xenografts in immunodeficient mice, pretreatment with calcitriol or calcitriol analogues followed by paclitaxel results in enhanced antitumor effects.[119,120] In vivo studies also indicate that the antitumor effects of calcitriol can be potentiated by agents that inhibit calcitriol metabolism. Azole antagonists of the primary catabolic enzyme (CYP24A1) responsible for vitamin D breakdown enhance the antitumor effects of calcitriol in vitro and in vivo.[114,116,121] Ketoconazole is the most readily available of such agents and this drug has significant utility in the treatment of men with prostate cancer in whom disease progression has occurred despite androgen deprivation (so-called androgen-independent or castra-tion-resistant PCa). The activity of ketoconazole in tumor cells (prostate and nonpros-tate) that are apparently unresponsive to androgens, supports the hypothesis that there are extra-androgenic mechanisms underlying ketoconazole activity.[116,122] There are more specific inhibitors of CYP24 than azoles and secosteroid vitamin D analogues. These agents have antitumor activity in in vitro and in vivo models and potentiate the antitumor activity of calcitriol.[123,124]

CLINICAL STUDIES
Single-Agent Calcitriol Trials: Phase I Studies and Toxicity

Most anticancer clinical trials of vitamin D analogues have been conducted with calci-triol because it is readily available as an injectable (Calcijex, Abbott Pharmaceuticals, Abbott Park, IL, USA) or oral (Rocaltrol, Hoffman-Roche Laboratories Inc, Nutley, NJ, USA) formulation. As described earlier, preclinical studies indicate that calcitriol has substantial antitumor activity when used in high doses. Most discussions of the role of vitamin D in cancer therapy express the concern that high-dose calcitriol is too toxic to be administered to patients with cancer. There are now many clinical studies that clearly establish that calcitriol can be safely administered in very high doses if an intermittent treatment schedule is used. Administration of oral calcitriol on a daily schedule (1.5–2.5 µg/d, weekly dose intensity ~10.5–17.5 µg/wk) is associ-ated with a 20% to 30% frequency of hypercalcemia in men with PCa and in postmen-opausal women.[125–128] However, in in vivo settings demonstrating calcitriol efficacy, high-dose intermittent administration schedules are used (see later).

Calcitriol administered by mouth daily for 3 days every week (28 µg daily for 3 days) + dexamethasone (4 mg daily for 4 days) weekly is very safe and well tolerated in men with advanced PCa.[120] We have conducted studies of escalating doses of calcitriol (QDX3 weekly) + paclitaxel (80 mg/kg weekly for 4 weeks), as well as calcitriol (QD X3 monthly) + carboplatin (320 mg/sqm, monthly). In these 2 studies, doses of calci-triol of 38 µg every day for 3 days weekly and 28 µg every day for 3 days monthly were safely administered together with paclitaxel and carboplatin, respectively.[129] Pharma-cokinetic studies in these trials demonstrated that calcitriol as Rocaltrol was unsuit-able for high-dose administration because of inconvenience (38 µg requires the administration of 76 caplets) and unsuitable pharmacokinetics.[130] Administration of high doses of this formulation does not lead to a proportional increase in serum levels or systemic exposure. Similar findings were noted by Beer and colleagues,[131] who studied a once weekly oral regimen. Novacea Pharmaceuticals undertook the devel-opment of a more suitable formulation. Their drug, DN-101, did have a linear relation-ship between dose and exposure up to doses of 165 µg.[132,133] Fakih and colleagues[134] studied intravenous calcitriol (Calcijex, Roche Pharmaceutical Corpora-tion) weekly + gefitinib and reported that very high doses of calcitriol can be administered safely. The dose-limiting toxicity of weekly intravenous calcitriol + gefitinib was grade 3 hypercalcemia at a dose of 98 µg/wk. The phase II dose of this regimen is 77 µg weekly alone and 98 µg/kg weekly when calcitriol is combined with high-dose dexamethasone.[134,135] The systemic exposure of calcitriol following 98 µg is approximately 30 ng/h/24 h which is in the range of exposure we have reported in murine models in which calcitriol has clear-cut antitumor activity.[136]

Beer and colleagues[131] have studied high-dose oral calcitriol (as Rocaltrol) and concluded that 0.5 µg/kg, weekly is very safe. Studies with DN-101 demonstrated that 45 µg weekly was safe and well tolerated and that 165 µg given on week 1, followed by 45 µg weekly produced no toxicity.[133] A linear relationship between dose of DN-101 administered and area under the curve (AUC) was maintained up to 165 µg. Studies using an intermittent schedule of administration (weekly or every day for 3 days weekly) have encountered dose-limiting hypercalcemia only at doses ~100 µg following intravenous administration; transient increase in serum calcium (11–13 mg/dL) does occur 1 to 3 days after completion of a single or daily for 3 days schedule. However, only at doses achieving AUC more than ~30 ng/h/ml has dose-limiting hypercalcemia been encountered. Hypercalciuria is universal following administration of high-dose calcitriol. Dietary calcium restriction is very difficult for patients to maintain and there is little evidence that it reduces hypercalciuria. There has been no deterioration of renal function in patients receiving high-dose intermittent calcitriol for more than 12 months. Radiographic monitoring for urinary tract stones (ultrasound or computed tomography) in our studies suggests that newly discovered urinary tract stones may occur in 1% to 3% of patients.[129,130]

Trials of single-agent calcitriol and other vitamin D analogues in PCa have resulted in a few partial responses and prostate-specific antigen (PSA) responses have been seen. However, important clinical antitumor effects are quite infrequent. Very few studies of calcitriol or any other analogue have been conducted using doses approaching the maximum tolerated dose (MTD). In view of the many unresolved questions regarding the MTD, optimal biologic dose, optimal schedule, and pharmaceutical concerns about the available vitamin D formulations, it is not surprising that thus far limited antitumor activity has been seen in phase I and II trials.

Other Calcitriol Analogues

There is only limited information regarding the use of other vitamin D analogues as cancer therapy. EB1089 (seocalcitol),[137–139] 1-alpha-vitamin D_2,[140–142] inecalcitol (19-nor-, 14-epi-, 23-yne, 1,25-dihydroxyvitamin D_3),[143] and paricalcitol (19-nor, 1-alpha, 25-dihdroxyvitamin D_2, Zemplar)[144] have each been studied, but always at relatively low doses and on schedules that would be predicted to make high-dose therapy impossible. No consistent and convincing evidence of antitumor activity has been seen in any of these studies.

Combination studies: phase I studies and toxicity

Several phase I clinical trials of calcitriol in combination with cytotoxic agents have been completed. Interpretation of the results of phase I and II clinical trials are hampered by the same challenges that limit our knowledge with regard to the interpretation of studies of calcitriol used as a single agent: lack of clear delineation of an optimal biologic dose and limited data on the MTD of calcitriol. Beer and colleagues[145] studied the combination of calcitriol + docetaxel with the intent of applying these studies to the treatment of men with advanced PCa progressing despite castration. These investigators used the commercially available oral formulation of calcitriol (Rocaltrol). They conducted a phase II trial of weekly doce-taxel (36 mg/m², weekly for 6 weeks) on day 2 + their phase II dose of calcitriol (0.5 µg/kg orally weekly) on day 1. No unusual toxicity was seen in this trial and PSA response (>50% reduction on 2 successive measurements maintained for >28 days) was seen in 30 of 37 patients (81%; 95% confidence interval [CI], 68%–94%). Pharmacokinetics of calcitriol and docetaxel were indistinguishable from those expected from single-agent therapy. These results were encouraging and provided the rationale for Novacea Company to develop a new formulation of calcitriol (DN-101) and to undertake 2 studies: first, a large randomized, double-blind trial of docetaxel ± DN-101 (ASCENT I = AIPC Study of Calcitriol Enhancing Taxotere)[146]; the end point of this trial was PSA response. ASCENT I enrolled 250 patients and the PSA response rates were 63% (DN-101) and 52% (placebo), P = .07. Patients in the DN-101 group had a hazard ratio for death of 0.67 (P = .04) in a secondary multivariate analysis that included baseline hemo-globin and performance status.[146] Median survival was not reached for the DN-101 arm and was estimated to be 24.5 months, compared with 16.4 months for placebo. Clinically important adverse events occurred in 58% of DN-101 patients and in 70% of placebo-treated patients (P = .07). Neither significant hypercal-cemia nor renal dysfunction was seen. The addition of weekly DN-101 did not increase the toxicity of weekly docetaxel and might even have decreased it.[146] These preliminary results showing increased survival in the DN-101 arm were very encouraging and led to ASCENT II, a 900-patient randomized, double-blinded, placebo-controlled phase III trial, in which survival was the end point. The goal of ASCENT II was to define any survival difference associated with cal-citriol treatment in combination with docetaxel with the goal of achieving approval from the US Food and Drug Administration (FDA) of this combination. Unfortu-nately, in designing ASCENT II, 2 issues were unaddressed that ultimately proved to be problematic in the interpretation of ASCENT II:

1. ASCENT II was designed as a randomized study comparing docetaxel (every 3 weeks, 75 mg/m², the FDA-approved regimen) + prednisone (daily, 10 mg) + placebo versus docetaxel (weekly, 36 mg/m², a regimen that at the time ASCENT II was initiated had been shown to be inferior to the weekly every 3 weeks docetaxel regimen) + prednisone (daily, 10 mg) + calcitriol (DN-101, 0.5 µg/kg 1 day before docetaxel). This asymmetric design violates 1 of the primary tenets of randomized trial design; that is, to eliminate all variables between standard and experimental arms, except 1.
2. There are no data that define either the optimal or maximal dose of oral calcitriol. The 0.5 µg/kg weekly oral dose was a dose of convenience. A dose of approxi-mately 77 µg (>1 µg/kg in a 70-kg patient) of calcitriol intravenously is required to achieve the AUC that is associated with antitumor effects in mice.

With these concerns in mind, perhaps it is not surprising that ASCENT II was halted in November 2007 when the data safety monitoring committee noted that the death rate in the investigational arm (weekly docetaxel + calcitriol + prednisone) was greater than in the standard therapy arm (every 3 weeks docetaxel + placebo + prednisone). Subsequent analysis of this trial to June 2008 indicated that all deaths in this study were caused by progressive prostate cancer and there was no excess of toxicity related to administration of calcitriol (John Curd, MD, personal communication, 2008). The result of ASCENT II is a discouraging finding in the quest to define a role for high-dose calcitriol in cancer therapy. However, there are several unaddressed questions in the development of calcitriol as a cancer therapy. The negative findings in ASCENT II may be related to inappropriate trial design and drug dose rather than failure of the overall concept.

There are considerable data indicating the synergistic potential of calcitriol and a variety of antitumor agents. Clinical trials of calcitriol and paclitaxel, docetaxel, carboplatin, and gefitinib have been conducted; no unusual toxicity was seen and antitumor responses were documented.[134,147,148] However, the drug formulations used did not allow dose escalation to doses near the MTD, except in the trial with gefitinib.

Although there are preclinical data that would support the study of combinations of calcitriol and several other antitumor agents including antimetabolites (methotrexate, cytosine arabinoside, gemcitabine), anthracyclines and anthracenediones, and topoisomerase inhibitors, no clinical trials of such combinations have been conducted.

SUMMARY

Considerable data described in the first part of this review suggest that there is a role for vitamin D in cancer therapy and prevention. Although the preclinical data are persuasive and the epidemiologic data intriguing, no well-designed clinical trial of optimal administration of vitamin D as a cancer therapy has ever been conducted. Had there been the opportunity and insight to develop calcitriol as any other cancer drug, the following studies would have been completed:

1. Definition of the MTD
2. Definition of a phase II dose, as a single agent and in combination with cytotoxic agents
3. Studies to define a biologically optimal dose
4. Phase II (probably randomized phase II) studies of calcitriol alone and chemotherapy ± calcitriol
5. Then, randomized phase III trials would be conducted and designed such that the only variable was the administration of calcitriol.

Prerequisites 1 to 5 have not been completed for calcitriol. Preclinical data provide considerable rationale for continued development of vitamin D analogue-based cancer therapies. However, design of future studies should be informed by good clinical trials design principles and the mistakes of the past not repeated. Such studies may finally provide compelling data to prove whether or not there is a role for vitamin D analogues in cancer therapy.

REFERENCES

1. Feldman D, Malloy PJ, Krishnan AV, et al. Vitamin D: biology, action and clinical implications. In: Marcus R, Feldman D, Nelson DA, et al, editors. 3rd edition, Osteoporosis, vol. 1. San Diego (CA): Academic Press; 2007. p. 317–82.
2. Deeb KK, Trump DL, Johnson CS. Vitamin D signalling pathways in cancer: potential for anticancer therapeutics. Nat Rev Cancer 2007;7(9):684–700.
3. Garland CF, Garland FC. Do sunlight and vitamin D reduce the likelihood of colon cancer? Int J Epidemiol 1980;9(3):227–31.
4. Hanchette CL, Schwartz GG. Geographic patterns of prostate cancer mortality. Evidence for a protective effect of ultraviolet radiation. Cancer 1992;70(12): 2861–9.
5. Schwartz GG, Hulka BS. Is vitamin D deficiency a risk factor for prostate cancer? (Hypothesis). Anticancer Res 1990;10(5A):1307–11.

6. Garland CF, Garland FC, Gorham ED, et al. The role of vitamin D in cancer prevention. Am J Public Health 2006;96(2):252–61.
7. Giovannucci E. Vitamin D status and cancer incidence and mortality. Adv Exp Med Biol 2008;624:31–42.
8. Garland CF, Gorham ED, Mohr SB, et al. Vitamin D and prevention of breast cancer: pooled analysis. J Steroid Biochem Mol Biol 2007;103(3–5):708–11.
9. Wei MY, Garland CF, Gorham ED, et al. Vitamin D and prevention of colorectal adenoma: a meta-analysis. Cancer Epidemiol Biomarkers Prev 2008;17(11): 2958–69.
10. Yin L, Grandi N, Raum E, et al. Meta-analysis: longitudinal studies of serum vitamin D and colorectal cancer risk. Aliment Pharmacol Ther 2009;30(2): 113–25.
11. Ng K, Meyerhardt JA, Wu K, et al. Circulating 25-hydroxyvitamin D levels and survival in patients with colorectal cancer. J Clin Oncol 2008;26(18):2984–91.
12. Ding EL, Mehta S, Fawzi WW, et al. Interaction of estrogen therapy with calcium and vitamin D supplementation on colorectal cancer risk: reanalysis of Women's Health Initiative randomized trial. Int J Cancer 2008;122(8):1690–4.
13. Corder EH, Friedman GD, Vogelman JH, et al. Seasonal variation in vitamin D, vitamin D-binding protein, and dehydroepiandrosterone: risk of prostate cancer in black and white men. Cancer Epidemiol Biomarkers Prev 1995; 4(6):655–9.
14. Corder EH, Guess HA, Hulka BS, et al. Vitamin D and prostate cancer: a pre-diagnostic study with stored sera. Cancer Epidemiol Biomarkers Prev 1993; 2(5):467–72.
15. Ahn J, Peters U, Albanes D, et al. Serum vitamin D concentration and prostate cancer risk: a nested case-control study. J Natl Cancer Inst 2008;100(11): 796–804.
16. Platz EA, Leitzmann MF, Hollis BW, et al. Plasma 1,25-dihydroxy- and 25-hydroxyvitamin D and subsequent risk of prostate cancer. Cancer Causes Control 2004;15(3):255–65.
17. Ahonen MH, Tenkanen L, Teppo L, et al. Prostate cancer risk and prediagnostic serum 25-hydroxyvitamin D levels (Finland). Cancer Causes Control 2000;11(9): 847–52.
18. Garland CF, Comstock GW, Garland FC, et al. Serum 25-hydroxyvitamin D and colon cancer: eight-year prospective study. Lancet 1989;2(8673):1176–8.
19. Skinner HG, Michaud DS, Giovannucci E, et al. Vitamin D intake and the risk for pancreatic cancer in two cohort studies. Cancer Epidemiol Biomarkers Prev 2006;15(9):1688–95.
20. Chiang KC, Chen TC. Vitamin D for the prevention and treatment of pancreatic cancer. World J Gastroenterol 2009;15(27):3349–54.
21. Colston KW, Welsh J. Vitamin D and breast cancer. In: Feldman D, Pike JW, Glorieux FH, editors. Vitamin D, vol. 2. San Diego (CA): Elsevier Academic Press; 2005. p. 1663–77.
22. Cross HS. Vitamin D and colon cancer. In: Feldman D, Pike JW, Glorieux FH, editors. Vitamin D. vol. 2. San Diego (CA): Elsevier Academic Press; 2005. p. 1709–25.
23. Gombart AF, Luong QT, Koeffler HP. Vitamin D compounds: activity against microbes and cancer. Anticancer Res 2006;26(4A):2531–42.
24. Gonzalez-Sancho JM, Larriba MJ, Ordonez-Moran P, et al. Effects of 1alpha, 25-dihydroxyvitamin D3 in human colon cancer cells. Anticancer Res 2006; 26(4A):2669–81.

25. Gross MD. Vitamin D and calcium in the prevention of prostate and colon cancer: new approaches for the identification of needs. J Nutr 2005;135(2): 326–31.

26. Krishnan AV, Peehl DM, Feldman D. Inhibition of prostate cancer growth by vitamin D: regulation of target gene expression. J Cell Biochem 2003;88(2):363–71.

27. Krishnan AV, Peehl DM, Feldman D. Vitamin D and prostate cancer. In: Feldman D, Pike JW, Glorieux FH, editors. 2nd edition. Vitamin D. vol. 2. San Diego (CA): Elsevier Academic Press; 2005. p. 1679–707.

28. Luong QT, Koeffler HP. Vitamin D compounds in leukemia. J Steroid Biochem Mol Biol 2005;97(1–2):195–202.

29. Schwartz GG, Skinner HG. Vitamin D status and cancer: new insights. Curr Opin Clin Nutr Metab Care 2007;10(1):6–11.

30. Stewart LV, Weigel NL. Vitamin D and prostate cancer. Exp Biol Med (Maywood) 2004;229(4):277–84.

31. Welsh J. Targets of vitamin D receptor signaling in the mammary gland. J Bone Miner Res 2007;22(Suppl 2):V86–90.

32. Campbell MJ, Elstner E, Holden S, et al. Inhibition of proliferation of prostate cancer cells by a 19-nor-hexafluoride vitamin D3 analogue involves the induction of p21waf1, p27kip1 and E-cadherin. J Mol Endocrinol 1997; 19(1):15–27.

33. Yang ES, Burnstein KL. Vitamin D inhibits G1 to S progression in LNCaP prostate cancer cells through p27Kip1 stabilization and Cdk2 mislocalization to the cytoplasm. J Biol Chem 2003;278(47):46862–8.

34. Blutt SE, Allegretto EA, Pike JW, et al. 1,25-Dihydroxyvitamin D3 and 9-cis-retinoic acid act synergistically to inhibit the growth of LNCaP prostate cells and cause accumulation of cells in G1. Endocrinology 1997;138(4):1491–7.

35. Jensen SS, Madsen MW, Lukas J, et al. Inhibitory effects of 1alpha,25-dihydroxyvitamin D(3) on the G(1)-S phase-controlling machinery. Mol Endocrinol 2001; 15(8):1370–80.

36. Ma Y, Yu WD, Hershberger PA, et al. 1alpha,25-Dihydroxyvitamin D3 potentiates cisplatin antitumor activity by p73 induction in a squamous cell carcinoma model. Mol Cancer Ther 2008;7(9):3047–55.

37. Boyle BJ, Zhao XY, Cohen P, et al. Insulin-like growth factor binding protein-3 mediates 1 alpha,25-dihydroxyvitamin d(3) growth inhibition in the LNCaP prostate cancer cell line through p21/WAF1. J Urol 2001;165(4):1319–24.

38. Peng L, Malloy PJ, Feldman D. Identification of a functional vitamin D response element in the human insulin-like growth factor binding protein-3 promoter. Mol Endocrinol 2004;18:1109–19.

39. Gocek E, Studzinski GP. Vitamin D and differentiation in cancer. Crit Rev Clin Lab Sci 2009;46(4):190–209.

40. Blutt SE, McDonnell TJ, Polek TC, et al. Calcitriol-induced apoptosis in LNCaP cells is blocked by overexpression of Bcl-2. Endocrinology 2000;141(1):10–7.

41. Narvaez CJ, Welsh J. Role of mitochondria and caspases in vitamin D-mediated apoptosis of MCF-7 breast cancer cells. J Biol Chem 2001;276(12):9101–7.

42. Ylikomi T, Laaksi I, Lou YR, et al. Antiproliferative action of vitamin D. Vitam Horm 2002;64:357–406.

43. Park WH, Seol JG, Kim ES, et al. Induction of apoptosis by vitamin D3 analogue EB1089 in NCI-H929 myeloma cells via activation of caspase 3 and p38 MAP kinase. Br J Haematol 2000;109(3):576–83.

44. Posner GH, Crawford KR, Peleg S, et al. A non-calcemic sulfone version of the vitamin D(3) analogue seocalcitol (EB 1089): chemical synthesis, biological

evaluation and potency enhancement of the anticancer drug adriamycin. Bioorg Med Chem 2001;9(9):2365–71.

45. Sundaram S, Sea A, Feldman S, et al. The combination of a potent vitamin D3 analog, EB 1089, with ionizing radiation reduces tumor growth and induces apoptosis of MCF-7 breast tumor xenografts in nude mice. Clin Cancer Res 2003;9(6):2350–6.

46. Getzenberg RH, Light BW, Lapco PE, et al. Vitamin D inhibition of prostate adenocarcinoma growth and metastasis in the Dunning rat prostate model system. Urology 1997;50(6):999–1006.

47. Nakagawa K, Kawaura A, Kato S, et al. 1 alpha,25-Dihydroxyvitamin D(3) is a preventive factor in the metastasis of lung cancer. Carcinogenesis 2005; 26(2):429–40.

48. Koli K, Keski-Oja J. 1alpha,25-dihydroxyvitamin D3 and its analogues down-regulate cell invasion-associated proteases in cultured malignant cells. Cell Growth Differ 2000;11(4):221–9.

49. Gonzalez-Sancho JM, Alvarez-Dolado M, Munoz A. 1,25-Dihydroxyvitamin D3 inhibits tenascin-C expression in mammary epithelial cells. FEBS Lett 1998; 426(2):225–8.

50. Sung V, Feldman D. 1,25-Dihydroxyvitamin D3 decreases human prostate cancer cell adhesion and migration. Mol Cell Endocrinol 2000;164(1–2): 133–43.

51. Bao BY, Yeh SD, Lee YF. 1alpha,25-dihydroxyvitamin D3 inhibits prostate cancer cell invasion via modulation of selective proteases. Carcinogenesis 2006;27(1): 32–42.

52. Allavena P, Garlanda C, Borrello MG, et al. Pathways connecting inflammation and cancer. Curr Opin Genet Dev 2008;18(1):3–10.

53. De Marzo AM, Platz EA, Sutcliffe S, et al. Inflammation in prostate carcinogenesis. Nat Rev Cancer 2007;7(4):256–69.

54. Mantovani A, Allavena P, Sica A, et al. Cancer-related inflammation. Nature 2008;454(7203):436–44.

55. Lucia MS, Torkko KC. Inflammation as a target for prostate cancer chemoprevention: pathological and laboratory rationale. J Urol 2004;171(2 Pt 2):S30–4 [discussion: S35].

56. Mantovani A, Pierotti MA. Cancer and inflammation: a complex relationship. Cancer Lett 2008;267(2):180–1.

57. Angelo LS, Kurzrock R. Vascular endothelial growth factor and its relationship to inflammatory mediators. Clin Cancer Res 2007;13(10):2825–30.

58. Kundu JK, Surh YJ. Inflammation: gearing the journey to cancer. Mutat Res 2008;659(1–2):15–30.

59. Moran EM. Epidemiological and clinical aspects of nonsteroidal anti-inflammatory drugs and cancer risks. J Environ Pathol Toxicol Oncol 2002;21(2): 193–201.

60. Thun MJ, Henley SJ, Patrono C. Nonsteroidal anti-inflammatory drugs as anticancer agents: mechanistic, pharmacologic, and clinical issues. J Natl Cancer Inst 2002;94(4):252–66.

61. Krishnan AV, Shinghal R, Raghavachari N, et al. Analysis of vitamin D-regulated gene expression in LNCaP human prostate cancer cells using cDNA microarrays. Prostate 2004;59(3):243–51.

62. Peehl DM, Shinghal R, Nonn L, et al. Molecular activity of 1,25-dihydroxyvitamin D3 in primary cultures of human prostatic epithelial cells revealed by cDNA microarray analysis. J Steroid Biochem Mol Biol 2004;92(3):131–41.

63. McCarty MF. Targeting multiple signaling pathways as a strategy for managing prostate cancer: multifocal signal modulation therapy. Integr Cancer Ther 2004; 3(4):349–80.

64. Maeda S, Omata M. Inflammation and cancer: role of nuclear factor-kappaB activation. Cancer Sci 2008;99(5):836–42.

65. Moreno J, Krishnan AV, Swami S, et al. Regulation of prostaglandin metabolism by calcitriol attenuates growth stimulation in prostate cancer cells. Cancer Res 2005;65(17):7917–25.

66. Srinivas S, Feldman D. A phase II trial of calcitriol and naproxen in recurrent prostate cancer. Anticancer Res 2009;29(9):3605–10.

67. Nonn L, Peng L, Feldman D, et al. Inhibition of p38 by vitamin D reduces inter-leukin-6 production in normal prostate cells via mitogen-activated protein kinase phosphatase 5: implications for prostate cancer prevention by vitamin D. Cancer Res 2006;66(8):4516–24.

68. Culig Z, Steiner H, Bartsch G, et al. Interleukin-6 regulation of prostate cancer cell growth. J Cell Biochem 2005;95(3):497–505.

69. Finley DS, Calvert VS, Inokuchi J, et al. Periprostatic adipose tissue as a modu-lator of prostate cancer aggressiveness. J Urol 2009;182(4):1621–7.

70. Karin M, Lin A. NF-kappaB at the crossroads of life and death. Nat Immunol 2002;3(3):221–7.

71. Ghosh S, Karin M. Missing pieces in the NF-kappaB puzzle. Cell 2002; 109(Suppl):S81–96.

72. Palayoor ST, Youmell MY, Calderwood SK, et al. Constitutive activation of Ikap-paB kinase alpha and NF-kappaB in prostate cancer cells is inhibited by ibuprofen. Oncogene 1999;18(51):7389–94.

73. Sovak MA, Bellas RE, Kim DW, et al. Aberrant nuclear factor-kappaB/Rel expression and the pathogenesis of breast cancer. J Clin Invest 1997; 100(12):2952–60.

74. Yu XP, Bellido T, Manolagas SC. Down-regulation of NF-kappa B protein levels in activated human lymphocytes by 1,25-dihydroxyvitamin D3. Proc Natl Acad Sci U S A 1995;92(24):10990–4.

75. Harant H, Wolff B, Lindley IJ. 1Alpha,25-dihydroxyvitamin D3 decreases DNA binding of nuclear factor-kappaB in human fibroblasts. FEBS Lett 1998; 436(3):329–34.

76. Stio M, Martinesi M, Bruni S, et al. The vitamin D analogue TX 527 blocks NF-kappaB activation in peripheral blood mononuclear cells of patients with Crohn's disease. J Steroid Biochem Mol Biol 2007;103(1):51–60.

77. Sun J, Kong J, Duan Y, et al. Increased NF-kappaB activity in fibroblasts lacking the vitamin D receptor. Am J Physiol Endocrinol Metab 2006;291(2): E315–22.

78. Schwab M, Reynders V, Loitsch S, et al. Involvement of different nuclear hormone receptors in butyrate-mediated inhibition of inducible NF kappa B signalling. Mol Immunol 2007;44(15):3625–32.

79. Bao BY, Yao J, Lee YF. 1alpha, 25-Dihydroxyvitamin D3 suppresses interleukin-8-mediated prostate cancer cell angiogenesis. Carcinogenesis 2006;27(9): 1883–93.

80. Jogie-Brahim S, Feldman D, Oh Y. Unraveling IGFBP-3 actions in human disease. Endocr Rev 2009;30(5):417–37.

81. Criswell T, Leskov K, Miyamoto S, et al. Transcription factors activated in mammalian cells after clinically relevant doses of ionizing radiation. Oncogene 2003;22(37):5813–27.

82. Kimura K, Bowen C, Spiegel S, et al. Tumor necrosis factor-alpha sensitizes prostate cancer cells to gamma-irradiation-induced apoptosis. Cancer Res 1999;59(7):1606–14.

83. Xu Y, Fang F, St Clair DK, et al. Suppression of RelB-mediated manganese superoxide dismutase expression reveals a primary mechanism for radiosensitization effect of 1alpha,25-dihydroxyvitamin D(3) in prostate cancer cells. Mol Cancer Ther 2007;6(7):2048–56.

84. De Marzo AM, DeWeese TL, Platz EA, et al. Pathological and molecular mechanisms of prostate carcinogenesis: implications for diagnosis, detection, prevention, and treatment. J Cell Biochem 2004;91(3):459–77.

85. De Marzo AM, Marchi VL, Epstein JI, et al. Proliferative inflammatory atrophy of the prostate: implications for prostatic carcinogenesis. Am J Pathol 1999;155(6): 1985–92.

86. Zha S, Gage WR, Sauvageot J, et al. Cyclooxygenase-2 is up-regulated in proliferative inflammatory atrophy of the prostate, but not in prostate carcinoma. Cancer Res 2001;61(24):8617–23.

87. Herszenyi L, Miheller P, Tulassay Z. Carcinogenesis in inflammatory bowel disease. Dig Dis 2007;25(3):267–9.

88. Itzkowitz SH, Yio X. Inflammation and cancer IV. Colorectal cancer in inflammatory bowel disease: the role of inflammation. Am J Physiol Gastrointest Liver Physiol 2004;287(1):G7–17.

89. Seril DN, Liao J, Yang GY, et al. Oxidative stress and ulcerative colitis-associated carcinogenesis: studies in humans and animal models. Carcinogenesis 2003;24(3):353–62.

90. Whittemore AS, Cirillo PM, Feldman D, et al. Prostate specific antigen levels in young adulthood predict prostate cancer risk: results from a cohort of black and white Americans. J Urol 2005;174(3):872–6 [discussion: 876].

91. Gupta S, Adhami VM, Subbarayan M, et al. Suppression of prostate carcinogenesis by dietary supplementation of celecoxib in transgenic adenocarcinoma of the mouse prostate model. Cancer Res 2004;64(9):3334–43.

92. Alagbala A, Moser MT, Johnson CS, et al. Prevention of prostate cancer progression with vitamin D compounds in the transgenic adenocarcinoma of the mouse prostate (TRAMP) model. Presented at the 4th Annual AACR International Conference on Frontiers in Cancer Prevention Research. Baltimore (MD), October 30 to November 2, 2005.

93. Alagbala AA, Moser MT, Johnson CS, et al. 1a,25-Dihydroxyvitamin D$_3$ and its analog (QW-1624F2-2) prevent prostate cancer progression. Presented at 13th Workshop on Vitamin D. Victoria, BC (Canada), April 8–12, 2006.

94. Banach-Petrosky W, Ouyang X, Gao H, et al. Vitamin D inhibits the formation of prostatic intraepithelial neoplasia in Nkx3.1;Pten mutant mice. Clin Cancer Res 2006;12(19):5895–901.

95. Folkman J. Angiogenesis in cancer, vascular, rheumatoid and other disease. Nat Med 1995;1(1):27–31.

96. Sakamoto S, Ryan AJ, Kyprianou N. Targeting vasculature in urologic tumors: mechanistic and therapeutic significance. J Cell Biochem 2008;103(3): 691–708.

97. Giaccia A, Siim BG, Johnson RS. HIF-1 as a target for drug development. Nat Rev Drug Discov 2003;2(10):803–11.

98. Rankin EB, Giaccia AJ. The role of hypoxia-inducible factors in tumorigenesis. Cell Death Differ 2008;15(4):678–85.

99. Majewski S, Skopinska M, Marczak M, et al. Vitamin D3 is a potent inhibitor of tumor cell-induced angiogenesis. J Investig Dermatol Symp Proc 1996;1(1): 97–101.
100. Mantell DJ, Owens PE, Bundred NJ, et al. 1 alpha,25-Dihydroxyvitamin D(3) inhibits angiogenesis in vitro and in vivo. Circ Res 2000;87(3):214–20.
101. Ben-Shoshan M, Amir S, Dang DT, et al. 1alpha,25-Dihydroxyvitamin D3 (calcitriol) inhibits hypoxia-inducible factor-1/vascular endothelial growth factor pathway in human cancer cells. Mol Cancer Ther 2007;6(4):1433–9.
102. Bernardi RJ, Johnson CS, Modzelewski RA, et al. Antiproliferative effects of 1alpha,25-dihydroxyvitamin D(3) and vitamin D analogs on tumor-derived endothelial cells. Endocrinology 2002;143(7):2508–14.
103. Chung I, Han G, Seshadri M, et al. Role of vitamin D receptor in the antiproliferative effects of calcitriol in tumor-derived endothelial cells and tumor angiogenesis in vivo. Cancer Res 2009;69(3):967–75.
104. Fukuda R, Kelly B, Semenza GL. Vascular endothelial growth factor gene expression in colon cancer cells exposed to prostaglandin E2 is mediated by hypoxia-inducible factor 1. Cancer Res 2003;63(9):2330–4.
105. McElwain MC, Dettelbach MA, Modzelewski RA, et al. Antiproliferative effects in vitro and in vivo of 1,25-dihydroxyvitamin D3 and a vitamin D3 analog in a squamous cell carcinoma model system. Mol Cell Differ 1995;3(1):31–50.
106. Zhang X, Jiang F, Li P, et al. Growth suppression of ovarian cancer xenografts in nude mice by vitamin D analogue EB1089. Clin Cancer Res 2005; 11(1):323–8.
107. Colston KW, Chander SK, Mackay AG, et al. Effects of synthetic vitamin D analogues on breast cancer cell proliferation in vivo and in vitro. Biochem Pharmacol 1992;44(4):693–702.
108. Welsh J, Wietzke JA, Zinser GM, et al. Vitamin D-3 receptor as a target for breast cancer prevention. J Nutr 2003;133(Suppl 7):2425S–33S.
109. Ma Y, Yu WD, Trump DL, et al. 1,25D3 enhances antitumor activity of gemcitabine and cisplatin in human bladder cancer models. Cancer 2010, in press.
110. Colston KW, James SY, Ofori-Kuragu EA, et al. Vitamin D receptors and antiproliferative effects of vitamin D derivatives in human pancreatic carcinoma cells in vivo and in vitro. Br J Cancer 1997;76(8):1017–20.
111. Moore TB, Koeffler HP, Yamashiro JM, et al. Vitamin D3 analogs inhibit growth and induce differentiation in LA-N-5 human neuroblastoma cells. Clin Exp Metastasis 1996;14(3):239–45.
112. Chung I, Wong MK, Flynn G, et al. Differential antiproliferative effects of calcitriol on tumor-derived and Matrigel-derived endothelial cells. Cancer Res 2006; 66(17):8565–73.
113. Chung I, Karpf AR, Muindi JR, et al. Epigenetic silencing of CYP24 in tumor-derived endothelial cells contributes to selective growth inhibition by calcitriol. J Biol Chem 2007;282(12):8704–14.
114. Ly LH, Zhao XY, Holloway L, et al. Liarozole acts synergistically with 1alpha,25-dihydroxyvitamin D3 to inhibit growth of DU 145 human prostate cancer cells by blocking 24-hydroxylase activity. Endocrinology 1999; 140(5):2071–6.
115. Miller GJ, Stapleton GE, Hedlund TE, et al. Vitamin D receptor expression, 24-hydroxylase activity, and inhibition of growth by 1alpha,25-dihydroxyvitamin D3 in seven human prostatic carcinoma cell lines. Clin Cancer Res 1995;1(9): 997–1003.

116. Peehl DM, Seto E, Hsu JY, et al. Preclinical activity of ketoconazole in combination with calcitriol or the vitamin D analogue EB 1089 in prostate cancer cells. J Urol 2002;168(4 Pt 1):1583–8.

117. Hershberger PA, McGuire TF, Yu WD, et al. Cisplatin potentiates 1,25-dihydroxyvitamin D3-induced apoptosis in association with increased mitogen-activated protein kinase kinase kinase 1 (MEKK-1) expression. Mol Cancer Ther 2002; 1(10):821–9.

118. Moffatt KA, Johannes WU, Miller GJ. 1alpha,25-Dihydroxyvitamin D3 and platinum drugs act synergistically to inhibit the growth of prostate cancer cell lines. Clin Cancer Res 1999;5(3):695–703.

119. Hershberger PA, Yu WD, Modzelewski RA, et al. Calcitriol (1,25-dihydroxycholecalciferol) enhances paclitaxel antitumor activity in vitro and in vivo and accelerates paclitaxel-induced apoptosis. Clin Cancer Res 2001;7(4):1043–51.

120. Trump DL, Hershberger PA, Bernardi RJ, et al. Anti-tumor activity of calcitriol: pre-clinical and clinical studies. J Steroid Biochem Mol Biol 2004;89–90(1–5): 519–26.

121. Muindi JR, Yu WD, Ma Y, et al. CYP24A1 inhibition enhances the antitumor activity of calcitriol. Submitted for publication, 2010.

122. Rochlitz CF, Damon LE, Russi MB, et al. Cytotoxicity of ketoconazole in malignant cell lines. Cancer Chemother Pharmacol 1988;21(4):319–22.

123. Kahraman M, Sinishtaj S, Dolan PM, et al. Potent, selective and low-calcemic inhibitors of CYP24 hydroxylase: 24-sulfoximine analogues of the hormone 1alpha,25-dihydroxyvitamin D(3). J Med Chem 2004;47(27):6854–63.

124. Lechner D, Manhardt T, Bajna E, et al. A 24-phenylsulfone analog of vitamin D inhibits 1alpha,25-dihydroxyvitamin D(3) degradation in vitamin D metabolism-competent cells. J Pharmacol Exp Ther 2007;320(3):1119–26.

125. Gallagher JC. Metabolic effects of synthetic calcitriol (Rocaltrol) in the treatment of postmenopausal osteoporosis. Metabolism 1990;39(4 Suppl 1):27–9.

126. Gallagher JC, Goldgar D. Treatment of postmenopausal osteoporosis with high doses of synthetic calcitriol. A randomized controlled study. Ann Intern Med 1990;113(9):649–55.

127. Gross C, Stamey T, Hancock S, et al. Treatment of early recurrent prostate cancer with 1,25-dihydroxyvitamin D3 (calcitriol). J Urol 1998;159(6):2035–9 [discussion: 2039–40].

128. Osborn JL, Schwartz GG, Smith DC, et al. 1,25-Dihydroxyvitamin D (calcitriol) in hormone refractory prostate cancer. Urol Oncol 1995;1(5):195–8.

129. Muindi JR, Peng Y, Potter DM, et al. Pharmacokinetics of high-dose oral calcitriol: results from a phase 1 trial of calcitriol and paclitaxel. Clin Pharmacol Ther 2002;72(6):648–59.

130. Muindi JR, Potter DM, Peng Y, et al. Pharmacokinetics of liquid calcitriol formulation in advanced solid tumor patients: comparison with caplet formulation. Cancer Chemother Pharmacol 2005;56(5):492–6.

131. Beer TM, Munar M, Henner WD. A phase I trial of pulse calcitriol in patients with refractory malignancies: pulse dosing permits substantial dose escalation. Cancer 2001;91(12):2431–9.

132. Beer TM, Javle M, Lam GN, et al. Pharmacokinetics and tolerability of a single dose of DN-101, a new formulation of calcitriol, in patients with cancer. Clin Cancer Res 2005;11(21):7794–9.

133. Beer TM, Javle MM, Ryan CW, et al. Phase I study of weekly DN-101, a new formulation of calcitriol, in patients with cancer. Cancer Chemother Pharmacol 2007;59(5):581–7.

134. Fakih MG, Trump DL, Muindi JR, et al. A phase I pharmacokinetic and pharma-codynamic study of intravenous calcitriol in combination with oral gefitinib in patients with advanced solid tumors. Clin Cancer Res 2007;13(4):1216–23.

135. Muindi JR, Johnson CS, Trump DL, et al. A phase I and pharmacokinetics study of intravenous calcitriol in combination with oral dexamethasone and gefitinib in patients with advanced solid tumors. Cancer Chemother Pharmacol 2009;65(1): 33–40.

136. Muindi JR, Modzelewski RA, Peng Y, et al. Pharmacokinetics of 1alpha,25-dihydroxyvitamin D3 in normal mice after systemic exposure to effective and safe antitumor doses. Oncology 2004;66(1):62–6.

137. Dalhoff K, Dancey J, Astrup L, et al. A phase II study of the vitamin D analogue Seocalcitol in patients with inoperable hepatocellular carcinoma. Br J Cancer 2003;89(2):252–7.

138. Evans TR, Colston KW, Lofts FJ, et al. A phase II trial of the vitamin D analogue Seocalcitol (EB1089) in patients with inoperable pancreatic cancer. Br J Cancer 2002;86(5):680–5.

139. Gulliford T, English J, Colston KW, et al. A phase I study of the vitamin D analogue EB 1089 in patients with advanced breast and colorectal cancer. Br J Cancer 1998;78(1):6–13.

140. Attia S, Eickhoff J, Wilding G, et al. Randomized, double-blinded phase II eval-uation of docetaxel with or without doxercalciferol in patients with metastatic, androgen-independent prostate cancer. Clin Cancer Res 2008;14(8):2437–43.

141. Liu G, Oettel K, Ripple G, et al. Phase I trial of 1alpha-hydroxyvitamin D(2) in patients with hormone refractory prostate cancer. Clin Cancer Res 2002;8(9): 2820–7.

142. Liu G, Wilding G, Staab MJ, et al. Phase II study of 1alpha-hydroxyvitamin D(2) in the treatment of advanced androgen-independent prostate cancer. Clin Cancer Res 2003;9(11):4077–83.

143. Medioni J, Eickhoff J, Wilding G, et al. Dose finding and safety analysis of inecal-citol in combination with a docetaxel-prednisone regimen in hormone-refractory prostate cancer (HRPC) patients. J Clin Oncol 2009;27:15s[Suppl abstr: 151].

144. Schwartz GG, Hall MC, Stindt D, et al. Phase I/II study of 19-nor-1alpha-25-dihy-droxyvitamin D2 (paricalcitol) in advanced, androgen-insensitive prostate cancer. Clin Cancer Res 2005;11(24 Pt 1):8680–5.

145. Beer TM, Eilers KM, Garzotto M, et al. Weekly high-dose calcitriol and docetaxel in metastatic androgen-independent prostate cancer. J Clin Oncol 2003;21(1): 123–8.

146. Beer TM, Ryan CW, Venner PM, et al. Double-blinded randomized study of high-dose calcitriol plus docetaxel compared with placebo plus docetaxel in androgen-independent prostate cancer: a report from the ASCENT investiga-tors. J Clin Oncol 2007;25(6):669–74.

147. Beer TM, Garzotto M, Katovic NM. High-dose calcitriol and carboplatin in meta-static androgen-independent prostate cancer. Am J Clin Oncol 2004;27(5): 535–41.

148. Flaig TW, Barqawi A, Miller G, et al. A phase II trial of dexamethasone, vitamin D, and carboplatin in patients with hormone-refractory prostate cancer. Cancer 2006;107(2):266–74.

Vitamin D and Diabetes

Tatiana Takiishi, MSc, Conny Gysemans, PhD,
Roger Bouillon, MD, PhD*, Chantal Mathieu, MD, PhD

KEYWORDS

- Vitamin D • Type 1 diabetes • Type 2 diabetes • β Cells
- Deficiency • Immune system

Diabetes mellitus is one of the most common endocrine diseases, characterized by an increase in plasma glucose. Different forms of diabetes with very distinct pathogenesis exist. Over time, diabetes can lead to blindness, kidney failure, and nerve damage. Diabetes is also an important factor in accelerating atherosclerosis, leading to stroke, coronary heart disease, and other large blood vessel diseases, all ultimately associated with increased mortality risks.

The most prevalent form of diabetes is type 2 diabetes (T2D), currently affecting more than 300 million people worldwide.[1] T2D is characterized by the combination of insulin resistance and failing β-cell function.[2] Type 1 diabetes (T1D), on the other hand, is an autoimmune disease in which the body's own immune system mistakenly attacks and destroys the insulin-producing β cell in the pancreas.[3] T1D typically occurs in young, lean individuals, but older patients can also be affected. This subgroup is referred to as latent autoimmune diabetes in adults (LADA). LADA is a slow, progressive form of T1D. Other forms of diabetes include gestational diabetes (GD), secondary diabetes due to pancreatic diseases or surgery, and genetic forms of diabetes.[4–6]

Vitamin D is a secosteroid that is generated from 7-dehydrocholesterol in skin under the influence of UV light. Therefore, by definition, vitamin D cannot be considered a true vitamin but rather a prohormone, as the natural source of vitamin D in evolution of vertebrates and primates is photosynthesis in the skin. Indeed, the normal human diet is usually poor in vitamin D except for fatty fish. Regardless of the source of vitamin D, it needs to be hydroxylated twice to become biologically active.[7] Vitamin D is first hydroxylated in the liver by 25-hydroxylases (25(OH)ase), consisting of

This work was supported by a postdoctoral fellowship for C.G. and a clinical fellowship for C.M. from the Flemish research fund "FWO Vlaanderen." T.T. received an SBA scholarship from the Katholieke Universiteit Leuven.

Laboratory for Experimental Medicine and Endocrinology (LEGENDO), Katholieke Universiteit Leuven, UZ Gasthuisberg, O&N I Herestraat 49 - bus 902, 3000, Leuven, Belgium
* Corresponding author.
E-mail address: Roger.bouillon@med.kuleuven.be

cytochrome P450 (CYP) isoforms (the mitochondrial CYP27A1 and the microsomal CYP2R1 [the most critical enzyme], CYP3A4, and CYPJ3) into 25-hydroxyvitamin D (25(OH)D). The second hydroxylation occurs in the kidney, by 1α-hydroxylase (1α(OH)ase, CYP27B1), as this tissue is normally the only one capable of the secretion of its end product, $1,25(OH)_2D$, into the blood circulation. Vitamin D and its metabolites are bound to a carrier protein (vitamin D binding protein; DBP) when transported through the circulation. Another multifunctional hydroxylase, 24-hydroxylase (24(OH)ase, CYP24A1), catabolizes vitamin D metabolites. Vitamin D exerts its action via a nuclear receptor (vitamin D receptor; VDR), present in nearly all nucleated cells, but with the highest concentration in the epithelial cells of the gut. However, most of these enzymes and proteins essential for the action of vitamin D are also present in many tissues not related to bone and calcium metabolism, such as the immune system.[7,8]

Over many years, links between vitamin D status and diabetes mellitus have been identified. As early as the 1980s, it was shown that vitamin D deficiency in rodents and rabbits inhibits pancreatic insulin secretion, indicating that vitamin D is essential for the function of the endocrine pancreas.[9] Later, the connection between vitamin D and diabetes was reinforced by the discovery of the VDR and DBP in pancreatic tissue (more specifically in the insulin-producing β cells) and also in various cell types of the immune system. Thus, vitamin D has been proposed as a possible therapeutic agent in the prevention and treatment of T1D and T2D.[8]

TYPE 1 DIABETES

T1D is a chronic autoimmune disease that results from the immune-mediated destruction of pancreatic β cells, thus resulting in insulin deficiency. The autoimmune process most commonly initiates in childhood and progresses for a variable period of months and even years before it leads to hyperglycemia and, thus, diagnosis. By the time of diagnosis only 10% to 30% of functional β-cell mass remains.[10,11] T1D is the second most common chronic disease in children, second only to asthma, and is considered as a complex genetic trait; not only do numerous genetic loci contribute to susceptibility, but environmental factors also play an important role in determining risk.

Vitamin D and Genetic Predisposition to T1D

In T1D the major genetic determinant is located in the major histocompatibility complex (MHC) region on chromosome 6p21,[12] although multiple non-MHC genes also contribute to T1D disease susceptibility.[13] Refining genetic mapping particularly of the non-MHC loci may improve the ability to predict the risk of T1D and facilitate the testing of more aggressive preventive therapies.[14] In this context, associations of T1D with polymorphisms in the CYP27B1 gene on chromosome 12q13.1-q13.3[15–17] may be useful. It is hypothesized that presence of polymorphisms in the CYP27B1 gene may reduce the (local) expression of 1α(OH)ase and consequently the conversion of 25(OH)D to $1,25(OH)_2D$, leading to increased predisposition to T1D.

In the past, it has been shown that allelic variations in the VDR gene are an important determinant for the amount of VDR expressed,[18] and which in turn may influence the immune-modulatory function of the VDR. Several authors have demonstrated that VDR polymorphisms are able to influence the immune response in either healthy individuals or T1D patients.[19,20] In epidemiologic studies, clear associations between VDR polymorphisms and T1D have been reported in South Indian, German, and Taiwanese populations,[21–23] but were not found in a large combined population sample of British,

Portuguese, and Finnish origin.[24–26] In a recent study it was shown that specific VDR polymorphisms interact with the predisposing HLA DRB1 allele through vitamin D response element present in the promoter region of the DRB1*0301 allele,[27] which may be detrimental for the manifestation of T1D, particularly in the case of vitamin D deficiency in early childhood due to poor expression of DRB1 0301 in the thymus.

1,25(OH)$_2$D is biologically inactivated through a series of events starting with 24-hydroxylation. The 24(OH)ase enzyme is encoded by the CYP24A1 gene located on chromosome 20q13.2-q13.3. At present, no associations between CYP24A1 gene polymorphisms and T1D have been found.[17]

Vitamin D as an Environmental Risk Factor

T1D has been linked to a clear north-south gradient as well as to a deficiency in vitamin D concentrations. Indeed, the incidence of T1D is higher in countries of northern latitude,[28–30] this trend being reversed in the southern hemisphere.[31] Latitude itself is unlikely to be an independent risk factor for T1D onset. On the other hand, UV-B irradiation, which follows a north-south gradient, is known to convert 7-dehydrocholesterol to vitamin D in the skin, and has protective properties against autoimmunity.[32] A more significant correlation of T1D has been observed with erythemal UV-B irradiation than with latitude. Recently, Mohr and colleagues[33] assessed the T1D incidence data for children younger than 14 years during 1990 to 1994 in 51 regions worldwide. This investigation found that incidence rates of T1D approached zero in regions worldwide with high UV-B irradiance. Furthermore, seasonality of T1D onset is well known.[34,35] Kahn and colleagues[36] reported that spring births were associated with increased likelihood of T1D, which might reflect insufficient maternal/neonatal vitamin D levels during a critical fetal/neonatal programming period. Indeed, vitamin D has been shown to have a role in development and function of the immune system.[37] In fact, inadequate vitamin D and other nutrients during immune system development (from gestation up to the second year of life) may play a critical role in the development of autoimmune diseases. Therefore, it is thought that restoration of vitamin D levels (either by supplementation with vitamin D or by administration of [less hypercalcemic analogues of] the active hormone 1,25(OH)$_2$D) may reduce the risk of T1D. How vitamin D interferes with the pathogenesis of T1D is still not fully elucidated, though some possible mechanisms have been suggested (**Fig. 1**).

Vitamin D as an Immune System Modulator

There is increasing evidence that active vitamin D (1,25(OH)$_2$D) acts as a modulator of the immune system. One of the first indications for this role was the finding of VDR expression in a wide range of immune cells (eg, monocytes, activated lymphocytes).[38,39] Also, activation of the nuclear VDR is known to modify transcription via several intracellular pathways and influence proliferation and differentiation of immune cells.[40,41]

Antigen-presenting cells: dendritic cells

Dendritic cells (DCs), which are highly specialized antigen-presenting cells, are known to be important for the priming of CD4$^+$ T cells. DCs act as sentinels in lymphoid and nonlymphoid organs, capturing and processing antigens; once the antigen is captured the DCs will mature, increasing the expression of costimulatory molecules.[42] For activation of T cells, appropriate interaction between the T-cell receptor and antigen/MHC complex as well as costimulatory signals are necessary. However, when there is a disruption in these interactions, T cells become anergic.[43] There is increasing evidence that by hampering the costimulatory capacity of DCs, a shift from

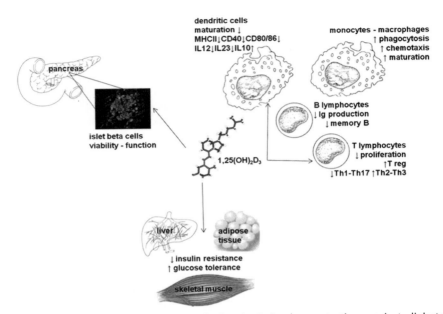

Fig. 1. Mechanisms of action of (active) vitamin D in the protection against diabetes. $1,25(OH)_2D_3$ plays an important role in glucose homeostasis via different mechanisms. $1,25(OH)_2D_3$ not only enhances and improves the β-cell function but also improves insulin sensitivity of the target cells (liver, skeletal muscle, and adipose tissue). In addition, $1,25(OH)_2D_3$ protects the β-cell from detrimental immune attacks, directly by its action on the β-cell but also indirectly by acting on different immune cells, including inflammatory macrophages, dendritic cells, and a variety of T cells. In addition, macrophages, as well as dendritic cells, T lymphocytes, and B lymphocytes can synthesize $1,25(OH)_2D_3$, all contributing to the regulation of local immune responses.

immunogenicity to tolerance can be achieved. $1,25(OH)_2D$ has dramatic effects on antigen presentation, whereby it reduces antigen presentation by suppressing the expression of MHC-II molecules as well as costimulatory molecules.[44–46] Many studies have shown the immunosuppressive properties of $1,25(OH)_2D_3$ on DCs. For instance, in vitro exposure of the cultured immature DCs to $1,25(OH)_2D_3$ can inhibit their maturation, decrease their production of interleukin (IL)-12, and increase the production of IL-10, thus leading to an immune-modulatory DC. $1,25(OH)_2D_3$ not only inhibits maturation of DCs but also increases the apoptosis of mature DCs.[47] Furthermore, coculture of $1,25(OH)_2D_3$-treated DCs with autoreactive T-cell clones isolated from T1D patients inhibited T-cell proliferation and showed selective apoptosis of the autoreactive T cells.[48] Extensive proteomic analysis of DCs treated with TX527, a 14-epivitamin D_3 analogue, showed that DCs are not merely locked in an immature state but adopt a tolerogenic phenotype with special migratory and endocytic properties compared with mature or immature DCs.[49] Furthermore, these $1,25(OH)_2D_3$-treated DCs may induce Treg cells and inhibit autoimmune diseases such as T1D.[50,51] However, most of these studies do not exclude that $1,25(OH)_2D_3$ could have a direct action on T-cell modulation as well.

T lymphocytes

VDR expression was first described in activated T cells, and early work suggested that vitamin D exerted its immune-modulatory effects on these cells. In the 1980s, several studies reported that $1,25(OH)_2D_3$ could inhibit proliferation of mitogen-stimulated T-cell cultures.[52–55] In 1987, Rigby and colleagues[56] described that $1,25(OH)_2D_3$ treatment inhibited IL-2 and interferon (IFN)-γ production by human T cells. Others demonstrated inhibition of the aforementioned cytokines as well as IL-12, a known T-cell stimulating factor that is involved in the differentiation of naïve T cells into Th0 cells, which further develop into either Th1 cells or Th2 cells. In addition, an enhancement of Th2-related cytokines (IL-4, IL-5, and IL-10) was observed.[57,58] As already mentioned, $1,25(OH)_2D_3$ can also induce Treg cells in vitro and in vivo.[51,59,60]

Until recently, most of these studies were performed on peripheral blood mononuclear cells (PBMC) consisting of lymphocytes and monocytes. As such, direct effects of $1,25(OH)_2D_3$ on T cells could not be proven.[61,62] Work by Jeffery and colleagues[63] on isolated $CD4^+$ cells demonstrated that $1,25(OH)_2D_3$ can directly modulate T-cell responses. $1,25(OH)_2D_3$ inhibited the production of IFN-γ, IL-17, and IL-21 inflammatory cytokines by $CD4^+$ T cells, and induced development of Treg cells expressing CTLA-4 and FoxP3. T cells cultured in the presence of both $1,25(OH)_2D_3$ and IL-2 expressed the highest levels of CTLA-4 and FoxP3, and possessed the ability to suppress proliferation of resting $CD4^+$ T cells. Of interest, a different study showed that exposure of the skin to the topical vitamin D analogue calcipotriol before immunization with ovalbumin (OVA) and CpG DNA as an immune-stimulatory adjuvant induces Treg cells that prevent consequent antigen-specific $CD8^+$ T-cell proliferation and IFN-γ production.[60]

B lymphocytes

Resting B lymphocytes normally do not express VDR.[39] On activation, however, VDR expression has been reported.[64] Administration of $1,25(OH)_2D_3$ decreases proliferation and immunoglobulin (Ig) production, and induces apoptosis.[64] Although $1,25(OH)_2D_3$ has potent direct effects on B lymphocytes in vitro, indirect mediation by T cells and monocytes or macrophages has been suggested as its most important mechanism of action.[64,65]

Cytokines

Active vitamin D has also been reported to down-regulate the production of several cytokines, in particular, inflammatory cytokines such as IL-2, IL-6, IL-12, IFN-γ, tumor necrosis factor (TNF)-α, and TNF-β, while enhancing anti-inflammatory cytokines such as IL-4, IL-10, and TGF-β.[66,67] This finding is of great relevance for the pathogenesis of T1D, as especially IFN-γ and IL-12, which are markers of Th1 immune responses, are known to enhance inflammatory processes and participate in immune-mediated destruction of insulin-producing β cells.[68] Recently, low-intensity chronic inflammation related to obesity has been linked to insulin resistance, the major cause of T2D. It is suggested that the relationship between vitamin D and low-intensity chronic inflammation and insulin resistance in T2D can be mediated in part by the immune-modulating properties of $1,25(OH)_2D_3$.[69]

Vitamin D and the β cell

Exposure of pancreatic β cells to proinflammatory cytokines induces endoplasmic reticulum stress, leading to death by apoptosis.[70] Treatment of β cells with $1,25(OH)_2D$ has been reported to directly protect against β-cell death by reducing expression of MHC class I molecules,[71] inducing expression of antiapoptotic A20 protein and decreasing expression of Fas.[72,73] The latter is a transmembrane cell surface receptor, transducing an apoptotic death signal and contributing to the pathogenesis of several autoimmune diseases including T1D. Of note, in vitro treatment of pancreatic islets with $1,25(OH)_2D_3$ was also shown to decrease IL-1β and IL-15 cytokine as well as IP-10 chemokine (IFN-γ inducible protein 10) expression in pancreatic β cells, indicating that $1,25(OH)_2D_3$ treatment could reduce the migration and recruitment of effector T cells and macrophages to the islets.[74]

Animal Models

The immune-modulatory properties of active vitamin D suggest that vitamin D (metabolites or analogues) could be potential therapeutic agents for the prevention or cure of T1D. Treatment of NOD mice, an animal model for T1D, with high doses of $1,25(OH)_2D_3$ (5 μg/kg/2 d) showed a decrease in insulitis and diabetes development.[75,76] Decreased numbers of effector T cells, as well as induction of Treg cells, was shown to be the basis for this protection.[59] Later, the authors demonstrated that the arrest of insulitis and block of T-cell infiltration into the pancreas by treatment of prediabetic NOD mice with $1,25(OH)_2D_3$ was associated with reduced chemokine production by islet cells.[74] Treatment of prediabetic NOD mice with $1,25(OH)_2D_3$ increased deletion of T lymphocytes in the thymus, allowing activation-induced cell death (AICD)-sensitive T lymphocytes to reach the periphery.[77] Culture of DCs and thymic T lymphocytes from $1,25(OH)_2D_3$-treated animals separately, however, demonstrated that both cell types needed to be exposed to $1,25(OH)_2D_3$ to obtain the apoptosis-restorative effect. Moreover, transfer experiments demonstrated that T lymphocytes from $1,25(OH)_2D_3$-treated NOD mice were not able to transfer diabetes into young irradiated NOD mice, in contrast to age-matched untreated mice.[78] The latter indicates that $1,25(OH)_2D_3$ is able to directly modulate immune cell responses. The authors also found that $1,25(OH)_2D_3$ is a potent inducer of thymic DC differentiation in NOD mice, consisting in modulation toward a more pronounced lymphoid phenotype and up-regulation of CD86.[77] Moreover, NOD DCs generated from bone marrow in the presence of in vitro $1,25(OH)_2D_3$ exhibit dedifferentiation features of tolerogenic DCs.[46]

Unfortunately, the doses needed for disease prevention in NOD mice lead to hypercalcemia and bone decalcification.[37] This issue can be (partially) solved by using structural analogues of $1,25(OH)_2D_3$.[37] In fact, administration of vitamin D_3 analogues, specifically selected for their enhanced immune effects and decreased calcemic effects, was shown to delay or even inhibit the development of insulitis and the onset of T1D in NOD mice.[79] The proposed mechanism of action was a restoration of suppressor-cell functionality.

In the streptozotocin-induced diabetes model, which is an inflammation-driven model of diabetes, $1,25(OH)_2D_3$ also induced a reduction in the incidence of diabetes.[80] In the case of overt diabetes, $1,25(OH)_2D_3$ has little effect in reverting the disease. It is possible that at this point the number of remaining β-cell mass is simply not sufficient to restore insulin needs.[81] Therefore, an alternative option to insulin therapy is islet or β-cell transplantation. In that regard, it has been shown that overtly diabetic NOD mice that received syngeneic islets and were treated with KH1060 (a 20-epivitamin D_3 analogue) together with cyclosporine displayed a significant prolongation of islet graft survival compared with untreated controls.[82] The authors also demonstrated that this analogue in combination with cyclosporine was able to prevent early graft failure and delay graft rejection of xenogeneic islets transplanted in spontaneously diabetic NOD mice.[83] More recently, a combination therapy using TX527, a 14-epivitamin D_3 analogue, with cyclosporine or IFN-β also induced a significant delay in diabetes recurrence after syngeneic islet transplantation, with an increase of IL-10 expression in islet grafts.[84] Work by Adorini[50] in an allogeneic islet transplantation model also confirmed that $1,25(OH)_2D_3$ treatment in combination with mycophenolate mofetil was able to reduce graft rejection, possibly by inducing tolerogenic DCs and/or Treg cells. Taken together, 1,25(OH)$_2$D$_3$ and its structural analogues display attractive anti-inflammatory properties that open new avenues for the primary, secondary, or tertiary prevention of T1D and other autoimmune diseases.

Nevertheless, despite all the work showing the beneficial effects of vitamin D in T1D prevention, data from VDR knockout mice show conflicting results. Zeitz and colleagues[85] showed in their model that mice presented higher concentrations of blood glucose and lower levels of circulating insulin, whereas Mathieu and colleagues[83] and Gysemans and colleagues[86] did not observe major alterations in glucose tolerance or diabetes incidence in their VDR knockout mouse models. However, these contradictory data could result from the different genetic background of the mice or the control of serum calcium homeostasis, but could also point toward redundancy of vitamin D signaling pathways, and may suggest that compensatory mechanisms are taking place when VDR is completely abrogated from early life onwards.

Clinical Interventions

Large-scale trials evaluating the efficacy of vitamin D in the prevention of T1D are still lacking, but interesting data can be obtained from epidemiologic observations and small-scale trials.

Several retrospective studies found beneficial effects of supplementation with regular vitamin D in early life on the later lifetime risk of T1D. Hypponen and colleagues[87] found a significantly reduced risk of T1D development in a birth-cohort study when high doses of vitamin D supplementation (up to 2000 IU/d) were given during infancy. In addition, 2 studies by Stene and colleagues[88,89] showed that use of cod liver oil, which is rich in vitamin D, during the first year of life was associated with a lower risk of developing T1D later in life. Finally, the European Community–sponsored Concerted Action on the Epidemiology and Prevention of Diabetes showed a 33% reduction of T1D in children who received vitamin D supplementation early in life.[90] A meta-analysis of data from 4 case-control studies and one cohort study revealed lately that the risk of T1D was significantly reduced (29% reduction) in infants who were supplemented with vitamin D as compared with those who were not supplemented (pooled odds ratio 0.71, 95% confidence interval [CI] 0.60–0.84).[91] There was also some evidence of a dose-response effect, with those using higher amounts of vitamin D being at lower risk of developing T1D. Some studies were not able to show an association with a reduced T1D risk, but none of them were associated with an increased risk.

Vitamin D supplementation during pregnancy has also yielded contradictory results. In 2000, Stene and colleagues[88] documented in a pilot case-control study that cod liver oil, taken by the mother during pregnancy, was associated with a lower risk of T1D in their offspring. In a larger case-control study, Stene and colleagues[89] could not confirm their initial results and were unable to find an association between the use of cod liver oil or other vitamin D supplements during pregnancy and T1D risk. Nevertheless, Fronczak and colleagues[92] reported lower levels of anti-islet cell auto-antibodies in almost two-thirds of children whose mothers had higher vitamin D intake during the third trimester. Taking into account that T1D susceptibility has been linked to certain HLA genotypes, Wicklow and Taback intend to pursue a trial using 2000 IU of regular vitamin D per day in newborn babies with increased HLA-associated risk. So far they have shown in a few babies that this dose of supplementation seems safe, and did not cause alterations in serum and urine calcium measurements[93] (**Table 1**).

Table 1
Reported effects of vitamin D supplementation in humans and etiology of T1D

Intervention	Subjects' Characteristics	Study Results	Ref.
Vitamin D supplements (first year of life)	1429 cases; 5026 controls Age <14 y	Risk T1D ↓ (OR = 0.83) age <5 y Risk T1D ↓ (OR = 0.81) age 5–9 y Risk T1D ↓ (OR = 0.47) age 10–14 y	90
Cod liver oil (pregnancy) (first year of life)	78 cases; 980 controls Pregnant women Offspring <15 y	Risk of T1D ↓ offspring (OR = 0.63) Risk of T1D ↓ cod-liver oil fed-infants (OR = 0.82)	88
2000 IU/d (first year of life)	81 cases; 10,285 controls Age 1–31 y	Insulin and C-peptide ↑ Risk of T1D ↓ (RR = 0.22)	87
Cod liver oil (first year of life)	95 cases; 346 controls Age <15 y	Risk of T1D ↓ Supplementation during 7–12 mo (OR = 0.55) Supplementation during 0–6 mo (OR = 0.80)	89
Vitamin D (food) (pregnancy)	Offspring Age <5 y	Insulin autoantibodies ↓ (OR = 0.49)	92
0.25 μg 1,25(OH)$_2$D$_3$ every 2 d or 25 mg nicotinamide/kg/d (1 y)	70 Recently diagnosed T1D Age >5 y	Insulin needs ↓ 1,25(OH)$_2$D$_3$- treated group at 3–6 mo	94
Vitamin D supplements (lactation)	159 cases; 318 controls Age 0–29 y	Risk of T1D ↓ (OR = 0.33)	95
0.5 μg 1α(OH)D$_3$/d (1 y)	35 LADA Adults	C-peptide ↑ β-Cell function ↑	96
2000 IU vitamin D first year of life	7 newborns HLA-associated T1D risk Age >1 y	Serum and urine calcium =	93

In column 1, intervention period is given in parentheses.
Abbreviations: OR, odds ratio; RR, relative risk.

Data on intervention with active vitamin D (1,25(OH)$_2$D) starting when β-cell damage is already present are disappointing. A small intervention trial in which newly-onset diabetic children were given a small dose (0.25 μg) of 1,25(OH)$_2$D or nicotinamide showed that although insulin requirements decreased in the group treated with 1,25(OH)$_2$D, they had no improvement in C-peptide levels.[94] LADA is considered to be a subtype of T1D, in which the clinical manifestation begins and progresses slowly in adulthood. As in T1D, patients with LADA exhibit the presence of autoantibodies to the islets, especially those against glutamic acid decarboxylase.[95] Li and colleagues[96] described results of a pilot study in which LADA patients were given a synthetic analogue of vitamin D$_3$, 1α(OH)D$_3$, in addition to insulin treatment. The patients who received the analogue exhibited a better ability to preserve β-cell function in comparison with patients treated with insulin alone (see **Table 1**).

TYPE 2 DIABETES

T2D is a disorder that results from defects in both insulin secretion and insulin sensitivity, and accounts for 90% of all diabetes cases. The growing rate of T2D is worrisome, with in the United States alone an estimated 1 million new cases every year.[97] Initially, patients counteract their increased insulin resistance and stabilize circulating glucose levels through increased insulin production by pancreatic β cells. As the disease progresses and functional alterations are accentuated, patients show decreased insulin secretion, and eventually they can also present loss of β-cell mass.[4,98] The exact mechanisms involving T2D development are still unknown, but lifestyle (eg, obesity, sedentary lifestyle, and unhealthy eating habits) and genetic components (eg, PPARγ and CAPN10 genes, and a whole set of gene polymorphisms each with small contributing effects) seem to be involved. This disease is most prevalent in obese, sedentary individuals with a concomitant elevation in free fatty acids and proinflammatory cytokines, and relatives of T2D patients also have an increased probability of developing this disease.[99]

Vitamin D and Lifestyle in T2D

The number one risk factor for T2D is obesity. However, weight loss is difficult to achieve and maintain in a long term. Identification of easily modifiable risk factors is, therefore, urgently needed for primary prevention of T2D. It is interesting that obesity is often related to hypovitaminosis D.[4,100] Indeed, the absolute fat mass has an inverse relation with the serum 25(OH)D concentration and correlates positively with the serum parathyroid hormone (PTH) level. This relationship may be caused by the great capacity of adipose tissue of storing vitamin D, thus making it biologically unavailable. An increased PTH level and a decreased amount of serum $25(OH)D_3$ as well as $1,25(OH)_2D_3$ can increase intracellular calcium in adipocytes, which then stimulates the lipogenesis and predisposes to further weight gain. Therefore, it is presently unclear whether (mild) vitamin D deficiency is contributing to or is the consequence of obesity.

Vitamin D deficiency has been associated with higher risks for metabolic syndrome and T2D.[101–103] Population studies suggest that vitamin D (and calcium) may play a significant role in promoting β-cell function and insulin sensitivity, important issues in the pathogenesis of T2D. The National Health and Nutrition Examination Survey (NHANES), a large cross-sectional study, showed an inverse correlation between serum 25(OH)D and incidence of T2D and insulin resistance.[102,104] In a prospective examination of the Medical Research Council Ely Study 1990 to 2000, an inverse relationship between 25(OH)D and glycemic status was found.[105] Supporting these data, a positive correlation between plasma 25(OH)D and insulin sensitivity in healthy subjects subjected to glucose tolerance tests was also reported.[103] On the other hand, prolonged treatment of osteomalacia with vitamin D can increase insulin secretion and improve glucose tolerance.[106,107]

Vitamin D deficiency in obese patients has been linked to secondary hyperparathyroidism, which can contribute to T2D development, as elevated levels of PTH have been associated to glucose intolerance and cardiovascular complications.[4] Current data suggest that T2D patients with vitamin D insufficiency have increased C-reactive protein, fibrinogen, and hemoglobin A1c compared with healthy controls,[108] indicating that inflammation provoked by immune cells (eg, macrophages) are implicated in insulin resistance and T2D. The authors reported that administration of vitamin D ameliorates markers of systemic inflammation, which are typically found in T2D patients, thereby possibly improving β-cell survival.[109]

Another intriguing observation is that insulin resistance in skeletal muscle has a positive correlation with T2D,[110] for which a possible explanation has recently been proposed.[111] Oh and colleagues[112] observed that up-regulation of caveolin-1 (highly likely to be involved in nongenomic vitamin D signaling[113]) significantly improved insulin sensitivity and improved glucose uptake in the skeletal muscle. Therefore, it would be interesting to investigate whether vitamin D supplementation in the nonobese T2D mouse model would improve insulin sensitivity and whether this would be correlated to caveolin-1 expression.

Vitamin D and Genetic Predisposition to T2D

T2D is a polygenic disorder, but monogenic disorders closely related to T2D also exist. Monogenic forms of T2D are rare and include subtypes of maturity onset diabetes (MODY). The majority of proteins that are linked to MODY are transcription factors (such as HNF-4α, HNF-1α, IPF-1, HNF-1β, and NEUROD1).[114] On the other hand, causative genes in the more common polygenic forms of T2D are harder to be identified. However, there are several indications that polymorphisms of the DBP and VDR are related to impaired glucose tolerance and obesity. Even though these correlations vary according to age, lifestyle, and ethnicity of the subjects, there seems to be a fair amount of evidence to support this theory.

The DBP protein (also known as group-specific component protein, or GC) located on chromosome 4q12 is a highly polymorphic serum protein, mainly produced in the liver, with 3 common alleles (Gc1F, Gc1S, and Gc2) and more than 120 rare variants.[115] Few studies have examined DBP polymorphisms and the risk of vitamin D–related diseases. In this regard, the DPB protein has been linked to abnormalities in glucose metabolism and obesity-related traits in different populations. Hirai and colleagues[116] evaluated the variations of the DBP gene (Gc1F, Gc1S, and Gc2) in Japanese individuals with normal glucose tolerance. These investigators demonstrated that people with Gc1S/Gc2 and Gc1S/Gc1S had significantly higher fasting plasma concentrations than those with Gc1F/Gc1F. The same group also reported that Japanese T2D patients had higher frequencies of the Gc1S/Gc2 genotype and lower frequencies of the Gc1F allele in comparison with control subjects.[117] Other studies in Caucasian patients of American or European origin could not confirm the relation between genetic variants of the DBP gene and the susceptibility to T2D.[118,119] It has been suggested that DBP polymorphisms can perhaps influence bioactive 25(OH)D levels through changes in the ratio of free/bound hormones, by a differential affinity, or through effects on concentrations of the DBP/25(OH)D complex that can be internalized by receptor-mediated endocytosis and activate the VDR pathway.[120]

The VDR gene is located on chromosome 12q13.11 and consists of 11 exons. Most VDR polymorphisms are located at the 3′ untranslated region of the VDR gene, such as the BsmI, ApaI, and TaqI restriction fragment length polymorphisms.[121] Several observational studies have reported associations between VDR polymorphisms and T2D, fasting glucose, glucose intolerance, insulin sensitivity, insulin secretion, and calcitriol levels.[4,122,123] In the Rancho Bernardo study, polymorphism in ApaI, BsmI, and TaqI in older Caucasian men was verified. The investigators observed that the frequency of aa genotype of ApaI polymorphism was marginally higher in T2D patients. Also, fasting plasma glucose and prevalence of glucose intolerance were significantly higher in nondiabetic persons with aa genotype compared with those with AA genotype. Moreover, the bb genotype of BsmI polymorphism was associated with insulin resistance.[124] Ortlepp and colleagues[125] investigated the association of fasting glucose, low physical activity, and BsmI VDR polymorphism. In this study, males with low physical activity and gene carriers with the genotype BB had significantly higher levels of fasting glucose than gene carriers with the genotype Bb or bb. Of note, this effect was not seen in individuals with high physical activity. A recent study found that the BsmI polymorphism seems to influence body mass index (BMI;

weight in kilograms divided by height in meters squared), whereas the FokI seems to affect insulin sensitivity and serum high-density lipoprotein cholesterol (cHDL) level. It was found that BB carriers tend to have higher BMI and waist circumference compared with the bb genotypes. Similarly, FF and Ff carriers had higher fasting insulin levels than the ff carriers, and lower cHDL levels in comparison with ff genotypes.[126] Ye and colleagues[127] also describe a correlation between BMI/obesity and VDR polymorphism. This study found that T2D patients who were diagnosed at 45 years or younger with T-allele of TaqI and the b-allele of BsmI had higher BMI. More recently, Dilmec and colleagues[128] could not find a correlation between VDR polymorphisms (ie, ApaI and TaqI) and T2D risk in a study of 241 individuals (72 patients with T2DM and 169 healthy individuals). Regarding the matter of ethnicity, studies are inconclusive, as associations between VDR polymorphisms and the risk of T2D in different ethnic populations have produced variable results.[129,130]

The pathophysiological mechanisms of these associations remain unexplained, but there seems to be a relation between the VDR genotype and certain traits of susceptibility to T2D. For instance, VDR polymorphisms are linked to obesity, and vitamin D itself has been reported to participate in adipocyte differentiation and metabolism. Moreover, polymorphisms of VDR might play a role in the pathogenesis of T2D by influencing the secretory capacity of β cells.[131] The VDR genotype was associated with altered fasting glucose, confirming the importance of vitamin D in the modulation of insulin secretion (see next section).

Vitamin D and the β cell

There is strong evidence that vitamin D is important for glucose homeostasis and that this could be mediated by its direct action on β-cell function. Several studies in animals and humans indicate a positive correlation between vitamin D deficiency and glucose intolerance as well as impaired insulin secretion.[132–135] Further, this deficiency seems to have a specific effect on insulin and not on other islet hormones such as glucagon.[136] For instance, experiments on glucose- and sulfonylurea-stimulated islets obtained from rats kept on a vitamin D–deficient diet showed impaired insulin secretion and glucose tolerance. These defects were partially corrected by vitamin D replenishment.[132,137,138] However, whether these defects are directly caused by lack of vitamin D or indirectly by hypocalcemia is not clear.

More convincing data on the beneficial effects of vitamin D on insulin secretion were obtained in experiments demonstrating that synthesis and release of insulin by islets isolated from normal animals could be enhanced by glucose challenge in the presence of high doses of $1,25(OH)_2D_3$.[139,140] Stimulation of islets by $1,25(OH)_2D_3$ was shown to significantly increase the levels of cytosolic Ca^{2+}, indicating that this could be a mechanism by which $1,25(OH)_2D_3$ is able to stimulate insulin secretion.[141–143] Ca^{2+} is known to be important for the exocytosis of insulin from the β cell and for β-cell glycolysis, which participates in translating circulating glucose levels.[144,145] Moreover, vitamin D could regulate insulin secretion and synthesis by facilitating the conversion of proinsulin to insulin, which is known to be dependent on the cleavage by β-cell calcium-dependent endopeptidases.[146,147] It is also possible that high intracellular Ca^{2+} improves the binding of calmodulin to the insulin receptor substrate-1, thereby interfering with insulin-stimulated tyrosine phosphorylation and phosphoinositide-3 kinase activation.[148,149] In this regard, PTH has been found to be inversely associated with insulin sensitivity.[150] Another possible mechanism that has been suggested is that vitamin D could directly modulate β-cell growth and differentiation.[151,152]

The effects of $1,25(OH)_2D_3$ and its analogues have been examined regarding binding to nuclear VDR and membrane VDR, through which they induce genomic and nongenomic responses, respectively. Among these studies, Sergeev and Rhoten[153] have reported that the administration of $1,25(OH)_2D_3$ evoked oscillations of intracellular Ca^{2+} in a pancreatic β-cell line within a few minutes. Later, Kajikawa and colleagues[154] demonstrated that the 6-s-*cis* analogue, $1,25(OH)_2$lumisterol$_3$, has a rapid insulinotropic effect, through nongenomic signal transduction via putative membrane VDR, which would be dependent on the augmentation of Ca^{2+} influx through voltage-dependent Ca^{2+} channels on the plasma membrane, being also linked to metabolic signals derived from glucose in pancreatic β cells.

As T2D has been recently associated with systemic inflammation, which is linked primarily to insulin resistance, vitamin D may also improve insulin sensitivity and β-cell function by directly modulating the generation and effects of inflammatory cytokines, as discussed previously.[155]

Animal Studies

Experimental studies in animal models also suggest a role for vitamin D in the pathogenesis of T2D. Animal studies reveal that vitamin D deficiency is associated with impaired insulin sensitivity, while insulin secretion increases through vitamin D supplementation.

Chang-Quan and colleagues[156] reported that T2D was associated with an abnormal vitamin D metabolism that was characterized by deficiency in $1,25(OH)_2D$ and was related to renal injury. In the ob/ob mouse model, treatment with $1\alpha(OH)D$ improved hyperglycemia, hyperinsulinemia, and fat tissue responsiveness to hormones.[157] Anderson and Rowling[158] demonstrated in Zucker Diabetic Fatty rats that vitamin D status was compromised due to poor vitamin D reabsorption in the kidney.

Considering that obesity seems to be an important risk factor to T2D, it was investigated whether vitamin D_3 had a beneficial effect on blood glucose in obese SHR and Wistar rats. Although vitamin D_3 supplementation in SHR rats did not alter the blood glucose levels in all rats, 40% of those rats had a reduction in glucose by 60%. In Wistar rats, a significant reduction in glucose levels in all animals supplemented with vitamin D_3 was found.[159] In addition, feeding of cod liver oil to streptozotocin-induced diabetic rats partially improved their blood glucose levels as well as their cardiovascular and metabolic abnormalities.[160] In another study, vitamin D_3 supplementation of spontaneously hypertensive rats normalized the membrane potential and contractility of aorta.[161]

Clinical Interventions

In view of the cellular, preclinical data and observational studies in man, it seems reasonable to consider that vitamin D status influences the incidence of T2D and that vitamin D supplementation could prevent or ameliorate the disease, at least in cases of (mild) vitamin D deficiency. Despite this, trials in patients have yielded conflicting results (**Table 2**).

Vitamin D_3 supplementation of vitamin D–deficient T2D patients tended to reduce insulin requirements and lower serum triglycerides.[177] Boucher and colleagues[167] showed transient improvement of insulin secretion and C-peptide levels in at-risk patients treated with intramuscular vitamin D. In support to these findings, a small study in which a group of T2D women received 1332 IU of vitamin D_3 daily for 1 month showed an improvement on first-phase insulin secretion and a trend toward decreased insulin resistance.[172] Moreover, the Nurses' Health Study, which included 1,580,957 women over a period of more than 20 years with no history of diabetes, cardiovascular disease, or cancer at baseline, showed that a combined daily intake of greater than 1200 mg calcium and greater than 800 IU vitamin D was associated

Table 2
Reported effects of vitamin D supplementation in humans and etiology of T2D

Intervention	Subjects' Characteristics	Study Results	Refs.
2000 IU vitamin D_3/d (2 y), n = 25 0.25 µg $1\alpha(OH)D_3$/d (2 y), n = 23 >0.25 µg $1,25(OH)_2D_3$/d (1 y), n = 40	n = 238 Postmenopausal women Age 45–54 y	Fasting glucose levels =	[162]
2 µg $1\alpha(OH)D_3$/d (3 wk)	7 cases; 7 controls T2D Japanese patients Age ~54 y	Insulin secretion ↑ Free fatty acid ↓	[163]
2000 IU vitamin D_3/d (6 mo)	4 cases; 10 controls Vitamin D deficient subjects Age ~32 y	Insulin secretion ↑	[164]
0.75 µg $1\alpha(OH)D_3$/d (3 mo)	65 Caucasian vitamin D sufficient men with impaired glucose tolerance Age 61–65 y	Glucose levels = Insulin secretion = Body weight ↓ Urinary calcium ↑	[165]
2000 IU vitamin D/d (1 mo)	1 Vitamin D deficient hypocalcemic woman Age ~65 y	Glucose tolerance ↑ β-Cell function ↑	[166]
Single IV injection of 100,000 IU vitamin D_3	22 Vitamin D deficient subjects Age ~45 y	Insulin and C-peptide ↑	[167]
500 mg Ca^{2+} and/or 0.5 µg $1,25(OH)_2D_3$/d (21 d)	17 Uremic men and women Age ~50 y	First-phase insulin secretion and insulin sensitivity ↑	[168]
Oral 1 µg $1,25(OH)_2D_3$/d (4 d)	20 T2D men and women Age ~60 y	Insulin secretion and C-peptide ↑ Urinary calcium ↑ in patients with short duration of diabetes	[169]
1.5 µg $1,25(OH)_2D_3$/d (7 d)	18 Healthy young men Age ~26 y	PTH concentration ↓ Urinary calcium ↑	[170]
Single IM injection 300,000 IU vitamin D_2	3 T2D men and women	Insulin resistance ↑	[171]
1332 IU vitamin D_3/d (1 mo)	10 T2D women Age ~54 y	First-phase insulin secretion ↑	[172]
Vitamin D and/or calcium supplementation	4843 cases; 1,576,114 controls Female nurses Age ~46 y	23% ↓ risk of T2D when vitamin D consumption/d is ≥800 IU compared with <200 IU/d	[173]
500 mg calcium and 700 IU vitamin D_3/d (3 y)	314 Nondiabetic Caucasians Age ~71 y	Rise glycemia and insulin resistance ↓ in patients with impaired fasting glucose levels	[174]
1000 mg Calcium and 400 IU vitamin D_3/d (6 y)	2291 cases; 31,660 controls Postmenopausal women Age 50–79 y	Insulin or glucose levels = Diabetes incidence =	[175]
3 doses of 120,000 IU vitamin D_3/fortnight (6 wk)	1000 healthy, centrally obese males Age ≥35 y	Insulin secretion = Insulin sensitivity ↑	[176]

In column 1, intervention period is given in parentheses.

with a 33% lower risk of T2D compared with an intake of less than 600 mg and 400 IU calcium and vitamin D.[173] In 2008, 2 nested case-control studies, collected by the Finnish Mobile Clinic from 1973 to 1980, were pooled for analysis. These results supported the hypothesis that high vitamin D status provides protection against T2D.[178] Recently, a New Zealand study found that South Asian women with insulin resistance improved markedly after taking vitamin D supplements.[179] Optimal vitamin D concentrations for reducing insulin resistance were shown to be 80 to 119 nmol/L, providing further evidence for an increase in the recommended adequate levels.

On the other hand, some studies show no effect of vitamin D supplementation and improvement of T2D. For instance, the Women's Health Initiative, in which low-dose calcium and 400 IU/d of vitamin D supplementation were given, did not show protection against diabetes.[175] It was recently reported that daily oral administration of 800 IU (20 μg) vitamin D_3 alone or in association with 1000 mg calcium to older people also failed to prevent T2D.[180] In one study, Asian T2D patients with vitamin D deficiency even had a worsening of their condition through increased insulin resistance and deterioration of glycemic control.[171] Another point to note is that, in general, no benefits in glucose tolerance have been seen with vitamin D supplementation in patients who are not vitamin D deficient.[108] Of importance is that some of these studies reported elevation in calcium urinary excretion in vitamin D–supplemented individuals.[165,169,170] The contradictory results of vitamin D supplementation in T2D suggest that dose and method of supplementation, as well as the genetic background and baseline vitamin D status of individuals, appear to be important for the efficacy of vitamin D supplementation against development of T2D.

GESTATIONAL DIABETES

GD is defined by β-cell dysfunction and insulin resistance during pregnancy. Women who have had GD have a 20% to 50% chance of developing T2D within 5 to 10 years.

Several studies demonstrated that pregnant women are more susceptible to hypovitaminosis D[181,182] and can suffer from insulin resistance.[4,183] Studies on the role of vitamin D and the regulation of glucose homeostasis in pregnancy are scarce, and data are not always consistent. Nevertheless, Zhang and colleagues[184] reported that each 5 ng/mL decrease in 25(OH)D levels relates to a 1.29-fold increase in GD risk. In addition, vitamin D depletion during pregnancy, aside from the classically known consequences such as decreased bone density and development of rickets in offspring, has also been associated with nonclassic consequences such as reduced fetal growth, disturbed brain development, and induction of T1D development.[185]

A study by Rudnicki and Molsted-Pederson,[186] in which they injected pregnant GD-diagnosed women intravenously with 1,25(OH)$_2$D, showed that these women had a transient decrease in fasting glucose levels but surprisingly also a decrease in insulin levels. These apparent contradictory results suggest that vitamin D could directly increase cellular glucose absorption by increasing insulin sensitivity.

VITAMIN D AND DIABETES COMPLICATIONS
Kidney Failure

Over time, hyperglycemia can have a damaging effect on the kidneys. Zhang and colleagues[187] reported that the prodrug vitamin D analogue, doxercalciferol (1α(OH)D$_2$), may protect kidneys in mice with diabetic nephropathy. This result suggests that vitamin D might be useful and preventative for the kidneys. The NHANES survey found that 25(OH)D levels were significantly lower in persons with severely decreased glomerular filtration rate when compared with healthy individuals.

In addition, persons with higher levels of 25(OH)D had decreased glucose homeostasis model assessment of insulin resistance (HOMA-IR), but 25(OH)D levels did not correlate with β-cell function (also estimated by HOMA).[188] In a cross-sectional analysis of the 2001 to 2006 NHANES study, diabetic patients with nephropathy had a high prevalence of vitamin D deficiency and insufficiency.[189] This finding may be worrisome, as recent work by Wolf and colleagues[190] suggested that vitamin D deficiency in hemodialysis patients was associated with increased mortality risks. Of note, an independent association between vitamin D deficiency and insufficiency with the presence of diabetic nephropathy was seen.[189] Given these findings, the improvement of the vitamin D status or pharmacologic intervention with vitamin D analogues for the prevention or treatment of renal failure needs further study.

Vision Loss and Blindness

Although not a sudden process, subjects with diabetes face a very real threat of vision loss, including blindness (diabetic retinopathy). Diabetes also increases the risk of developing cataracts (clouding of the eyes lenses) and glaucoma (damage to the optic nerves). In T2D patients, severity of retinopathy was inversely correlated with serum $1,25(OH)_2D_3$ levels.[191] Age-related macular degeneration (AMD) occurs when the macula, the area at the back of the retina that produces the sharpest vision, deteriorates over time. AMD is the most common cause of blindness among individuals older than 50 years. Levels of serum vitamin D were inversely associated with early AMD.[192] These data suggest that vitamin D supplementation might have a beneficial effect on eye health.

Hypertension, Heart Attack, and Stroke

As many as 65% of diabetic patients will eventually die of heart failure or stroke. A wealth of recent data suggests a central role of the vitamin D endocrine system on blood pressure regulation and cardiovascular health. For this important topic, recent reviews discussing a potential link between low 25(OH)D levels and cardiovascular disease and the possible mechanisms mediating it have been published.[193–195] Here it was summarized that severe vitamin D deficiency or resistance caused hypertension in animal models. In addition, mild vitamin D deficiency was associated with higher blood pressure in Caucasians, Hispanics, and African Americans.[196] In recent years, Pilz and colleagues[197] have demonstrated a clear association between low levels of 25(OH)D as well as of $1,25(OH)_2D$ with prevalent myocardial dysfunction, deaths due to heart failure, and sudden cardiac death. In the Multi-Ethnic Study of Atherosclerosis, low 25(OH)D levels were linked to increased risk for developing incident coronary artery calcification.[198] Also, direct effects of vitamin D on the cardiovascular system may be involved. Because various tissues such as cardiomyocytes,[199] vascular smooth muscle cells,[200] and endothelial cells express the VDR and vitamin D affects inflammation as well as cellular proliferation and differentiation, vitamin D may lower the risk of developing cardiovascular disease. A recent meta-analysis of 18 independent randomized controlled trials for vitamin D, including 57,311 participants, described that intake of regular vitamin D supplements (from 300 IU to 2000 IU) was associated with reduced mortality risk (relative risk 0.93; 95% CI, 0.87–0.99).[201] Interventional trials are warranted to elucidate whether vitamin D replenishment is useful for prevention or treatment of cardiovascular diseases and other health outcomes.

Nerve Damage and Dementia

Neuropathy is a common complication in diabetic patients, with a hallmark of sensory neuropathy being the loss of sensation in feet, a risk factor for limb amputation.

Recently, diabetic neuropathy has been linked with low levels of 25(OH)D.[202] In this study, a total of (only) 51 patients with T2D (all vitamin D insufficient) with typical neuropathic pain were included and given vitamin D_3 treatment (mean dose, approximately 2000 IU). Serum concentrations of 25(OH)D increased from 18 to 30 ng/mL, and the intervention was associated with significant pain reduction. Whether vitamin D can be useful as therapeutic application for neuropathic pain needs to be elucidated in adequately powered prospective clinical studies.

Diabetes also increases the risk of Alzheimer disease and vascular dementia.[203] There is ample biologic evidence to support a role for vitamin D in neuroprotection and reducing inflammation, and moreover to put forward a role for vitamin D in brain development and function.[30] Whether vitamin D can reduce the risk of diseases linked to dementia, such as vascular and metabolic diseases like diabetes, needs further investigation.

Bone Fractures

Large cross-sectional studies have indicated that patients with T2D have significantly increased risk of bone fractures, predominantly hip fractures.[204] This group of patients frequently displayed loss of vision caused by diabetic eye disease, peripheral neuropathy, arterial hypertension, orthostatic hypotonia, and ischemic disease of the brain, heart, and lower extremities—conditions that predispose to falls. Lately, frequently used drugs in T2D (thiazolidinediones) have been implicated in an increase in bone fractures. Implication of the vitamin D system in this issue is unlikely, but data are scarce. The ADOPT (A Diabetes Outcome Progression Trial) group recently reported slightly reduced vitamin D levels in rosiglitazone-treated patients compared with metformin-treated patients.[205] Moreover, as vitamin D exerts a direct action on skeletal muscle function,[206] it was suggested that T2D patients might benefit from eliminating unfavorable diet and environmental factors, such as low physical action and low vitamin D intake. Several meta-analyses of randomized controlled trials showed that vitamin D supplementation (>400 IU/d) reduces the risk of nonvertebral fractures by 20% and hip fractures by 18%.[207,208] These studies also pointed out that vitamin D deficiency is common in patients with hip fractures, and truly contributes to the risk of fracture.

SUMMARY

There is no doubt that vitamin D deficiency is the cause of several metabolic bone diseases, but vitamin D status is also linked to many major human diseases including immune disorders. Mounting data strengthen the link between vitamin D and diabetes, in particular T1D and T2D. Despite some inconsistencies between studies that associate serum 25(OH)D levels with the risk of developing T1D or T2D, there seems to be an overall trend for an inverse correlation between levels of 25(OH)D and both disorders. There is also compelling evidence that $1,25(OH)_2D$ regulates β-cell function by different mechanisms, such as influencing insulin secretion by regulating intracellular levels of Ca^{2+}, increasing β-cell resistance to apoptosis, and perhaps also increasing β-cell replication.

The capacity of vitamin D, more specifically $1,25(OH)_2D$, to modulate immune responses is of particular interest for both the therapy and prevention of diabetes. In the case of T1D, vitamin D supplementation in prediabetic individuals could help prevent or reduce the initiation of autoimmune processes possibly by regulating thymic selection of the T-cell repertoire, decreasing the numbers of autoreactive T cells, and inducing Treg cells. Although immune modulation is generally discussed for the treatment of T1D, it is also relevant for T2D. Indeed, recent studies have shown that T2D patients have increased systemic inflammation and that this state can induce β-cell dysfunction and death.

Supplementation trials with regular vitamin D for the protection against the development of T1D and T2D have generated some contradictory data, but many weaknesses can be identified in these trials as most were underpowered or open-labeled. However, the overwhelming strength of preclinical data and of the observational studies make vitamin D or its analogues strong candidates for the prevention or treatment of diabetes or its complications. However, proof of causality needs well-designed clinical trials and if positive, adequate dosing, regimen, and compound studies are needed to define the contribution of vitamin D status and therapy in the global diabetes problem. There are many confounding factors that need to be taken into consideration when translating successful vitamin D therapies in animal models into humans, for example, gender, age, lifestyle, and genetic background. To come to solid conclusions on the potential of vitamin D or its analogues in the prevention of or therapy for all forms of diabetes, it is clear that large prospective trials with carefully selected populations and end points will be needed, but should also receive high priority.

REFERENCES

1. IDF diabetes atlas. 4th edition. International Diabetes Federation; 2009. Available at: http://www.diabetesatlas.org/. Accessed November 11, 2009.
2. LeRoith D. Beta-cell dysfunction and insulin resistance in type 2 diabetes: role of metabolic and genetic abnormalities. Am J Med 2002;113(Suppl 6A):3S–11S.
3. Knip M, Siljander H. Autoimmune mechanisms in type 1 diabetes. Autoimmun Rev 2008;7(7):550–7.
4. Palomer X, Gonzalez-Clemente JM, Blanco-Vaca F, et al. Role of vitamin D in the pathogenesis of type 2 diabetes mellitus. Diabetes Obes Metab 2008;10(3): 185–97.
5. Wilkin TJ. Changing perspectives in diabetes: their impact on its classification. Diabetologia 2007;50(8):1587–92.
6. Resmini E, Minuto F, Colao A, et al. Secondary diabetes associated with principal endocrinopathies: the impact of new treatment modalities. Acta Diabetol 2009;46(2):85–95.
7. Bouillon R, Carmeliet G, Verlinden L, et al. Vitamin D and human health: lessons from vitamin D receptor null mice. Endocr Rev 2008;29(6):726–76.
8. Mathieu C, Gysemans C, Giulietti A, et al. Vitamin D and diabetes. Diabetologia 2005;48(7):1247–57.
9. Nyomba BL, Auwerx J, Bormans V, et al. Pancreatic secretion in man with subclinical vitamin D deficiency. Diabetologia 1986;29(1):34–8.
10. Harris SS. Vitamin D in type 1 diabetes prevention. J Nutr 2005;135(2):323–5.
11. Knip M. Natural course of preclinical type 1 diabetes. Horm Res 2002;57(Suppl 1):6–11.
12. Barrett JC, Clayton DG, Concannon P, et al. Genome-wide association study and meta-analysis find that over 40 loci affect risk of type 1 diabetes. Nat Genet 2009;41(6):703–7.
13. Steck AK, Zhang W, Bugawan TL, et al. Do non-HLA genes influence development of persistent islet autoimmunity and type 1 diabetes in children with high-risk HLA-DR, DQ genotypes? Diabetes 2009;58(4):1028–33.

14. Concannon P, Rich SS, Nepom GT. Genetics of type 1A diabetes. N Engl J Med 2009;360(16):1646–54.
15. Lopez ER, Regulla K, Pani MA, et al. CYP27B1 polymorphisms variants are associated with type 1 diabetes mellitus in Germans. J Steroid Biochem Mol Biol 2004;89–90(1–5):155–7.
16. Pani MA, Regulla K, Segni M, et al. Vitamin D 1alpha-hydroxylase (CYP1alpha) polymorphism in Graves' disease, Hashimoto's thyroiditis and type 1 diabetes mellitus. Eur J Endocrinol 2002;146(6):777–81.
17. Bailey R, Cooper JD, Zeitels L, et al. Association of the vitamin D metabolism gene CYP27B1 with type 1 diabetes. Diabetes 2007;56(10):2616–21.
18. Ogunkolade BW, Boucher BJ, Prahl JM, et al. Vitamin D receptor (VDR) mRNA and VDR protein levels in relation to vitamin D status, insulin secretory capacity, and VDR genotype in Bangladeshi Asians. Diabetes 2002;51(7):2294–300.
19. van Etten E, Verlinden L, Giulietti A, et al. The vitamin D receptor gene FokI polymorphism: functional impact on the immune system. Eur J Immunol 2007;37(2): 395–405.
20. Garcia D, Angel B, Carrasco E, et al. VDR polymorphisms influence the immune response in type 1 diabetic children from Santiago, Chile. Diabetes Res Clin Pract 2007;77(1):134–40.
21. Pociot F, McDermott MF. Genetics of type 1 diabetes mellitus. Genes Immun 2002;3(5):235–49.
22. Pani MA, Knapp M, Donner H, et al. Vitamin D receptor allele combinations influence genetic susceptibility to type 1 diabetes in Germans. Diabetes 2000;49(3): 504–7.
23. Chang TJ, Lei HH, Yeh JI, et al. Vitamin D receptor gene polymorphisms influence susceptibility to type 1 diabetes mellitus in the Taiwanese population. Clin Endocrinol (Oxf) 2000;52(5):575–80.
24. Guo SW, Magnuson VL, Schiller JJ, et al. Meta-analysis of vitamin D receptor polymorphisms and type 1 diabetes: a HuGE review of genetic association studies. Am J Epidemiol 2006;164(8):711–24.
25. Lemos MC, Fagulha A, Coutinho E, et al. Lack of association of vitamin D receptor gene polymorphisms with susceptibility to type 1 diabetes mellitus in the Portuguese population. Hum Immunol 2008;69(2):134–8.
26. Turpeinen H, Hermann R, Vaara S, et al. Vitamin D receptor polymorphisms: no association with type 1 diabetes in the Finnish population. Eur J Endocrinol 2003;149(6):591–6.
27. Israni N, Goswami R, Kumar A, et al. Interaction of vitamin D receptor with HLA DRB1 0301 in type 1 diabetes patients from North India. PLoS One 2009;4(12): e8023.
28. Karvonen M, Viik-Kajander M, Moltchanova E, et al. Incidence of childhood type 1 diabetes worldwide. Diabetes Mondiale (DiaMond) Project Group. Diabetes Care 2000;23(10):1516–26.
29. Geographic patterns of childhood insulin-dependent diabetes mellitus. Diabetes Epidemiology Research International Group. Diabetes 1988;37(8): 1113–9.
30. Sloka S, Grant M, Newhook LA. The geospatial relation between UV solar radiation and type 1 diabetes in Newfoundland. Acta Diabetol 2010;47(1):73–8.
31. Staples JA, Ponsonby AL, Lim LL, et al. Ecologic analysis of some immune-related disorders, including type 1 diabetes, in Australia: latitude, regional ultraviolet radiation, and disease prevalence. Environ Health Perspect 2003;111(4): 518–23.

32. Cantorna MT, Mahon BD. Mounting evidence for vitamin D as an environmental factor affecting autoimmune disease prevalence. Exp Biol Med (Maywood) 2004;229(11):1136–42.
33. Mohr SB, Garland CF, Gorham ED, et al. The association between ultraviolet B irradiance, vitamin D status and incidence rates of type 1 diabetes in 51 regions worldwide. Diabetologia 2008;51(8):1391–8.
34. Karvonen M, Jantti V, Muntoni S, et al. Comparison of the seasonal pattern in the clinical onset of IDDM in Finland and Sardinia. Diabetes Care 1998;21(7): 1101–9.
35. Neu A, Kehrer M, Hub R, et al. Incidence of IDDM in German children aged 0-14 years. A 6-year population-based study (1987–1993). Diabetes Care 1997; 20(4):530–3.
36. Kahn HS, Morgan TM, Case LD, et al. Association of type 1 diabetes with month of birth among U.S. youth: the SEARCH for Diabetes in Youth Study. Diabetes Care 2009;32(11):2010–5.
37. Bouillon R, Verstuyf A, Branisteanu D, et al. [Immune modulation by vitamin D analogs in the prevention of autoimmune diseases]. Verh K Acad Geneeskd Belg 1995;57(5):371–7 [in Dutch].
38. Provvedini DM, Tsoukas CD, Deftos LJ, et al. 1,25-dihydroxyvitamin D_3 receptors in human leukocytes. Science 1983;221(4616):1181–3.
39. Veldman CM, Cantorna MT, DeLuca HF. Expression of 1,25-dihydroxyvitamin D_3 receptor in the immune system. Arch Biochem Biophys 2000;374(2): 334–8.
40. Dong X, Lutz W, Schroeder TM, et al. Regulation of relB in dendritic cells by means of modulated association of vitamin D receptor and histone deacetylase 3 with the promoter. Proc Natl Acad Sci U S A 2005;102(44): 16007–12.
41. Muthian G, Raikwar HP, Rajasingh J, et al. 1,25 Dihydroxyvitamin-D_3 modulates JAK-STAT pathway in IL-12/IFNgamma axis leading to Th1 response in experimental allergic encephalomyelitis. J Neurosci Res 2006;83(7): 1299–309.
42. Guery JC, Adorini L. Dendritic cells are the most efficient in presenting endogenous naturally processed self-epitopes to class II-restricted T cells. J Immunol 1995;154(2):536–44.
43. Schwartz RH. A cell culture model for T lymphocyte clonal anergy. Science 1990;248(4961):1349–56.
44. Griffin MD, Lutz WH, Phan VA, et al. Potent inhibition of dendritic cell differentiation and maturation by vitamin D analogs. Biochem Biophys Res Commun 2000;270(3):701–8.
45. van Halteren AG, van Etten E, de Jong EC, et al. Redirection of human autoreactive T-cells upon interaction with dendritic cells modulated by TX527, an analog of 1,25 dihydroxyvitamin D3. Diabetes 2002;51(7):2119–25.
46. van Etten E, Dardenne O, Gysemans C, et al. 1,25-Dihydroxyvitamin D_3 alters the profile of bone marrow-derived dendritic cells of NOD mice. Ann N Y Acad Sci 2004;1037:186–92.
47. Penna G, Adorini L. 1 Alpha,25-dihydroxyvitamin D_3 inhibits differentiation, maturation, activation, and survival of dendritic cells leading to impaired alloreactive T cell activation. J Immunol 2000;164(5):2405–11.
48. van Halteren AG, Tysma OM, van Etten E, et al. 1alpha,25-dihydroxyvitamin D_3 or analogue treated dendritic cells modulate human autoreactive T cells via the selective induction of apoptosis. J Autoimmun 2004;23(3):233–9.

49. Ferreira GB, van Etten E, Lage K, et al. Proteome analysis demonstrates profound alterations in human dendritic cell nature by TX527, an analogue of vitamin D. Proteomics 2009;9(14):3752–64.

50. Adorini L. Tolerogenic dendritic cells induced by vitamin D receptor ligands enhance regulatory T cells inhibiting autoimmune diabetes. Ann N Y Acad Sci 2003;987:258–61.

51. Penna G, Roncari A, Amuchastegui S, et al. Expression of the inhibitory receptor ILT3 on dendritic cells is dispensable for induction of CD4+Foxp3+ regulatory T cells by 1,25-dihydroxyvitamin D_3. Blood 2005;106(10):3490–7.

52. Bhalla AK, Amento EP, Serog B, et al. 1,25-Dihydroxyvitamin D_3 inhibits antigen-induced T cell activation. J Immunol 1984;133(4):1748–54.

53. Rigby WF, Stacy T, Fanger MW. Inhibition of T lymphocyte mitogenesis by 1,25-dihydroxyvitamin D_3 (calcitriol). J Clin Invest 1984;74(4):1451–5.

54. Nunn JD, Katz DR, Barker S, et al. Regulation of human tonsillar T-cell proliferation by the active metabolite of vitamin D_3. Immunology 1986;59(4):479–84.

55. Matsui T, Nakao Y, Koizumi T, et al. 1,25-Dihydroxyvitamin D_3 regulates proliferation of activated T-lymphocyte subsets. Life Sci 1985;37(1):95–101.

56. Rigby WF, Denome S, Fanger MW. Regulation of lymphokine production and human T lymphocyte activation by 1,25-dihydroxyvitamin D_3. Specific inhibition at the level of messenger RNA. J Clin Invest 1987;79(6):1659–64.

57. Boonstra A, Barrat FJ, Crain C, et al. 1alpha,25-Dihydroxyvitamin D_3 has a direct effect on naïve CD4(+) T cells to enhance the development of Th2 cells. J Immunol 2001;167(9):4974–80.

58. Willheim M, Thien R, Schrattbauer K, et al. Regulatory effects of 1alpha,25-dihydroxyvitamin D_3 on the cytokine production of human peripheral blood lymphocytes. J Clin Endocrinol Metab 1999;84(10):3739–44.

59. Gregori S, Giarratana N, Smiroldo S, et al. 1alpha,25-dihydroxyvitamin D_3 analog enhances regulatory T-cells and arrests autoimmune diabetes in NOD mice. Diabetes 2002;51(5):1367–74.

60. Ghoreishi M, Bach P, Obst J, et al. Expansion of antigen-specific regulatory T cells with the topical vitamin D analog calcipotriol. J Immunol 2009;182(10):6071–8.

61. Hewison M, Gacad MA, Lemire J, et al. Vitamin D as a cytokine and hematopoetic factor. Rev Endocr Metab Disord 2001;2(2):217–27.

62. Baeke F, van Etten E, Gysemans C, et al. Vitamin D signaling in immune-mediated disorders: evolving insights and therapeutic opportunities. Mol Aspects Med 2008;29(6):376–87.

63. Jeffery LE, Burke F, Mura M, et al. 1,25-Dihydroxyvitamin D_3 and IL-2 combine to inhibit T cell production of inflammatory cytokines and promote development of regulatory T cells expressing CTLA-4 and FoxP3. J Immunol 2009;183(9):5458–67.

64. Chen S, Sims GP, Chen XX, et al. Modulatory effects of 1,25-dihydroxyvitamin D_3 on human B cell differentiation. J Immunol 2007;179(3):1634–47.

65. Shiozawa S, Shiozawa K, Tanaka Y, et al. 1 alpha,25-Dihydroxyvitamin D_3 inhibits proliferative response of T- and B-lymphocytes in a serum-free culture. Int J Immunopharmacol 1987;9(6):719–23.

66. Imazeki I, Matsuzaki J, Tsuji K, et al. Immunomodulating effect of vitamin D_3 derivatives on type-1 cellular immunity. Biomed Res 2006;27(1):1–9.

67. van Etten E, Mathieu C. Immunoregulation by 1,25-dihydroxyvitamin D_3: basic concepts. J Steroid Biochem Mol Biol 2005;97(1–2):93–101.

68. Sia C. Imbalance in Th cell polarization and its relevance in type 1 diabetes mellitus. Rev Diabet Stud 2005;2(4):182–6.
69. Flores M. A role of vitamin D in low-intensity chronic inflammation and insulin resistance in type 2 diabetes mellitus? Nutr Res Rev 2005;18(2):175–82.
70. Eizirik DL, Cardozo AK, Cnop M. The role for endoplasmic reticulum stress in diabetes mellitus. Endocr Rev 2008;29(1):42–61.
71. Hahn HJ, Kuttler B, Mathieu C, et al. 1,25-Dihydroxyvitamin D_3 reduces MHC antigen expression on pancreatic beta-cells in vitro. Transplant Proc 1997; 29(4):2156–7.
72. Riachy R, Vandewalle B, Kerr Conte J, et al. 1,25-dihydroxyvitamin D_3 protects RINm5F and human islet cells against cytokine-induced apoptosis: implication of the antiapoptotic protein A20. Endocrinology 2002;143(12):4809–19.
73. Riachy R, Vandewalle B, Moerman E, et al. 1,25-Dihydroxyvitamin D_3 protects human pancreatic islets against cytokine-induced apoptosis via down-regulation of the Fas receptor. Apoptosis 2006;11(2):151–9.
74. Gysemans CA, Cardozo AK, Callewaert H, et al. 1,25-Dihydroxyvitamin D_3 modulates expression of chemokines and cytokines in pancreatic islets: implications for prevention of diabetes in nonobese diabetic mice. Endocrinology 2005;146(4):1956–64.
75. Mathieu C, Waer M, Laureys J, et al. Prevention of autoimmune diabetes in NOD mice by 1,25 dihydroxyvitamin D3. Diabetologia 1994;37(6):552–8.
76. Mathieu C, Laureys J, Sobis H, et al. 1,25-Dihydroxyvitamin D_3 prevents insulitis in NOD mice. Diabetes 1992;41(11):1491–5.
77. Decallonne B, van Etten E, Overbergh L, et al. 1Alpha,25-dihydroxyvitamin D_3 restores thymocyte apoptosis sensitivity in non-obese diabetic (NOD) mice through dendritic cells. J Autoimmun 2005;24(4):281–9.
78. Casteels K, Waer M, Bouillon R, et al. 1,25-Dihydroxyvitamin D_3 restores sensitivity to cyclophosphamide-induced apoptosis in non-obese diabetic (NOD) mice and protects against diabetes. Clin Exp Immunol 1998;112(2):181–7.
79. Mathieu C, Waer M, Casteels K, et al. Prevention of type I diabetes in NOD mice by nonhypercalcemic doses of a new structural analog of 1,25-dihydroxyvitamin D_3, KH1060. Endocrinology 1995;136(3):866–72.
80. Del Pino-Montes J, Benito GE, Fernandez-Salazar MP, et al. Calcitriol improves streptozotocin-induced diabetes and recovers bone mineral density in diabetic rats. Calcif Tissue Int 2004;75(6):526–32.
81. Keymeulen B, Vandemeulebroucke E, Ziegler AG, et al. Insulin needs after CD3-antibody therapy in new-onset type 1 diabetes. N Engl J Med 2005;352(25): 2598–608.
82. Casteels K, Waer M, Laureys J, et al. Prevention of autoimmune destruction of syngeneic islet grafts in spontaneously diabetic nonobese diabetic mice by a combination of a vitamin D_3 analog and cyclosporine. Transplantation 1998; 65(9):1225–32.
83. Mathieu C, Van Etten E, Gysemans C, et al. In vitro and in vivo analysis of the immune system of vitamin D receptor knockout mice. J Bone Miner Res 2001; 16(11):2057–65.
84. Gysemans C, Van Etten E, Overbergh L, et al. Treatment of autoimmune diabetes recurrence in non-obese diabetic mice by mouse interferon-beta in combination with an analogue of 1alpha,25-dihydroxyvitamin-D3. Clin Exp Immunol 2002;128(2):213–20.
85. Zeitz U, Weber K, Soegiarto DW, et al. Impaired insulin secretory capacity in mice lacking a functional vitamin D receptor. FASEB J 2003;17(3):509–11.

86. Gysemans C, van Etten E, Overbergh L, et al. Unaltered diabetes presentation in NOD mice lacking the vitamin D receptor. Diabetes 2008;57(1): 269–75.

87. Hypponen E, Laara E, Reunanen A, et al. Intake of vitamin D and risk of type 1 diabetes: a birth-cohort study. Lancet 2001;358(9292):1500–3.

88. Stene LC, Ulriksen J, Magnus P, et al. Use of cod liver oil during pregnancy associated with lower risk of type I diabetes in the offspring. Diabetologia 2000;43(9):1093–8.

89. Stene LC, Joner G. Use of cod liver oil during the first year of life is associated with lower risk of childhood-onset type 1 diabetes: a large, population-based, case-control study. Am J Clin Nutr 2003;78(6):1128–34.

90. Vitamin D supplement in early childhood and risk for type I (insulin-dependent) diabetes mellitus. The EURODIAB Substudy 2 Study Group. Diabetologia 1999; 42(1):51–4.

91. Zipitis CS, Akobeng AK. Vitamin D supplementation in early childhood and risk of type 1 diabetes: a systematic review and meta-analysis. Arch Dis Child 2008; 93(6):512–7.

92. Fronczak CM, Baron AE, Chase HP, et al. In utero dietary exposures and risk of islet autoimmunity in children. Diabetes Care 2003;26(12):3237–42.

93. Wicklow BA, Taback SP. Feasibility of a type 1 diabetes primary prevention trial using 2000 IU vitamin D3 in infants from the general population with increased HLA-associated risk. Ann N Y Acad Sci 2006;1079:310–2.

94. Pitocco D, Crino A, Di Stasio E, et al. The effects of calcitriol and nicotinamide on residual pancreatic beta-cell function in patients with recent-onset Type 1 diabetes (IMDIAB XI). Diabet Med 2006;23(8):920–3.

95. Pozzilli P, Di Mario U. Autoimmune diabetes not requiring insulin at diagnosis (latent autoimmune diabetes of the adult): definition, characterization, and potential prevention. Diabetes Care 2001;24(8):1460–7.

96. Li X, Liao L, Yan X, et al. Protective effects of 1-alpha-hydroxyvitamin D_3 on residual beta-cell function in patients with adult-onset latent autoimmune diabetes (LADA). Diabetes Metab Res Rev 2009;25(5):411–6.

97. Pittas AG, Harris SS, Eliades M, et al. Association between serum osteocalcin and markers of metabolic phenotype. J Clin Endocrinol Metab 2009;94(3): 827–32.

98. Guillausseau PJ, Meas T, Virally M, et al. Abnormalities in insulin secretion in type 2 diabetes mellitus. Diabetes Metab 2008;34(Suppl 2):S43–8.

99. Zimmet P, Alberti KG, Shaw J. Global and societal implications of the diabetes epidemic. Nature 2001;414(6865):782–7.

100. Zittermann A. Vitamin D in preventive medicine: are we ignoring the evidence? Br J Nutr 2003;89(5):552–72.

101. Scragg R. Vitamin D and type 2 diabetes: are we ready for a prevention trial? Diabetes 2008;57(10):2565–6.

102. Scragg R, Sowers M, Bell C. Serum 25-hydroxyvitamin D, diabetes, and ethnicity in the third national health and nutrition examination survey. Diabetes care 2004;27(12):2813–8.

103. Chiu KC, Chu A, Go VL, et al. Hypovitaminosis D is associated with insulin resistance and beta cell dysfunction. Am J Clin Nutr 2004;79(5): 820–5.

104. Ford ES, Ajani UA, McGuire LC, et al. Concentrations of serum vitamin D and the metabolic syndrome among U.S. adults. Diabetes Care 2005;28(5): 1228–30.

105. Forouhi NG, Luan J, Hennings S, et al. Incidence of Type 2 diabetes in England and its association with baseline impaired fasting glucose: the Ely study 1990–2000. Diabet Med 2007;24(2):200–7.

106. Clark SA, Stumpf WE, Sar M. Effect of 1,25 dihydroxyvitamin D_3 on insulin secretion. Diabetes 1981;30(5):382–6.

107. Boucher BJ. Inadequate vitamin D status: does it contribute to the disorders comprising syndrome 'X'? Br J Nutr 1998;79(4):315–27.

108. Cigolini M, Iagulli MP, Miconi V, et al. Serum 25-hydroxyvitamin D_3 concentrations and prevalence of cardiovascular disease among type 2 diabetic patients. Diabetes care 2006;29(3):722–4.

109. Giulietti A, van Etten E, Overbergh L, et al. Monocytes from type 2 diabetic patients have a pro-inflammatory profile. 1,25-Dihydroxyvitamin D(3) works as anti-inflammatory. Diabetes Res Clin Pract 2007;77(1):47–57.

110. DeFronzo RA, Tripathy D. Skeletal muscle insulin resistance is the primary defect in type 2 diabetes. Diabetes Care 2009;32(Suppl 2):S157–63.

111. Boucher BJ. Does vitamin D status contribute to caveolin-1-mediated insulin sensitivity in skeletal muscle? Diabetologia 2009;52(10):2240 author reply 2241–3.

112. Oh YS, Khil LY, Cho KA, et al. A potential role for skeletal muscle caveolin-1 as an insulin sensitivity modulator in ageing-dependent non-obese type 2 diabetes: studies in a new mouse model. Diabetologia 2008;51(6):1025–34.

113. Huhtakangas JA, Olivera CJ, Bishop JE, et al. The vitamin D receptor is present in caveolae-enriched plasma membranes and binds 1 alpha,25(OH)2-vitamin D_3 in vivo and in vitro. Mol Endocrinol 2004;18(11):2660–71.

114. Malecki MT. Genetics of type 2 diabetes mellitus. Diabetes Res Clin Pract 2005; 68(Suppl 1):S10–21.

115. Cooke NE, Haddad JG. Vitamin D binding protein (Gc-globulin). Endocr Rev 1989;10(3):294–307.

116. Hirai M, Suzuki S, Hinokio Y, et al. Variations in vitamin D-binding protein (group-specific component protein) are associated with fasting plasma insulin levels in Japanese with normal glucose tolerance. J Clin Endocrinol Metab 2000;85(5):1951–3.

117. Hirai M, Suzuki S, Hinokio Y, et al. Group specific component protein genotype is associated with NIDDM in Japan. Diabetologia 1998;41(6):742–3.

118. Klupa T, Malecki M, Hanna L, et al. Amino acid variants of the vitamin D-binding protein and risk of diabetes in white Americans of European origin. Eur J Endocrinol 1999;141(5):490–3.

119. Malecki MT, Klupa T, Wanic K, et al. Vitamin D binding protein gene and genetic susceptibility to type 2 diabetes mellitus in a Polish population. Diabetes Res Clin Pract 2002;57(2):99–104.

120. Sinotte M, Diorio C, Berube S, et al. Genetic polymorphisms of the vitamin D binding protein and plasma concentrations of 25-hydroxyvitamin D in premenopausal women. Am J Clin Nutr 2009;89(2):634–40.

121. Uitterlinden AG, Fang Y, van Meurs JB, et al. Vitamin D receptor gene polymorphisms in relation to Vitamin D related disease states. J Steroid Biochem Mol Biol 2004;89–90(1–5):187–93.

122. Uitterlinden AG, Fang Y, Van Meurs JB, et al. Genetics and biology of vitamin D receptor polymorphisms. Gene 2004;338(2):143–56.

123. Valdivielso JM, Fernandez E. Vitamin D receptor polymorphisms and diseases. Clin Chim Acta 2006;371(1–2):1–12.

124. Oh JY, Barrett-Connor E. Association between vitamin D receptor polymorphism and type 2 diabetes or metabolic syndrome in community-dwelling older adults: the Rancho Bernardo Study. Metabolism 2002;51(3):356–9.

125. Ortlepp JR, Metrikat J, Albrecht M, et al. The vitamin D receptor gene variant and physical activity predicts fasting glucose levels in healthy young men. Diabet Med 2003;20(6):451–4.

126. Filus A, Trzmiel A, Kuliczkowska-Plaksej J, et al. Relationship between vitamin D receptor BsmI and FokI polymorphisms and anthropometric and biochemical parameters describing metabolic syndrome. Aging Male 2008;11(3):134–9.

127. Ye WZ, Reis AF, Dubois-Laforgue D, et al. Vitamin D receptor gene polymorphisms are associated with obesity in type 2 diabetic subjects with early age of onset. Eur J Endocrinol 2001;145(2):181–6.

128. Dilmec F, Uzer E, Akkafa F, et al. Detection of VDR gene ApaI and TaqI polymorphisms in patients with type 2 diabetes mellitus using PCR-RFLP method in a Turkish population. J Diabetes Complications 2009. [Epub ahead of print].

129. Bid HK, Konwar R, Aggarwal CG, et al. Vitamin D receptor (FokI, BsmI and TaqI) gene polymorphisms and type 2 diabetes mellitus: a North Indian study. Indian J Med Sci 2009;63(5):187–94.

130. Malecki MT, Frey J, Moczulski D, et al. Vitamin D receptor gene polymorphisms and association with type 2 diabetes mellitus in a Polish population. Exp Clin Endocrinol Diabetes 2003;111(8):505–9.

131. Speer G, Cseh K, Winkler G, et al. Oestrogen and vitamin D receptor (VDR) genotypes and the expression of ErbB-2 and EGF receptor in human rectal cancers. Eur J Cancer 2001;37(12):1463–8.

132. Norman AW, Frankel JB, Heldt AM, et al. Vitamin D deficiency inhibits pancreatic secretion of insulin. Science 1980;209(4458):823–5.

133. Chertow BS, Sivitz WI, Baranetsky NG, et al. Cellular mechanisms of insulin release: the effects of vitamin D deficiency and repletion on rat insulin secretion. Endocrinology 1983;113(4):1511–8.

134. Cade C, Norman AW. Vitamin D_3 improves impaired glucose tolerance and insulin secretion in the vitamin D-deficient rat in vivo. Endocrinology 1986;119(1):84–90.

135. Kumar PD, Rajaratnam K. Renal diseases in diabetes mellitus. J Indian Med Assoc 1997;95(7):426–8.

136. Kadowaki T, Miyake Y, Hagura R, et al. Risk factors for worsening to diabetes in subjects with impaired glucose tolerance. Diabetologia 1984;26(1):44–9.

137. Chertow BS, Sivitz WI, Baranetsky NG, et al. Islet insulin release and net calcium retention in vitro in vitamin D-deficient rats. Diabetes 1986;35(7):771–5.

138. Cade C, Norman AW. Rapid normalization/stimulation by 1,25-dihydroxyvitamin D_3 of insulin secretion and glucose tolerance in the vitamin D-deficient rat. Endocrinology 1987;120(4):1490–7.

139. Ishida H, Seino Y, Seino S, et al. Effect of 1,25-dihydroxyvitamin D_3 on pancreatic B and D cell function. Life Sci 1983;33(18):1779–86.

140. d'Emden MC, Dunlop M, Larkins RG, et al. The in vitro effect of 1 alpha,25-dihydroxyvitamin D_3 on insulin production by neonatal rat islets. Biochem Biophys Res Commun 1989;164(1):413–8.

141. de Boland AR, Norman A. Evidence for involvement of protein kinase C and cyclic adenosine 3′,5′ monophosphate-dependent protein kinase in the 1,25-dihydroxy-vitamin D_3-mediated rapid stimulation of intestinal calcium transport, (transcaltachia). Endocrinology 1990;127(1):39–45.

142. Bourlon PM, Faure-Dussert A, Billaudel B. Modulatory role of 1,25 dihydroxyvitamin D_3 on pancreatic islet insulin release via the cyclic AMP pathway in the rat. Br J Pharmacol 1997;121(4):751–8.

143. Hoenderop JG, Dardenne O, Van Abel M, et al. Modulation of renal Ca^{2+} transport protein genes by dietary Ca^{2+} and 1,25-dihydroxyvitamin D_3 in 25-hydroxyvitamin D_3-1alpha-hydroxylase knockout mice. FASEB J 2002;16(11):1398–406.

144. Milner RD, Hales CN. The role of calcium and magnesium in insulin secretion from rabbit pancreas studied in vitro. Diabetologia 1967;3(1):47–9.

145. Hou JC, Min L, Pessin JE. Insulin granule biogenesis, trafficking and exocytosis. Vitam Horm 2009;80:473–506.

146. Rhodes CJ, Alarcon C. What beta-cell defect could lead to hyperproinsulinemia in NIDDM? Some clues from recent advances made in understanding the proinsulin-processing mechanism. Diabetes 1994;43(4):511–7.

147. Hitman GA, Mannan N, McDermott MF, et al. Vitamin D receptor gene polymorphisms influence insulin secretion in Bangladeshi Asians. Diabetes 1998;47(4):688–90.

148. Munshi HG, Burks DJ, Joyal JL, et al. Ca^{2+} regulates calmodulin binding to IQ motifs in IRS-1. Biochemistry 1996;35(49):15883–9.

149. Li Z, Joyal JL, Sacks DB. Binding of IRS proteins to calmodulin is enhanced in insulin resistance. Biochemistry 2000;39(17):5089–96.

150. McCarty MF, Thomas CA. PTH excess may promote weight gain by impeding catecholamine-induced lipolysis-implications for the impact of calcium, vitamin D, and alcohol on body weight. Med Hypotheses 2003;61(5–6):535–42.

151. Lee S, Clark SA, Gill RK, et al. 1,25-Dihydroxyvitamin D_3 and pancreatic beta-cell function: vitamin D receptors, gene expression, and insulin secretion. Endocrinology 1994;134(4):1602–10.

152. Huotari MA, Palgi J, Otonkoski T. Growth factor-mediated proliferation and differentiation of insulin-producing INS-1 and RINm5F cells: identification of betacellulin as a novel beta-cell mitogen. Endocrinology 1998;139(4):1494–9.

153. Sergeev IN, Rhoten WB. 1,25-Dihydroxyvitamin D3 evokes oscillations of intracellular calcium in a pancreatic beta-cell line. Endocrinology 1995;136(7):2852–61.

154. Kajikawa M, Ishida H, Fujimoto S, et al. An insulinotropic effect of vitamin D analog with increasing intracellular Ca^{2+} concentration in pancreatic beta-cells through nongenomic signal transduction. Endocrinology 1999;140(10):4706–12.

155. Larsen CM, Faulenbach M, Vaag A, et al. Sustained effects of interleukin-1 receptor antagonist treatment in type 2 diabetes. Diabetes Care 2009;32(9):1663–8.

156. Chang-Quan H, Bi-Rong D, Ping H, et al. Insulin resistance, renal injury, renal 1-alpha hydroxylase, and bone homeostasis in aged obese rats. Arch Med Res 2008;39(4):380–7.

157. Kawashima H, Castro A. Effect of 1 alpha-hydroxyvitamin D_3 on the glucose and calcium metabolism in genetic obese mice. Res Commun Chem Pathol Pharmacol 1981;33(1):155–61.

158. Anderson RL, Rowling MJ. Renal 25-hydroxycholecalciferol reabsorption is modulated in a type II diabetic rat model [1_meeting abstracts]. FASEB J 2009;23:736.1.

159. de Souza Santos R, Vianna LM. Effect of cholecalciferol supplementation on blood glucose in an experimental model of type 2 diabetes mellitus in spontaneously hypertensive rats and Wistar rats. Clin Chim Acta 2005;358(1–2):146–50.

160. Ceylan-Isik A, Hunkar T, Asan E, et al. Cod liver oil supplementation improves cardiovascular and metabolic abnormalities in streptozotocin diabetic rats. J Pharm Pharmacol 2007;59(12):1629–41.

161. Silva EG, Vianna LM, Okuyama P, et al. Effect of treatment with cholecalciferol on the membrane potential and contractility of aortae from spontaneously hypertensive rats. Br J Pharmacol 1996;118(6):1367–70.

162. Nilas L, Christiansen C. Treatment with vitamin D or its analogues does not change body weight or blood glucose level in postmenopausal women. Int J Obes 1984;8(5):407–11.

163. Inomata S, Kadowaki S, Yamatani T, et al. Effect of 1 alpha (OH)-vitamin D_3 on insulin secretion in diabetes mellitus. Bone Miner 1986;1(3):187–92.

164. Gedik O, Akalin S. Effects of vitamin D deficiency and repletion on insulin and glucagon secretion in man. Diabetologia 1986;29(3):142–5.

165. Ljunghall S, Lind L, Lithell H, et al. Treatment with one-alpha-hydroxycholecalciferol in middle-aged men with impaired glucose tolerance—a prospective randomized double-blind study. Acta Med Scand 1987;222(4):361–7.

166. Kumar S, Davies M, Zakaria Y, et al. Improvement in glucose tolerance and beta-cell function in a patient with vitamin D deficiency during treatment with vitamin D. Postgrad Med J 1994;70(824):440–3.

167. Boucher BJ, Mannan N, Noonan K, et al. Glucose intolerance and impairment of insulin secretion in relation to vitamin D deficiency in east London Asians. Diabetologia 1995;38(10):1239–45.

168. Allegra V, Luisetto G, Mengozzi G, et al. Glucose-induced insulin secretion in uremia: role of 1 alpha,25(HO)2-vitamin D3. Nephron 1994;68(1):41–7.

169. Orwoll E, Riddle M, Prince M. Effects of vitamin D on insulin and glucagon secretion in non-insulin-dependent diabetes mellitus. Am J Clin Nutr 1994;59(5): 1083–7.

170. Fliser D, Stefanski A, Franek E, et al. No effect of calcitriol on insulin-mediated glucose uptake in healthy subjects. Eur J Clin Invest 1997;27(7):629–33.

171. Taylor AV, Wise PH. Vitamin D replacement in Asians with diabetes may increase insulin resistance. Postgrad Med J 1998;74(872):365–6.

172. Borissova AM, Tankova T, Kirilov G, et al. The effect of vitamin D_3 on insulin secretion and peripheral insulin sensitivity in type 2 diabetic patients. Int J Clin Pract 2003;57(4):258–61.

173. Pittas AG, Dawson-Hughes B, Li T, et al. Vitamin D and calcium intake in relation to type 2 diabetes in women. Diabetes care 2006;29(3):650–6.

174. Pittas AG, Harris SS, Stark PC, et al. The effects of calcium and vitamin D supplementation on blood glucose and markers of inflammation in nondiabetic adults. Diabetes care 2007;30(4):980–6.

175. de Boer IH, Tinker LF, Connelly S, et al. Calcium plus vitamin D supplementation and the risk of incident diabetes in the Women's Health Initiative. Diabetes Care 2008;31(4):701–7.

176. Nagpal J, Pande JN, Bhartia A. A double-blind, randomized, placebo-controlled trial of the short-term effect of vitamin D_3 supplementation on insulin sensitivity in apparently healthy, middle-aged, centrally obese men. Diabet Med 2009;26(1):19–27.

177. Pittas AG, Lau J, Hu FB, et al. The role of vitamin D and calcium in type 2 diabetes. A systematic review and meta-analysis. J Clin Endocrinol Metab 2007; 92(6):2017–29.

178. Knekt P, Laaksonen M, Mattila C, et al. Serum vitamin D and subsequent occurrence of type 2 diabetes. Epidemiology 2008;19(5):666–71.

179. von Hurst PR, Stonehouse W, Coad J. Vitamin D supplementation reduces insulin resistance in South Asian women living in New Zealand who are insulin resistant and vitamin D deficient - a randomised, placebo-controlled trial. Br J Nutr 2009;103(4):549–55.

180. Avenell A, Cook JA, MacLennan GS, et al. Vitamin D supplementation and type 2 diabetes: a substudy of a randomised placebo-controlled trial in older people (RECORD trial, ISRCTN 51647438). Age Ageing 2009;38(5):606–9.

181. Kazemi B, Seyed N, Moslemi E, et al. Insulin receptor gene mutations in Iranian patients with type II diabetes mellitus. Iran Biomed J 2009;13(3):161–8.

182. Holmes VA, Barnes MS, Alexander HD, et al. Vitamin D deficiency and insufficiency in pregnant women: a longitudinal study. Br J Nutr 2009;102(6):876–81.

183. Maghbooli Z, Hossein-Nezhad A, Karimi F, et al. Correlation between vitamin D_3 deficiency and insulin resistance in pregnancy. Diabetes Metab Res Rev 2008; 24(1):27–32.

184. Zhang C, Qiu C, Hu FB, et al. Maternal plasma 25-hydroxyvitamin D concentrations and the risk for gestational diabetes mellitus. PLoS One 2008;3(11):e3753.

185. Lapillonne A. Vitamin D deficiency during pregnancy may impair maternal and fetal outcomes. Med Hypotheses 2010;74(1):71–5.

186. Rudnicki PM, Molsted-Pedersen L. Effect of 1,25-dihydroxycholecalciferol on glucose metabolism in gestational diabetes mellitus. Diabetologia 1997;40(1): 40–4.

187. Zhang Y, Deb DK, Kong J, et al. Long-term therapeutic effect of vitamin D analog doxercalciferol on diabetic nephropathy: strong synergism with AT1 receptor antagonist. Am J Physiol Renal Physiol 2009;297(3):F791–801.

188. Chonchol M, Scragg R. 25-Hydroxyvitamin D, insulin resistance, and kidney function in the Third National Health and Nutrition Examination Survey. Kidney Int 2007;71(2):134–9.

189. Diaz VA, Mainous AG 3rd, Carek PJ, et al. The association of vitamin D deficiency and insufficiency with diabetic nephropathy: implications for health disparities. J Am Board Fam Med 2009;22(5):521–7.

190. Wolf M, Shah A, Gutierrez O, et al. Vitamin D levels and early mortality among incident hemodialysis patients. Kidney Int 2007;72(8):1004–13.

191. Aksoy H, Akcay F, Kurtul N, et al. Serum 1,25 dihydroxy vitamin D $(1,25(OH)_2D_3)$, 25 hydroxy vitamin D (25(OH)D) and parathormone levels in diabetic retinopathy. Clin Biochem 2000;33(1):47–51.

192. Parekh N, Chappell RJ, Millen AE, et al. Association between vitamin D and age-related macular degeneration in the Third National Health and Nutrition Examination Survey, 1988 through 1994. Arch Ophthalmol 2007;125(5):661–9.

193. Gouni-Berthold I, Krone W, Berthold HK. Vitamin D and cardiovascular disease. Curr Vasc Pharmacol 2009;7(3):414–22.

194. Judd SE, Tangpricha V. Vitamin D deficiency and risk for cardiovascular disease. Am J Med Sci 2009;338(1):40–4.

195. Bouillon R. Vitamin D as potential baseline therapy for blood pressure control. Am J Hypertens 2009;22(8):816.

196. Schmitz KJ, Skinner HG, Bautista LE, et al. Association of 25-hydroxyvitamin D with blood pressure in predominantly 25-hydroxyvitamin D deficient Hispanic and African Americans. Am J Hypertens 2009;22(8):867–70.

197. Pilz S, Marz W, Wellnitz B, et al. Association of vitamin D deficiency with heart failure and sudden cardiac death in a large cross-sectional study of patients referred for coronary angiography. J Clin Endocrinol Metab 2008;93(10): 3927–35.

198. de Boer IH, Kestenbaum B, Shoben AB, et al. 25-Hydroxyvitamin D levels inversely associate with risk for developing coronary artery calcification. J Am Soc Nephrol 2009;20(8):1805–12.

199. Tishkoff DX, Nibbelink KA, Holmberg KH, et al. Functional vitamin D receptor (VDR) in the t-tubules of cardiac myocytes: VDR knockout cardiomyocyte contractility. Endocrinology 2008;149(2):558–64.

200. Wu-Wong JR, Nakane M, Ma J, et al. VDR-mediated gene expression patterns in resting human coronary artery smooth muscle cells. J Cell Biochem 2007; 100(6):1395–405.

201. Autier P, Gandini S. Vitamin D supplementation and total mortality: a meta-analysis of randomized controlled trials. Arch Intern Med 2007;167(16):1730–7.

202. Lee P, Chen R. Vitamin D as an analgesic for patients with type 2 diabetes and neuropathic pain. Arch Intern Med 2008;168(7):771–2.

203. Xu W, Qiu C, Gatz M, et al. Mid- and late-life diabetes in relation to the risk of dementia: a population-based twin study. Diabetes 2009;58(1):71–7.

204. Miazgowski T, Krzyzanowska-Swiniarska B, Ogonowski J, et al. Does type 2 diabetes predispose to osteoporotic bone fractures? Endokrynol Pol 2008;59(3): 224–9.

205. Zinman B, Haffner SM, Herman WH, et al. Effect of rosiglitazone, metformin, and glyburide on bone biomarkers in patients with type 2 diabetes. J Clin Endocrinol Metab 2010;95(1):134–42.

206. Boland R, Norman A, Ritz E, et al. Presence of a 1,25-dihydroxy-vitamin D_3 receptor in chick skeletal muscle myoblasts. Biochem Biophys Res Commun 1985;128(1):305–11.

207. Bischoff-Ferrari HA, Willett WC, Wong JB, et al. Prevention of nonvertebral fractures with oral vitamin D and dose dependency: a meta-analysis of randomized controlled trials. Arch Intern Med 2009;169(6):551–61.

208. Boonen S, Lips P, Bouillon R, et al. Need for additional calcium to reduce the risk of hip fracture with vitamin D supplementation: evidence from a comparative metaanalysis of randomized controlled trials. J Clin Endocrinol Metab 2007; 92(4):1415–23.

Vitamin D Analogs

Glenville Jones, PhD

KEYWORDS

- Calcitriol • Vitamin D analogs
- Calcium and phosphate homeostasis
- Cell differentiation

Of late, vitamin D has gone through a renaissance with the association of vitamin D deficiency with a wide array of common diseases, including breast, colorectal, and prostate cancers; cardiovascular disease; autoimmune conditions; and infections.[1,2] As a result, vitamin D and its metabolites and analogs constitute a valuable group of compounds that can be used to regulate gene expression in functions as varied as calcium and phosphate homeostasis, as well as cell growth regulation and cell differentiation of a variety of cell types, such as enterocytes, keratinocytes, and epithelial cells of vasculature. The discovery of the metabolites, 25-hydroxyvitamin D_3 (25-OH-D_3) (calcidiol) and 1α,25-dihydroxyvitamin D_3 (1α,25-[OH]$_2D_3$) (calcitriol), in the early 1970s led to their chemical synthesis, and over the past 3 decades, the development of several generations of calcitriol analogs.[3] The pharmaceutical industry has attempted to separate the calcemic properties of 1α,25-(OH)$_2D_3$ from its cell-differentiating properties[4] to develop vitamin D analogs with specialized calcemic or noncalcemic (cell-differentiating) uses.[5,6] Several low-calcemic agents in the forms of calcipotriol, 22-oxacalcitriol (OCT), 19-nor-1α,25-(OH)$_2D_2$, and 1α-OH-D_2 have resulted, with widespread use in the treatment of psoriasis and secondary hyperparathyroidism. Research has also focused on the synthesis of vitamin D receptor (VDR) antagonists and cytochrome P450 (CYP) 24 inhibitors, which block VDR-mediated action or the catabolism of 25-OH-D and 1α,25-(OH)$_2$D to provide agents with possible use in metabolic bone diseases, osteoporosis, and cancer.[3,7] Perception of the importance of vitamin D/25-OH-D repletion has been modified by the concept that some 1α,25-(OH)$_2D_3$ is produced locally by target cells, making this molecule an endocrine and intracrine factor.[1,2] This review discusses the full spectrum of vitamin D compounds currently available, some of their possible uses, and potential mechanisms of action.

PHARMACOLOGICALLY IMPORTANT VITAMIN D COMPOUNDS

Vitamin D compounds can be subdivided into 4 major groups (**Figs. 1–4**).

The author is supported by the Canadian Institutes of Health Research.
Department of Biochemistry, Room 650, Botterell Hall, Queen's University, Kingston, Ontario, Canada K7L 3N6
E-mail address: gj1@queensu.ca

Endocrinol Metab Clin N Am 39 (2010) 447–472
doi:10.1016/j.ecl.2010.02.003
0889-8529/10/$ – see front matter © 2010 Elsevier Inc. All rights reserved.

endo.theclinics.com

Vitamin D Metabolites [Ring Structure][a]	Side Chain Structure	Site of Synthesis	Relative VDR-binding Affinity	Relative DBP-binding Affinity	References
Vitamin D₃ [1]	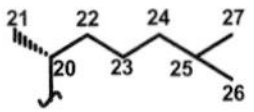	Skin	~0.001	3,180	Mellanby[131] McCollum et al[132]
25-OH-D₃ [1]	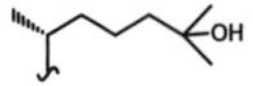	Liver	0.1	66,800	Blunt et al[133]
1α,25-(OH)₂D₃ [3]	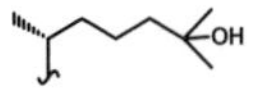	Kidney	100	100	Fraser and Kodicek[134] Holick et al[135]
24(R),25-(OH)₂D₃ [1]	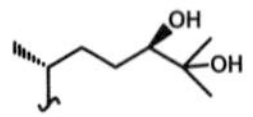	Kidney	0.02	33,900	Holick et al[136]
1α,24(R),25-(OH)₃D₃ [3]	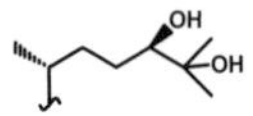	Target tissues[b]	10	21	Holick et al[137]
25(S),26-(OH)₂D₃ [1]	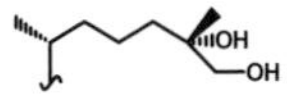	Liver ?	0.02	26,800	Suda et al[138]
25-OH-D₃-26,23-lactone [1]	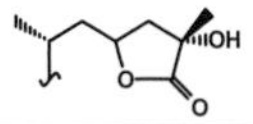	Kidney	0.01	250,000	Horst[139]

[a] Structure of the vitamin D nucleus (secosterol ring structure).
[b] Known target tissues included intestine, bone, kidney, skin, and the parathyroid gland.

Vitamin D Nucleus

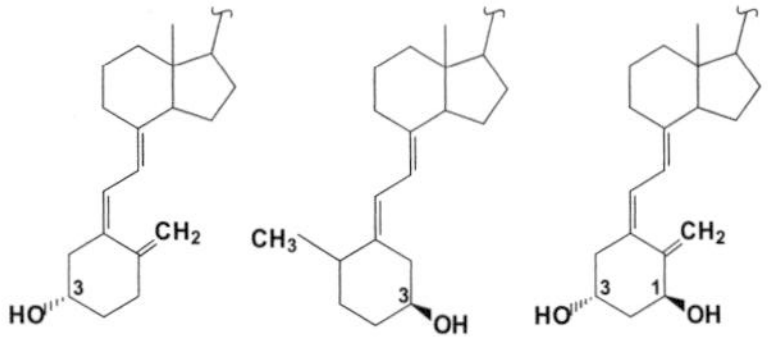

Fig. 1. Vitamin D and its natural metabolites.[131–139] (*Data from* Stern P. A monolog on analogs. In vitro effects of vitamin D metabolites and consideration of the mineralisation question. Calcif Tissue Int 1981;33:1–4; and Bishop JE, Collins ED, Okamura WH, et al. Profile of ligand specificity of the vitamin D binding protein for 1α,25-dihydroxyvitamin D₃ and its analogs. J Bone Miner Res 1994;9:1277–88.)

Vitamin D Prodrug [Ring Structure][a]	Side Chain Structure	Company	Status	Possible Target Diseases	Mode of delivery	References
1α-OH-D₃ [3]		Leo	In use Europe	Osteoporosis	Systemic	Barton et al[15]
1α-OH-D₂ [3]		Genzyme	In use USA	Secondary Hyperparathyroidism	Systemic	Paaren et al[16]
Dihydrotachysterol [2]		Duphar	Withdrawn	Renal failure	Systemic	Jones et al[27]
Vitamin D₂ [1]		Various	In use USA	Rickets Osteomalacia	Systemic Systemic	Park[140]
1α-OH-D₅ [3]		NCI	In use USA	Cancer	Systemic	Mehta et al[17]

[a] Structure of the vitamin D nucleus (secosterol ring structure).

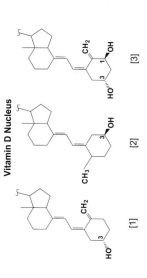

Vitamin D Nucleus

[1]   [2]   [3]

Fig. 2. Vitamin D prodrugs.[15–17,27,140]

Vitamin D Analog [Ring Structure][a]	Side Chain Structure	Company	Status	Possible Target Diseases	Mode of Delivery	References
Calcitriol, 1α,25-(OH)$_2$D$_3$ [3]		Roche, Duphar	In use worldwide	Hypocalcemia Psoriasis	Systemic Topical	Baggiolini et al[141]
26,27-F$_6$-1α,25-(OH)$_2$D$_3$ [3]		Sumitomo-Taisho	In use Japan	Osteoporosis Hypoparathyroidism	Systemic Systemic	Kobayashi et al[142]
19-Nor-1α,25-(OH)$_2$D$_2$ [5]		Abbott	In use USA	Secondary Hyperparathyroidism	Systemic	Perlman et al[143]
22-Oxacalcitriol (OCT) [3]		Chugai	In use Japan	Secondary Hyperparathyroidism Psoriasis	Systemic Topical	Murayama et al[144]
Calcipotriol (MC903) [3]		Leo	In use worldwide	Psoriasis Cancer	Topical Topical	Calverley[145]
1α,25-(OH)$_2$-16-ene-23-yne-D$_3$ (Ro 23-7553) [6]		Roche	Pre-clinical	Leukemia	Systemic	Baggiolini et al[32]
EB1089 [3]		Leo	Clinical trials	Cancer	Systemic	Binderup et al[146]
20-epi-1α,25-(OH)$_2$D$_3$ [3]		Leo	Pre-clinical	Immune diseases	Systemic	Calverley et al[147]
2-methylene-19-nor-20-epi-1α,25-(OH)$_2$D$_3$ (2MD) [7]		Deltanoids	Pre-clinical	Osteoporosis	Systemic	Shevde et al[37]
BXL-628 (formerly Ro-269228) [8]		Bioxell	Clinical trials	Prostate Cancer	Systemic	Marchiani et al[148]
ED71 [4]		Chugai	Clinical trials	Osteoporosis	Systemic	Nishii et al[30]
1α,24(S)-(OH)$_2$D$_2$ [3]		Genzyme	Pre-clinical	Psoriasis	Topical	Strugnell et al[31]
1α,24(R)-(OH)$_2$D$_3$ (TV-02) [3]		Teijin	In use Japan	Psoriasis	Topical	Morisaki et al[149]

[a]Structure of the vitamin D nucleus (secosterol ring structure).

Vitamin D Nucleus

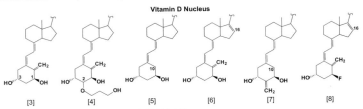

[3]   [4]   [5]   [6]   [7]   [8]

Fig. 3. Analogs of 1α,25-(OH)$_2$D$_3$.[30–32,37,141–149]

Vitamin D and Its Natural Metabolites

Fig. 1 shows the structures of vitamin D$_3$ and some of its important metabolites. Ironically, vitamin D$_3$, the natural form of vitamin D, is not approved for use as a drug in the United States, whereas it is found increasingly as an over-the-counter natural food supplement and is used in both roles in virtually every other country in the world.

Name	Structure	Name	Structure
LG190090 **Ligand Pharmaceuticals** Non-steroidal VDR agonist Boehm et al[40]	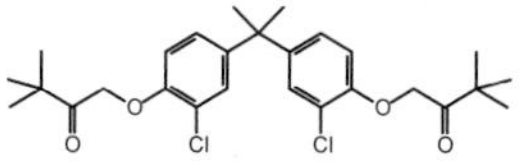	**LY2108491** **Eli Lilly** Non-steroidal VDR agonist Ma et al[41]	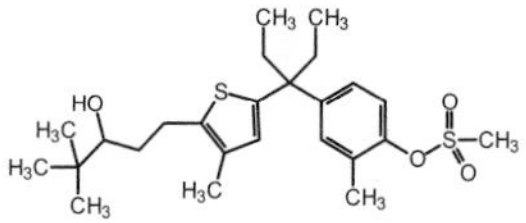
TEI-9647 **Teijin** VDR antagonist Dehydration product of 1α,25(R)-$(OH)_2D_3$- 26,23(S)-lactone Saito and Kittaka[43] Ochiai et al[150] Toell et al[44]	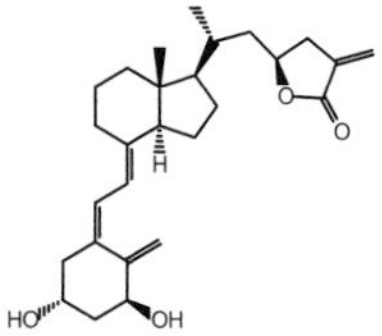	**ZK159222** **Schering** VDR antagonist Toell et al[44]	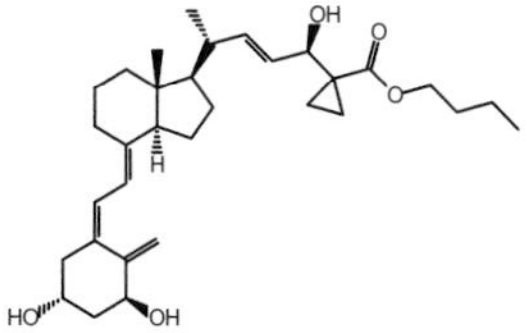
SDZ 89-443 **Sandoz/ Novartis** P450 inhibitor Schuster et al[46]	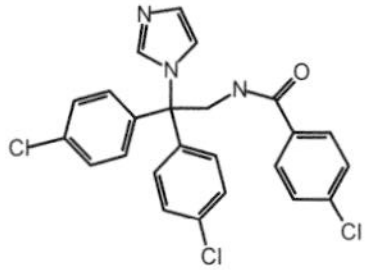	**VID400** **Sandoz/ Novartis** P450 inhibitor Schuster et al[46]	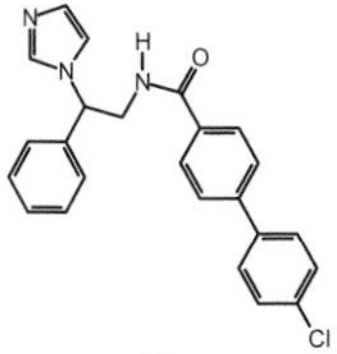
CTA016 Cytochroma CYP24A1 inhibitor Posner et al[47]	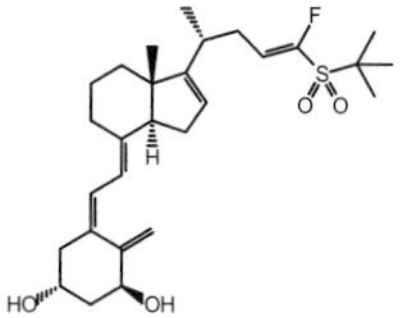	**ZG 1368** D-ring modified VDR agonist Verstuyf et al[34]	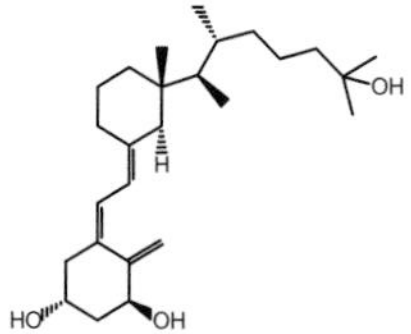
KS 176 C-ring modified VDR agonist Verstuyf et al[34]	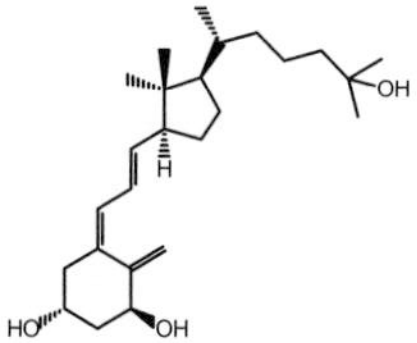	**SL 117** E-ring modified VDR agonist Verstuyf et al[34]	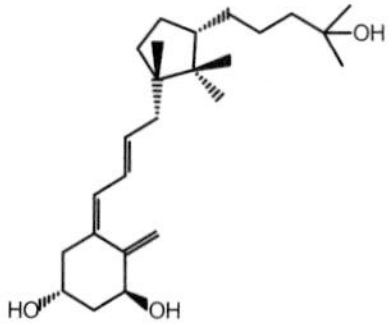

Fig. 4. Miscellaneous vitamin D compounds.[34,40,41,43,44,46,47,150]

During the late 1960s and early 1970s, most of the principal vitamin D metabolites were first isolated and identified by gas chromatography–mass spectrometry and their exact stereochemical structure determined.[3] This led to chemical synthesis of the naturally occurring isomer and its testing in various biologic assays in vitro and in vivo. All the major metabolites, namely, 25-OH-D_3 (Calderol), 1α,25-$(OH)_2D_3$ (Rocaltrol), and 24,25-dihydroxyvitamin D_3 24(R),25-$(OH)_2D_3$, Secalciferol) are currently or have been available for use as drugs globally.

Vitamin D Prodrugs

Fig. 2 lists some of the important prodrugs of vitamin D. All of these compounds require a step (or more) of activation in vivo before they are biologically active. Included here is vitamin D_2 (ergocalciferol), which is derived from the fungal sterol, ergosterol, by irradiation. When the nutritional basis of rickets and osteomalacia became apparent in the first half of the twentieth century, vitamin D (in particular vitamin D_2 because it was less expensive) became the treatment of choice for these diseases. In North America, low-dose prophylactic vitamin D (400 IU) in the form of dietary supplements or fortification of milk, margarine, bread, and other food products replaced much of the need for therapeutic vitamin D to abolish overt rickets and osteomalacia. Florid vitamin D deficiency rickets has become uncommon in North America because of adherence to public health guidelines and the fact that vitamin D fortification is required by law, in contrast to before fortification, and it is still more prevalent in the world where food fortification is not practiced. In the United States, vitamin D_2 is the form of vitamin D used exclusively in pharmaceutical preparations, whereas vitamin D_3 is increasingly incorporated in over-the-counter supplements. Vitamin D_2 differs only in that it possesses 2 specific modifications of the side chain (see **Fig. 2**) but these differences do not preclude the same series of activation steps as vitamin D_3, these hydroxylations giving rise to the metabolites 25-OH-D_2, 1α,25-$(OH)_2D_2$, and 24,25-$(OH)_2D_2$ respectively. Recently, there has been controversy regarding the relative usefulness of dietary vitamin D_2 and vitamin D_3 to raise the circulating 25-OH-D level.[8] Evidence suggests that oral pharmacologic doses of vitamin D_3 are significantly more effective than equivalent doses of vitamin D_2 for increasing the 25-OH-D level to the sufficient range (>40 ng/mL)[9] whereas there is ample evidence vitamin D_2 compounds are less toxic than their vitamin D_3 counterparts.[10,11] Alternatively, other studies using smaller, daily oral dosing of vitamins D_2 and D_3 suggest approximate bioequivalence.[12–14]

25-OH-D_3 was developed and approved as the pharmaceutical preparation Calderol in the 1970s but was withdrawn recently and is currently available only in Europe. Two other prodrugs, 1α-OH-D_3 and 1α-OH-D_2, were synthesized in the 1970s[15,16] as alternative sources of 1α,25-$(OH)_2D_3$ and 1α,25-$(OH)_2D_2$, respectively, that in the process circumvent the renal 1α-hydroxylase enzyme, which was shown to be tightly regulated and prone to damage in renal disease. The prodrug, 1α-OH-D_5, has been in clinical trials for the treatment of breast cancer.[17] The 1α-hydroxylated prodrugs have also been used in the treatment of osteoporosis. Although the etiology of this disease is complex and likely multifactorial,[18] there have been consistent claims that serum levels of 1α,25-$(OH)_2D_3$ are low in osteoporosis.[19] In addition, evidence that certain VDR genotypes correlate with bone mineral density[20,21] suggests some genetically inherited basis involving vitamin D exists leading to increased susceptibility to osteoporosis. As a consequence, it is not surprising that clinical trials of 1α-OH-D_3,[22] 1α-OH-D_2,[23] and 1α,25-$(OH)_2D_3$[24–26] have led to reports of modest gains in bone mineral density and reductions in fracture rates in osteoporotic patients, a topic reviewed by Seeman and colleagues.[18]

The final compound in **Fig. 2**, dihydrotachysterol (DHT) has a complex history as a prodrug. Originally it was believed to be active when converted to 25-OH-DHT by virtue of an A ring rotated 180° such that the 3β-hydroxyl function assumes a pseudo-1α-hydroxyl position.[27] The mechanism of action of DHT has become less clear with the description of the extrarenal metabolism of 25-OH-DHT to $1\alpha,25$-$(OH)_2$-DHT and $1\beta,25$-$(OH)_2$-DHT, 2 further metabolites that have greater biologic activity than the two 25-OH-DHT metabolites or DHT themselves.[28]

Calcitriol Analogs

Fig. 3 lists some of the most promising vitamin D analogs of $1\alpha,25$-$(OH)_2D_3$ approved by governmental agencies; currently under development by various industrial or university research groups; or abandoned at various stages of the development process. Because the number of vitamin D analogs synthesized now lists in the thousands, the table is provided mainly to give a flavor of the structures experimented with thus far, the worldwide scope of the companies involved, and the broad spectrum of target diseases and uses.

The first generation of calcitriol analogs included molecules with fluorine atoms placed at metabolically vulnerable positions in the side chain and resulted in highly stable and potent calcemic agents, such as $26,27$-F_6-$1\alpha,25$-$(OH)_2D_3$. A second generation of analogs focused on features that make the molecule more susceptible to clearance, such as in calcipotriol (MC903), where a C22-C23 double bond, a 24-hydroxyl function, and a cyclopropane ring have been introduced into the side chain or in OCT, where the 22-carbon has been replaced with an oxygen atom. Both modifications have given rise to highly successful analogs, calcipotriol and maxacalcitol, marketed in Europe and Japan, respectively.[29,30]

The C24 position is the chemists' favorite site for modification and many analogs contain 24-hydroxyl groups (eg, $1\alpha,24[S]$-$[OH]_2D_2$ and $1\alpha,24[R]$-$[OH]_2D_3$).[31] Other analogs contain multiple changes in the side chain in combination, including unsaturation; 20-epimerization; 22-oxa replacement; and homologation in the side-chain or terminal methyl groups. The resultant molecules, such as EB1089 and KH1060, attracted the strong attention of researchers because of their increased potency in vitro and were pursued as possible anticancer and immunomodulatory compounds, respectively, but their development seems to have been stalled.

Attempts have been made to modify the nucleus of calcitriol. The Roche compound, $1\alpha,25$-$(OH)_2$-16-ene-23-yne-D_3, touted as an antitumor compound in vivo, possesses a D-ring double bond.[32] Declercq and Bouillon[33] have made a novel 14-epi,19-nor-23-yne derivative with the same 23-yne feature, which also holds promise in cancer therapy (see **Fig. 3**), and the same researchers have introduced a series of biologically active analogs without 1 of the other of the C/D rings but with a rigid backbone to maintain the spatial arrangement of the A-ring hydroxyl groups and the side chain (see **Fig. 4**).[34] The A-ring–substituted 2-hydroxypropoxy-derivative, ED71, which by virtue of an A-ring substituent at C2 and tighter binding affinity to DBP has a longer half-life in the plasma,[30] has been tested as an antiosteoporosis drug. It has been claimed that ED71 has performed well at restoring bone mass without causing hypercalcemia in long-term studies involving ovariectomized rats and in phase I and II clinical trials.[35] Other bulky modifications at the C2 position of the A ring are accommodated well by the VDR, as indicated by modeling and biologic activity studies.[36,37] Another C-substituted bone-specific analog, 2MD,[37] is currently at an early stage of pharmaceutical development for the treatment of osteoporosis.

19-nor-$1\alpha,25$-$(OH)_2D_2$, lacks a 19-methylene group and is similar to the in vivo active metabolite, $1\alpha,25$-$(OH)_2DHT_2$, formed from dihydrotachysterol, because it lacks a functional group at the pseudo C19 position. Many other compounds have been developed with rigid or altered cis-triene structures or modifications of the 1α-, 3β-, or 25-hydroxyl functions for use as drugs but allow establishing minimal requirements for biologic activity in structure/activity studies.[5] BXL628 combines 1-flourination; 16-ene and 23-ene unsaturations; 26,27-homologation; and 20-epimerization, all found in earlier generations of analogs to make a antiproliferative agent currently in clinical trials for the treatment of prostate cancer and prostatitis.[38,39]

Miscellaneous Vitamin D Analogs and Associated Drugs

One series of compounds (depicted in **Fig. 4**) is the substituted biphenyls originally developed by Ligand, representing nonsteroidal scaffolds selected by high-throughput screening, which show weak VDR binding but good transactivation through vitamin D responsive element (VDRE)–driven, vitamin D–dependent genes and produce hypercalcemia in vivo.[40] This family has recently been extended by the synthesis of some highly potent, tissue-selective nonsecosteroidal VDR modulators with nanomolar affinity (eg, LY2109866).[41] This is the first class of vitamin D mimics that lack the conventional cis-triene secosteroid structure while maintaining the spatial separation of the A-ring and side-chain hydroxyl functions needed to bind to certain key residues of the ligand-binding pocket of the VDR. Although these nonsecosteroidal compounds are purported to exhibit an improvement of the therapeutic index over calcitriol in animal models, they are still to be tested clinically. In addition, **Fig. 4** shows the structures of 2 different classes of VDR/cacitriol antagonists. The former compounds, including TEI-9647, are dehydration products of the metabolite, $1α,25-(OH)_2D_3$-26,23-lactone (see **Fig. 1**), and are used in the treatment of Paget disease.[42–44]

Another group of compounds that has an impact on the vitamin D field that is under development are the CYP24A1 inhibitors. By blocking CYP24A1, the main catabolic pathway within the vitamin D target cell, these agents extend the life of the natural agonist, calcitriol, giving rise to a longer-lasting biologic effect.[45] Sandoz/Novartis developed a group of molecules that have greater specificity toward CYP24A1 and CYP27B1 from the general CYP inhibitor, ketoconazole, which showed usefulness in blocking cell proliferation in vitro but these compounds were discontinued after early clinical trials.[46] Cytochroma has developed a library of CYP24A1 inhibitors synthesized by Posner and colleagues[47] based on vitamin D templates; some of these are pure CYP24A1 inhibitors whereas others are mixed VDR agonist/CYP24A1 inhibitors (see **Fig. 4**). Some of these drugs have currently reached phase IIB human clinical trials for the treatment of psoriasis and are being tested systemically in the treatment of secondary hyperparathyroidism.[48] Their promise stems from their ability to block the attenuating action of CYP24 on calcitriol-mediated pre-pro-parathyroid hormone (PTH) gene suppression.

CLINICAL APPLICATIONS OF VITAMIN D COMPOUNDS

The clinical potential of vitamin D analogs has been discussed comprehensively in published reviews.[49,50] This article focuses on diseases currently treated with vitamin D analogs.

Secondary Hyperparathyroidism

Chronic kidney disease (CKD) is accompanied by a gradual fall in serum $1α,25-(OH)_2D$ levels over the 5-stage natural history of the disease, stages being defined by the decline in glomerular filtration rate (GFR). CKD culminates in the need for dialysis (stage 5). For 3 decades, this reduction in serum $1α,25-(OH)_2D$ was assumed the result of a decline in 1α-hydroxylase (CYP27B1) activity, due in turn to loss of the protein itself, but the recent elucidation of the FGF23-regulated phosphate homeostatic pathway has opened up an alternative explanation. Because FGF23 triggers down-regulation of 1α-hydroxylase (CYP27B1) and up-regulation of the catabolic 24-hydroxylase (CYP24A1), this hormone may also contribute to the progressive reduction in circulating $1\alpha,25$-$(OH)_2D$ levels.[51] Furthermore, FGF23 rises as early as CKD stage 1, preceding the decline in the 1α-hydroxylase activity that occurs in CKD stage 2 and well before the hypocalcemia and secondary hyperparathyroidism, which characterize the later stages of this disease. Unchecked, these biochemical events, together with the other sequelae of renal failure, such as phosphate retention, can result in renal osteodystrophy. Active vitamin D analogs, such as 1α-OH-D_3 and $1\alpha,25$-$(OH)_2D_3$, raise plasma Ca^{2+} concentrations and, in addition, lower PTH levels by direct suppression of PTH gene transcription at the level of the PTH gene promoter. Slatopolsky and colleagues[52] showed that intravenous infusion of active vitamin D preparations results in a more effective suppression of plasma PTH levels without such a profound increase in plasma (Ca^{2+}) in end-stage renal disease (ESRD). Subsequent work has used low-calcemic vitamin D analogs, such as 1α-OH-D_2 (doxercalciferol), OCT, or 19-nor-$1\alpha,25$-$(OH)_2D_2$ (paricalcitol), as substitutes for the more calcemic natural hormone. The Food and Drug Administration has approved oral and intravenous versions of these drugs for the treatment of secondary hyperparathyroidism at stages 3 and 4 of the disease as well as hemodialysis and peritoneal dialysis patients.

In 2003, a body of nephrologists released guidelines[53] recommending more aggressive use of vitamin D preparations and active vitamin D analogs in the treatment of secondary hyperparathyroidism in CKD. Kidney Disease Outcomes Quality Initiative (K/DOQI) guidelines suggested that treatment as early as stage 3 (GFR <60) might benefit patients by limiting the extreme rises in plasma PTH levels and preventing the parathyroid gland resistance to vitamin D treatment often observed in ESRD. K/DOQI guidelines also recognized the high frequency of vitamin D deficiency (25-OH-D <10 ng/mL) and vitamin D insufficiency (25-OH-D 10–30 ng/mL) in the CKD and ESRD populations[54] and made the opinion-based recommendation to make an initial attempt at vitamin D repletion with escalating doses of vitamin D_2 before administration of active vitamin D analog replacement therapy. This initial intervention to boost 25-OH-D levels has proved successful in stage 3 CKD patients in that it increases $1\alpha,25$-$(OH)_2D$ and mildly suppresses PTH, but the strategy failed to produce the desired effects in stage 4 CKD patients due to reduced renal 1α-hydroxylase activity.[55,56] Currently, oral and intravenous formulations of various active vitamin D analogs are available for use in stage 3–5 patients to take over when vitamin D repletion fails to regulate PTH levels.

The emergence of the potential importance of the extrarenal 1α-hydroxylase in normal human physiology has led to a re-evaluation of the vitamin D repletion and active hormone replacement arms of the CKD therapy.[2] The value of the vitamin D repletion is now seen as providing the substrate 25-OH-D for the renal 1α-hydroxylase, which is the main determinant of circulating $1\alpha,25$-$(OH)_2D_3$, and the extrarenal 1α-hydroxylase, which is postulated to augment $1\alpha,25$-$(OH)_2D_3$ synthesis for local or intracrine actions around the body. Although the decline of the renal enzyme during CKD is well established, the fate of the extrarenal 1α-hydroxylase in the face of uremia is largely a matter of conjecture. Evidence from anephric patients treated with large doses of 25-OH-D_3[57] suggests that the extrarenal enzyme survives in CKD patients, arguing that provision of a source of 25-OH-D to vitamin D–deficient and insufficient patients throughout all stages of CKD is warranted. The data from anephrics also argues for the more judicious use of active vitamin D analogs as hormone replacement therapy in addition to conventional vitamin D repletion therapy. Early attempts at this type of combined vitamin D/active vitamin D analog approach in a pediatric population have resulted in more efficient PTH control without many of the usual problems of soft tissue calcification observed in patients treated only with active vitamin D analogs.[58] The 3-fold higher susceptibility of CKD patients for cardiovascular disease[59,60] may also point to the deleterious effects of untreated vitamin D deficiency on the vasculature and highlight the beneficial effects of renally and locally produced $1\alpha,25$-$(OH)_2D$ for maintaining normal blood pressure, for antiproliferative effects on myocardial cell hypertrophy, and for direct suppressive effects on vascular epithelial cell osteoblastic gene expression (eg, Runx2 and osterix).[61,62]

Hyperproliferative Conditions: Psoriasis and Cancer

The demonstration that $1\alpha,25$-$(OH)_2D_3$ is an antiproliferative, prodifferentiating agent for certain cell types in vivo and many cell lines in vitro suggested that vitamin D analogs might offer some relief in hyperproliferative disorders, such as psoriasis and cancer. Early psoriasis trials with systemic $1\alpha,25$-$(OH)_2D_3$ were moderately successful but plagued with hypercalcemic side effects. Modifications to the protocol included (1) administration of calcitriol overnight when intestinal concentrations of $[Ca^{2+}]$ were low and (2) substitution of low-calcemic analogs for the calcitriol.

Although oral calcitriol can be an effective treatment for psoriasis when administered using an overnight protocol, the most popular treatment for psoriasis is the topical administration of the low-calcemic analog, calcipotriol, formulated as an ointment, which results in an improvement in more than 75% of patients.[29] $1\alpha,25$-$(OH)_2D_3$ and calcipotriol are effective in psoriasis because they block hyperproliferation of keratinocytes, increase differentiation of keratinocytes, and help suppress local inflammatory factors through their immunomodulatory properties. Calcipotriol has been marketed worldwide for use in psoriasis for more than 15 years.

Several thousands of vitamin D analogs have been tested in vitro and in vivo with some degree of success in controlling the growth of tumor cells, thus offering potential for use as anticancer drug therapies.[7] Many vitamin D compounds are effective antiproliferative or prodifferentiation agents in vitro acting through a variety of mechanisms involving alterations of cell cycle genes and proapototic genes to produce their effects. Preclinical studies in laboratory animals have also resulted in promising data.[7] With the analog EB1089, the promising antiproliferative effects observed in vitro and in the N-nitroso-N-methylurea (NMU)-induced mammary tumor and in LNCaP prostate cancer xenograft models[63] were also extended into the clinic. Early trials in limited numbers of breast cancer patients have been followed-up with more extensive ongoing phase II and phase III clinical trials in several different cancers.[64–66] Several other anlogs have entered clinical trials for the treatment of a variety of hyperproliferative diseases, usually involving VDR-positive tumors.[7]

Despite the promise of vitamin D analogs as anticancer agents, there is yet to result in an approved vitamin D analog for use in any type of cancer.[7] The principal problem in anticancer studies involving orally administered vitamin D compounds is hypercalcemia. Although the newer analogs seem less calcemic than calcitriol itself, they retain some ability to raise serum calcium; they are not noncalcemic as is sometimes claimed. Another problem emerging from experience with clinical trials is that effective doses needed to retard cell growth (approximately 1 nM or higher) cannot be attained in vivo due to low bioavailability.[67–69] One of the determinants of tumor cell vitamin D analog levels is the catabolic enzyme, CYP24A1, which is up-regulated in vitamin D target cells and limits the effective drug concentration reached. Thus, another approach to effective vitamin D therapy in cancer patients is the potential use of a CYP24 inhibitor (see **Fig. 4**) with or without calcitriol/calcitriol analog.[7] Nevertheless, it remains uncertain if a vitamin D compound can be developed that is sufficiently devoid of calcemic activity while retaining significant antiproliferative activity to be effective against tumors and also surviving the catabolic processes that operate in vivo.

CRITERIA THAT INFLUENCE PHARMACOLOGIC EFFECTS OF VITAMIN D COMPOUNDS

Three decades of work on vitamin D analogs have shown that several factors play a role in dictating the success of synthetic compounds to mimic some or all of the actions of calcitriol. These factors are discussed briefly.

Activating Enzymes

In vitro models show that some vitamin D compounds lacking 1α-hydroxylation (25-OH-D$_3$ and 24[R],25-[OH]$_2$D$_3$) are capable of interacting with VDR and transactivating reporter genes but this occurs only at high (μM) concentrations of ligand.[70] It seems unlikely that these concentrations will be reached in vivo except in hypervitaminosis D.[71] Consequently, most of the compounds described in **Figs. 1** and **2** lack vitamin D biologic activity unless they are activated in vivo. This is the case particularly for the parent vitamin D$_3$ itself; for its main circulating form, 25-OH-D$_3$; or for any of the prodrugs listed in **Fig. 2**. Vitamins D$_2$ and D$_3$ depend on the liver 25-hydroxylase and kidney 1α-hydroxylase enzyme systems to be activated, whereas most prodrugs require only a single step of activation. In particular, the 1α-OH-D drugs were designed to overcome the tightly regulated 1α-hydroxylase step, which is defective in chronic renal failure. In essence, prodrugs depend on the weakly regulated 25-hydroxylase step in the liver for activation. CYP27A1, the CYP originally thought responsible for 25-hydroxylation of vitamin D$_3$, has been shown to be a bifunctional enzyme that can execute activation of vitamin D$_3$ and the 27-hydroxylation of cholesterol during bile acid biosynthesis.[72] CYP27A1, however, has a low affinity for vitamin D, does not 25-hydroxylate vitamin D$_2$, and when mutated results in cerebrotendinous xanthomatosis, not rickets. Consequently, a more physiologically relevant 25-hydroxylase within the group of candidate orphan P450s[45] may be CYP2R1,[73] because this is a high-affinity microsomal enzyme with a known human mutation causing rickets and has been shown to 25-hydroxylate a vitamin D$_2$ prodrug, 1α-OH-D$_2$.[74] Recently, CYP2R1 was crystallized with several vitamin D substrates in the active site making it likely that it is the physiologically relevant isoform.[75]

The role of extrarenal tissues to 1α-hydroxylate various 25-hydroxylated metabolites and analogs in normal physiology has been controversial. It was widely accepted, however, that extrarenal 1α-hydroxylase activity is pathologically relevant in granulomatous conditions (eg, sarcoidosis).[76] In sarcoid patients, 25-OH-D can be converted to $1\alpha,25$-(OH)$_2$D in monocytes/macrophages, a step that, unlike in renal cases, is not subject to tight regulation, thus potentially more likely to result in hypercalcemia. Exposure of such patients to sunlight or administration of 25-OH-D can result in excessive plasma levels of $1\alpha,25$-(OH)$_2$D. After the cloning of the CYP representing the 1α-hydroxylase (officially named CYP27B1),[77,78] it was quickly shown that CYP27B1 can also be expressed extrarenally in skin, colon, and lung cancer cells.[79,80] Knowledge has been extended over the past decade with studies of CYP27B1 messenger RNA levels using real-time PCR and specific anti-CYP27B1 antibodies[81] to show a widespread distribution of this enzyme in many normal tissues as well as pathologic situations. As alluded to previously, the concept of the extrarenal 1α-hydroxylase suggests that this enzyme plays an important physiologic as well as pathologic role[2] and this has raised the level of importance given to ensuring mainte-nance of adequate 25-OH-D levels by vitamin D or direct 25-OH-D_3 supplementation.

Most of the calcitriol analogs listed in **Fig. 3** are thought to be active, not requiring any step of activation before their action on the transcriptional machinery or in nonge-nomic pathways.

Vitamin D Binding Protein

The vitamin D binding protein (DBP) provides transport for all lipid-soluble vitamin D compounds, from vitamin D to $1\alpha,25$-$(OH)_2D_3$, so it is not surprising that DBP also carries vitamin D analogs. Most of the analogs of calcitriol, designed to date, contain modifications to the side chain and this is usually detrimental to binding to DBP. Several analogs (eg, calcipotriol, OCT, and 19-nor-$1\alpha,25$-$[OH]_2D_2$) have weak affinities for DBP, reduced by as much as 2 to 3 orders of magnitude relative to $1\alpha,25$-$(OH)_2D_3$. This property has important implications for metabolic clearance rates, delivery to target cells, and tissue distribution.[82,83] Detailed studies with one analog, OCT, have shown it to bind primarily to β-lipoprotein and exhibit an abnormal tissue distri-bution in vivo, with disproportionally high concentrations (ng/g tissue) in the parathy-roid gland.[84] It was thus proposed that this unusual distribution may make OCT a useful systemically administered drug with a selective advantage in the treatment of hyperparathyroidism. Another vitamin D analog with a modified side chain is 20-epi-$1\alpha,25$-$(OH)_2D_3$, where the 20-S configuration of the side chain is opposite to the normal 20-R configuration. The DBP binding affinity of this analog is virtually unmea-surable as it does not displace [^{3}H]25-OH-D_3 from the plasma binding protein.[85] Reporter gene transactivation assays show that 20-epi-$1\alpha,25$-$(OH)_2D_3$ transactivates equally well in COS cells incubated in the presence and absence of fetal calf serum (as a source of DBP), whereas $1\alpha,25$-$(OH)_2D_3$–induced reporter gene expression is sensi-tive to DBP in the external growth medium, requiring 2-fold less hormone in the absence of DBP as in its presence.[85] It therefore seems that analogs that bind DBP less well than $1\alpha,25$-$(OH)_2D_3$ derive a target cell advantage over the natural hormone, if they are able to find alternative plasma carrier proteins to transport them to their target cells. These same alternative plasma carriers, however, presumably result in changes in the tissue distribution and hepatic clearance of analogs over the natural metabolites of vitamin D. The recent development of a DBP knockout mouse[86] suggests that 25-OH-D_3 clearance is more rapid in the absence of DBP.

VDR/RXR/VDRE Interactions

Three decades of work have established that $1\alpha,25$-$(OH)_2D_3$ is able to work through a VDR-mediated genomic mechanism to stimulate transcriptional activity at vitamin D–dependent genes.[87] Cloning of the VDR and elucidation of the 3-D structure of its ligand-binding domain have provided a huge boost to delineating the precise confor-mational changes that take place when the natural ligand binds to the VDR[88] and the nature of the postligand binding transcriptional events that occur thereafter, in partic-ular the nature of the coactivator proteins involved.[89] Basic knowledge of the mecha-nism of action of vitamin D has also been aided by the opportunity to observe the lack of effects of calcitriol and its analogs in the VDR knockout mouse.[90,91] These studies have largely refuted claims of alternative non–VDR-mediated mechanisms to produce physiologically relevant effects that might complicate understanding of the pharmaco-logic effects of vitamin D analogs.

Much evidence exists to support the viewpoint that vitamin D analogs mimic $1\alpha,25$-$(OH)_2D_3$ and use primarily a genomic mechanism. In early work, Stern[92] showed that there exists a strong correlation between chick intestinal VDR binding of an analog and its potency in a [^{45}Ca] rat bone resorption assay, suggesting that a vitamin D analog is only as good as its affinity for the VDR. More recent work has suggested that this a highly simplified viewpoint and that VDR binding affinity may not even be the major factor, transactivation activity arising from a series of additional parameters including conformation of the ligand/VDR complex, binding of the retinoid X receptor (RXR) partner, stability of the VDR/RXR/ligand complex, or even the nature of the coactivator proteins recruited to the complex. Recent data from the superagonist analogs[93–95] suggest that 20-epi compounds, including KH1060, are consistently only 1 to 2 orders of magnitude more potent than $1\alpha,25$-(OH)$_2$D$_3$ in gene transactivation assays or differentiation assays. Thus it seems that the quantitative advantages claimed for some of the calcitriol analogs are modest. Part of this advantage can be explained by other factors, such as differences in DBP binding or analog clearance.

Perhaps more important is whether or not analogs can be qualitatively different from $1\alpha,25$-(OH)$_2$D$_3$ in their actions and work selectively in calcium and phosphate homeostasis or cell differentiation. Freedman and coworkers[96,97] reported that the ability of a various analogs to transactivate vitamin D–dependent genes or to stimulate differentiation of cells is best correlated with their ability to recruit the coactivator, DRIP205, one of the many components of the DRIP complex isolated by Freedman and coworkers. Among the other coactivators/transcription factors implicated in vitamin D analog action is GRIP1/TIF2, which has been purported to have a particular propensity to interact with the analog OCT.[98] In another study, by Issa and colleagues,[99] a broad panel of vitamin D analogs showed that GRIP1 was more consistently recruited at levels closer to that of $1\alpha,25$-(OH)$_2$D$_3$ than was another coactivator, AIB1. Work by Peleg and colleagues[100] offers an insight into the purported bone tissue selectivity of the Roche analog, Ro 26-9228 (see **Fig. 3**), renamed BXL628, by showing recruitment of GRIP1 in osteoblasts but not in Caco-2 colon cancer cells, although paradoxically BXL628 is being pursued clinically in prostatic disease rather than osteoporosis. Nevertheless, it seems that there is a fairly strong basis for the hypothesis that differences in the biopotency advantage of certain vitamin D analogs over $1\alpha,25$-(OH)$_2$D$_3$ are due in part to changes in the recruitment of the RXR dimerization partner or coactivators (eg, see Eelen and colleagues[33]), but there is no consensus on which of these coactivator proteins is the important one or if these different coactivators can explain tissue/cell selectivity. Work using chromatin immunoprecipitation (CHIP) assays,[101] which shows temporal changes in coactivator recruitment at vitamin D–dependent gene promoters, may aid in understanding this complex transcriptional story.

Target Cell Catabolic Enzymes

Much evidence has accumulated to show that $1\alpha,25$-(OH)$_2$D$_3$ is subject to target cell catabolism and side-chain cleavage to calcitroic acid via a 24-oxidation pathway catalysed by the CYP, CYP24A1.[102] CYP24A1 is vitamin D inducible because its gene promoter contains a double VDRE; it performs multiple steps in side-chain modification process; it is present in most (if not all) vitamin D target cells,[45,103] and its role seems to desensitize the target cell to continuing hormonal stimulation by $1\alpha,25$-(OH)$_2$D$_3$.[104] The CYP24A1 knockout mouse shows 50% lethality at weaning; death results from hypercalcemia and nephrocalcinosis, and surviving mice show an inability to rapidly clear a bolus dose of $1\alpha,25$-(OH)$_2$D$_3$ from the bloodstream and tissues.[105,106] CYP24A1 knockout mice also exhibit a metabolic bone disease reminiscent of the excessive osteoid bone pathology observed in rodents given excessive amounts of $1\alpha,25$-(OH)$_2$D$_3$.[107] Moreover, recent work crossing the CYP24 knockout mouse with the VDR knockout mouse rescues this bone defect,[108] suggesting

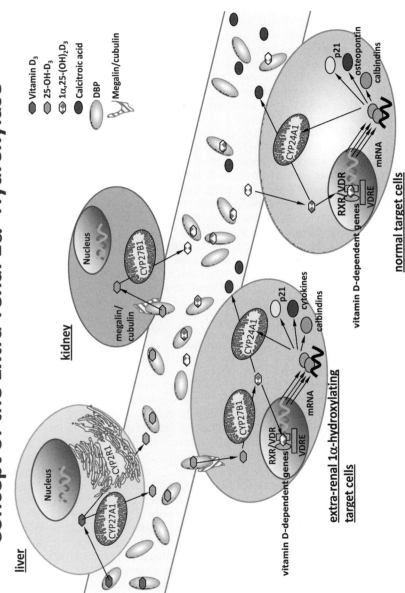

Concept of the Extra-renal 1α-Hydroxylase

excessive VDR-mediated signaling is the cause, although the bone lesion can also be relieved by administration of 24,25-$(OH)_2D_3$.[109]

The demonstrated importance of CYP24 to 1α,25-$(OH)_2D_3$ clearance leads the question of whether or not vitamin D analogs might be subject to the same catabolic processes that determine their pharmacokinetics. There are vitamin D analogs, such as calcipotriol, OCT, EB1089, and KH1060, that are metabolized by vitamin D target cells to clearly defined and unique metabolites,[94,110–112] which resemble products of the 24-oxidation pathway for 1α,25-$(OH)_2D_3$. Furthermore, some of these metabolites are products only of vitamin D target cells and are calcitriol inducible, suggesting that CYP24 is involved in their formation, this having been confirmed with some analogs, such as calcipotriol.[74] Even in the case of several analogs blocked at C24 and subject to metabolism elsewhere on the side chain, the involvement of CYP24 is strongly implicated or proved, including 23-hydroxylation of 26,27-hexafluro-1α,25-$(OH)_2D_3$; 26-hydroxylation of 24-difluro-1α,25-$(OH)_2D_3$; 26-hydroxylation of 1α,25-$(OH)_2$-16-ene-23-yne-D_3; and 26- and 28-hydroxylation of 1α,25-$(OH)_2D_2$. Because many of these same products are observed in vitro and in vivo and because pharmacokinetic parameters often parallel target cell metabolic parameters,[83] a conclusion is that target cell metabolism of vitamin D analogs must contribute to the pharmacokinetics and biologic activity observed in vitro and in vivo. Even studies, such as that of Eelen and colleagues,[33] which claimed differences in VDR-mediated

◄───

Fig. 5. Current concepts of the activation, mechanism of action, and catabolism of vitamin D. The model incorporates a plasma-binding protein (DBP), which acts as a carrier of vitamin D metabolites and analogs; activating enzymes (CYPs) involved in activation of vitamin D or prodrug; target cell transcriptional machinery (VDR, RXR, coactivators) involved in biologic actions of 1α,25-$(OH)_2D_3$ or its analogs; and target cell catabolic enzyme system (CYP24A1) involved in degradation of 1α,25-$(OH)_2D_3$ or its analog. The figure shows the metabolism of vitamin D in the context of the cells involved. (*Top left*) Hepatocyte showing some of the candidate CYPs shown to 25-hydroxylate vitamin D and its prodrugs; note that VDR is believed to be absent from liver cells. (*Top middle*) Proximal tubular cell showing the key elements in the uptake of 25-OH-D_3 and its conversion to 1α,25-$(OH)_2D_3$. Megalin/cubulin are cell surface receptors that execute endocytosis of the DBP/25-OH-D_3 complex, whereas CYP27B1 is the main component of the 1α-hydroxylase, responsible for synthesis of circulating 1α,25-$(OH)_2D_3$. (*Lower right*) Conventional target cell, which lacks megalin/cubulin and takes up only the free ligand, 1α,25-$(OH)_2D_3$, but not the DBP originally involved in transporting the ligand to the target cell. The key elements of the transcriptional machinery are shown, including VDR/RXR as well as representative gene products, such as cell division protein p21, the bone matrix protein osteopontin, the calcium transport protein calbindin, and the autoregulatory protein CYP24A1. The role of the highly inducible CYP24A1 is to convert the hormone (or analog) into inactive degradation products, such as calcitroic acid, which enter plasma and are excreted in bile. (*Lower left*) Target cell, which expresses extrarenal 1α-hydroxylase (CYP27B1) and the megalin/cubulin machinery to take up 25-OH-D_3, thus capable of making 1α,25-$(OH)_2D_3$ locally. The cell can also respond in a likewise manner to the conventional target cell because it also possesses the VDR and other transcriptional machinery. The expectation is that cells involved in cell differentiation or controlling cell division require higher concentrations of 1α,25-$(OH)_2D_3$ to modulate a different set of genes, and the CYP27B1 boosts local production to augment that circulating 1α,25-$(OH)_2D_3$ arriving from the kidney in the bloodstream. Under normal physiologic processes, locally produced 1α,25-$(OH)_2D_3$ does not enter the general circulation, although in pathologic conditions (eg, sarcoidosis) this could occur. At this time, it is not clear how many cell types can be considered simple target cells and how many possess the CYP27B1 and megalin/cubulin to allow for local production of hormone. (*Reproduced from* Jones G. Pharmacokinetics of vitamin D toxicity. Am J Clin Nutr 2008;88(Suppl):582S–6S; with permission.)

gene expression at the coactivator level, also show that a CYP24A1 inhibitor, VID400 (see **Fig. 4**), narrowed potency differences between 23-yne analogs and $1\alpha,25$-$(OH)_2D_3$ by blocking catabolism of the latter and reveal that analogs derive advantages at metabolic and transcriptional levels. Unfortunately, this metabolic blockade approach has not always been used in analog screening and there is little doubt that poor performance during in vivo testing is the result of poor metabolic stability of the studied analog.

Some of the calcitriol analogs with modifications in the vicinity of C23, namely, 20-epi-$1\alpha,25$-$(OH)_2D_3$,[85] $1\alpha,25$-$(OH)_2$-16ene-D_3,[113] and 20-methyl-$1\alpha,25$-$(OH)_2D_3$,[114] undergo 24-oxidation pathway metabolism that stalls at the level of the 24-oxo metabolite, seemingly because the enzyme CYP24A1 cannot efficiently carry out the usual 23-hydroxylation step and complete the catabolic sequence to the inactive cleaved product. The consequence, at least in vitro, is that the 24-oxo metabolite accumulates and there are claims that this metabolite retains significant biologic activity.[113] Recently, this hypothesis has received a boost with the work of Zella and colleagues,[95] who have found that the superagonist 20-epi-$1\alpha,25$-$(OH)_2D_3$ exhibits a prolonged duration of action on intestinal calcium regulating genes selectively and these researchers have proposed that this advantage over $1\alpha,25$-$(OH)_2D_3$ stems from a reduction in its catabolic rate.

Hepatic Clearance or Nonspecific Metabolism

The poor DBP binding properties of many side-chain–modified calcitriol analogs opens up the possibility of alternative plasma carriers and accelerated degradation. The liver plays a major role in such metabolic clearance and a few detailed studies performed to date have included in vitro incubation with liver preparations. Calcipotriol,[115] OCT,[111] EB1089,[116] and KH1060[117] are all subject to metabolism by liver enzymes. One such liver enzyme capable of 23- and 24-hydroxylation of $1\alpha,25$-$(OH)_2D_3$, and possibly some of its analogs, is the abundant cytochrome P450, CYP3A4.[118] This enzyme is up-regulated by $1\alpha,25$-$(OH)_2D_3$ in duodenum, suggesting a physiologically relevant loop exists.[119] Because over the years, there have been frequent reports of drug-induced osteomalacia associated with coincidental use of anticonvulsants (eg, diphenylhydantoin) or barbiturates and vitamin D preparations,[120] the direct association between CYP3A4 and $1\alpha,25$-$(OH)_2D_3$ is potentially important to explain the putative accelerated clearance of some vitamin D metabolites.[121] One such phenomenon that might be explained by intestinal CYP3A4 action is the purported lower toxicity of vitamin D_2 compounds as compared with their vitamin D_3 counterparts (discussed previously). Work using microsomes from an intestinal cell line and supersomes enriched in recombinant human CYP3A4 catabolize $1\alpha,25$-$(OH)_2D_2$ at a significantly faster rate than $1\alpha,25$-$(OH)_2D_3$.[122] The implication of this finding is that $1\alpha,25$-$(OH)_2D_2$ and possibly other synthetic analogs, such as the mixed VDR agonist/CYP24A1 inhibitor, CTA018,[48] are selectively broken down in intestine, potentially reducing their gene expression effects on intestinal calcium and phosphate absorption but not on other tissues.

MEMBRANE RECEPTORS AND NONGENOMIC EFFECTS OF VITAMIN D ANALOGS

The nongenomic actions of $1\alpha,25$-$(OH)_2D_3$ have been reviewed extensively elsewhere.[9,123] The membrane VDR initially described by Nemere and colleagues[124] and identified as annexin II[125] was postulated to be involved in mediating putative nongenomic effects. Further attempts to purify and identify the putative membrane receptor have resulted in a membrane-activated rapid response to steroids (MARRS) in chick intestinal cells[126] that may also explain rapid nongenomic actions.[123] Little work has been performed on the analog specificity of the vitamin D binding site of membrane VDR/annexin II or MARRS complex, however; thus, the possibility that the nongenomic actions/membrane VDR might explain other vitamin D analog actions seems premature and unproved.

PROPOSED MOLECULAR MECHANISMS OF ACTION OF VITAMIN D COMPOUNDS

Fig. 5 contains a general model to predict how vitamin D analogs work. It allows for consideration of prodrugs (those requiring 25-hydroxylation by CYP27A1 or CYP2R1 and those requiring 1α-hydroxylation by the kidney or extrarenal 1α-hydroxylase) and $1\alpha,25\text{-(OH)}_2D_3$ analogs. This model, therefore, makes a distinction between those target cells that express an extrarenal 1α-hydroxylase (CYP27B1) and, therefore, have the ability to make and respond their own local $1\alpha,25\text{-(OH)}_2D_3$ and those that simply respond through their VDR with altered transcription. This model features a conventional VDR-RXR heterodimer working through a VDRE in most genes. Crucial parameters for each new analog include

1. Affinity for DBP
2. Affinity for VDR
3. Ability to recruit RXR and coactivators followed by transactivation of genes
4. Rate of target cell metabolism (reflected partly in pharmacokinetic parameters)
5. Rate of hepatic or nonspecific clearance (reflected partly in pharmacokinetic parameters).

The author's view is that all listed parameters contribute significantly to the overall biologic activity of any given analog.

FUTURE PROSPECTS

The eludicidation of the genomic mechanism of action of $1\alpha,25\text{-(OH)}_2D_3$ will probably reveal new post-VDR coactivator-based approaches by which the vitamin D signaling cascade can be exploited. The significant progress made in characterizing the coactivator proteins and the rest of the transcriptional apparatus will continue and will benefit from parallel work on other transcriptional modulators (eg, other steroids).

Studies of the vitamin D binding pockets of VDR, DBP, and the 3 (or more) vitamin D–related CYPs will continue to be a major goal now that all these specific proteins have been cloned, overexpressed, and crystallized. Work on the ligand-binding domain of the VDR[88] will be extended to new analogs and coactivator complexes and the other major proteins in the vitamin D signal transduction pathway.

The wide availability of recombinant proteins for hundreds of CYPs from species across the phylogenetic tree, including 58 CYPs in the human genome, has allowed for the elucidation of some crystal structures and modeling studies of the enzymes involved in vitamin D metabolism.[127,128] Current models are starting to reveal key substrate side-chain contact residues (eg, Ala326 within CYP24A1) associated with hydroxylation.[129] The recent crystallization and structural determination of the microsomal CYP2R1, the putative vitamin D-25-hydroxylase, is a harbinger of what is to come in this field.[75]

Access to full-length CYP24A1 and CYP27B1 has also permitted a more efficient search for potential inhibitors. Specific inhibitors of CYP24A1 and CYP27B1[46,47,130] may be of value in blocking $1\alpha,25\text{-(OH)}_2D_3$ catabolism in certain clinical conditions where excessive breakdown is suspected. In general, modeling of VDR and CYPs is expected to lead to more rational vitamin D analog design to take advantage of structural idiosyncrasies of all of these key proteins. Meanwhile, the not-so-rational synthesis of new analogs is likely to continue. The list of applications for these new vitamin D analogs continues to increase,[1,2] making synthesis a worthwhile exercise.

ACKNOWLEDGMENTS

The author acknowledges the valuable contributions of Dr David Prosser to the compilation of the figures generated for this review article.

REFERENCES

1. Holick MF. Vitamin D deficiency. N Engl J Med 2007;357:266–81.
2. Jones G. Expanding role for vitamin D in chronic kidney disease: importance of blood 25-OH-D levels and extra-renal 1α-hydroxylase in the classical and non-classical actions of 1α,25-dihydroxyvitamin D_3. Semin Dial 2007;20: 316–24.
3. Jones G, Strugnell S, DeLuca HF. Current understanding of the molecular actions of vitamin D. Physiol Rev 1998;78:1193–231.
4. Miyaura C, Abe E, Kuribayashi T, et al. 1α,25-dihydroxyvitamin D_3 induces differentiation of human myeloid leukemia cells. Biochem Biophys Res Commun 1981;102:937–43.
5. Bouillon R, Okamura WH, Norman AW. Structure-function relationships in the vitamin D endocrine system. Endocr Rev 1995;16:200–57.
6. Jones G. Vitamin D and analogues. In: Bilezikian J, Raisz L, Rodan G, editors. Principles of bone biology. Third edition. Section: pharmacological mechanisms of therapeutics. San Diego (CA): Academic Press Inc; 2008. p.1777–99
7. Masuda S, Jones G. The promise of vitamin D analogs in the treatment of hyperproliferative conditions. Mol Cancer Ther 2006;5:797–808.
8. Vieth R. The pharmacology of Vitamin D, including fortification strategies. In: Feldman D, Pike JW, Glorieux FH, editors. Vitamin D. 2nd edition. New York: Elsevier Academic Press; 2005. p. 995–1015.
9. Armas LA, Hollis BW, Heaney RP. Vitamin D_2 is much less effective than vitamin D_3 in humans. J Clin Endocrinol Metab 2004;89:5387–91.
10. Roborgh JR, de Man T. The hypercalcemic activity of dihydrotachysterol-$_2$ and dihydrotachysterol-$_3$ and of the vitamins D_2 and D_3: comparative experiments in rats. Biochem Pharmacol 1960;2:1–6.
11. Sjöden G, Smith C, Lindgren U, et al. 1α-Hydroxyvitamin D_2 is less toxic than 1α-hydroxyvitamin D_3 in the rat. Proc Soc Exp Biol Med 1985;178:432–6.
12. Rapuri PB, Gallagher JC, Haynatzki G. Effect of vitamins D_2 and D_3 supplement use on serum 25OHD concentration in elderly women in summer and winter. Calcif Tissue Int 2004;74:150–6.
13. Holick MF, Biancuzzo RM, Chen TC, et al. Vitamin D_2 is as effective as vitamin D_3 in maintaining circulating concentrations of 25-hydroxyvitamin D. J Clin Endocrinol Metab 2008;93:677–81.
14. Thacher TD, Obadofin MO, O'Brien KO, et al. The effect of vitamin D_2 and vitamin D_3 on intestinal calcium absorption in Nigerian children with rickets. J Clin Endocrinol Metab 2009;94:3314–21.
15. Barton DH, Hesse RH, Pechet MM, et al. A convenient synthesis of 1α-hydroxyvitamin D_3. J Am Chem Soc 1973;95:2748–9.
16. Paaren HE, Hamer DE, Schnoes HK, et al. Direct C-1 hydroxylation of vitamin D compounds: convenient preparation of 1α-hydroxyvitamin D_3, 1α,25-dihydroxyvitamin D_3, and 1α-hydroxyvitamin D_2. Proc Natl Acad Sci U S A 1978;75:2080–1.

17. Mehta R, Hawthorne M, Uselding L, et al. Prevention of N-methyl-N-nitrosourea-induced mammary carcinogenesis in rats by 1alpha-hydroxyvitamin D_5. J Natl Cancer Inst 2000;92:1836–40.

18. Seeman E, Tsalamandris C, Bass S, et al. Present and future of osteoporosis therapy. Bone 1995;17:23S–9S.

19. Riggs BL, Melton LJ III. The prevention and treatment of osteoporosis. N Engl J Med 1992;327:620–7.

20. Morrison NA, Qi JC, Tokita A, et al. Prediction of bone density from vitamin D receptor alleles. Nature 1994;367:284–7.

21. Uitterlinden AG, Fang Y, van Meurs JBJ, et al. Analog metabolism. In: Feldman D, Pike W, Glorieux F, editors. Vitamin D. 2nd edition. San Diego (CA): Academic Press; 2005. p. 1121–58.

22. Orimo H, Shiraki M, Hayashi T, et al. Reduced occurrence of vertebral crush fractures in senile osteoporosis treated with 1α(OH)-vitamin D_3. Bone Miner 1987;3:47–52.

23. Gallagher JC, Bishop CW, Knutson JC, et al. Effects of increasing doses of 1α-hydroxyvitamin D_2 on calcium homeostasis in postmenopausal osteopenic women. J Bone Miner Res 1994;9:607–14.

24. Gallagher JC, Riggs BL, Recker RR, et al. The effect of calcitriol on patients with postmenopausal osteoporosis with special reference to fracture frequency. Proc Soc Exp Biol Med 1989;191:287–92.

25. Ott S, Chesnut CH. Calcitriol treatment is not effective in post-menopausal osteoporosis. Ann Intern Med 1989;110:267–74.

26. Tilyard MW, Spears GFS, Thomson J, et al. Treatment of post-menopausal osteoporosis with calcium. N Engl J Med 1992;326:357–62.

27. Jones G, Edwards N, Vriezen D, et al. Isolation and identification of seven metabolites of 25-hydroxydihydrotachysterol₃ formed in the isolated perfused rat kidney: a model for the study of side-chain metabolism of vitamin D. Biochemistry 1988;27:7070–9.

28. Qaw F, Calverley MJ, Schroeder NJ, et al. In vivo metabolism of the vitamin D analog, dihydrotachysterol. Evidence for formation of 1α,25-and 1β,25-dihydroxydihydrotachysterol metabolites and studies of their biological activity. J Biol Chem 1993;268:282–92.

29. Kragballe K, Gjertsen BT, De Hoop D, et al. Double-blind, right/left comparison of calcipotriol and betamethasone valerate in treatment of psoriasis vulgaris. Lancet 1991;337:193–6.

30. Nishii Y, Sato K, Kobayashi T. The development of vitamin D analogues for the treatment of osteoporosis. Osteoporos Int 1993;1(Suppl):S190–3.

31. Strugnell S, Byford V, Makin HLJ, et al. 1α,24(S)-dihydroxyvitamin D_2: a biologically active product of 1α-hydroxyvitamin D_2 made in the human hepatoma, Hep3B. Biochem J 1995;310:233–41.

32. Baggiolini EG, Partridge JJ, Shiuey S-J, et al. Cholecalciferol 23-yne derivatives, their pharmaceutical compositions, their use in the treatment of calcium related diseases, and their antitumor activity, US 4,804,502 [abstract]. Chem Abstr 1989;111:58160d.

33. Eelen G, Valle N, Sato Y, et al. Superagonistic fluorinated vitamin D_3 analogs stabilize helix 12 of the vitamin D receptor. Chem Biol 2008;15:1029–34.

34. Verstuyf A, Verlinden L, van Etten E, et al. Biological activity of CD-ring modified 1α,25-dihydroxyvitamin D analogues: C-ring and five-membered D-ring analogues. J Bone Miner Res 2000;15:237–52.

35. Matsumoto T, Kubodera N. ED-71, a new active vitamin D_3, increases bone mineral density regardless of serum 25(OH)D levels in osteoporotic subjects. J Steroid Biochem Mol Biol 2007;103:584–6.

36. Suhara Y, Nihei KI, Kurihara M, et al. Efficient and versatile synthesis of novel 2α-substituted $1\alpha,25$-dihydroxyvitamin D_3 analogues and their docking to vitamin D receptors. J Org Chem 2001;66:8760–71.

37. Shevde NK, Plum LA, Clagett-Dame M, et al. A potent analog of $1\alpha,25$-dihydroxyvitamin D_3 selectively induces bone formation. Proc Natl Acad Sci U S A 2002; 99:13487–91.

38. Crescioli C, Ferruzzi P, Caporali A, et al. Inhibition of prostate cell growth by BXL-628, a calcitriol analogue selected for a phase II clinical trial in patients with benign prostate hyperplasia. Eur J Endocrinol 2004;150: 591–603.

39. Adorini L, Penna G, Amuchastegui S, et al. Inhibition of prostate growth and inflammation by the vitamin D receptor agonist BXL-628 (elocalcitol). J Steroid Biochem Mol Biol 2007;103:689–93.

40. Boehm MF, Fitzgerald P, Zou A, et al. Novel nonsecosteroidal vitamin D mimics exert VDR-modulating activities with less calcium mobilization than 1,25-dihydroxyvitamin D_3. Chem Biol 1999;6:265–75.

41. Ma Y, Khalifa B, Yee YK, et al. Identification and characterization of noncalcemic, tissue-selective, nonsecosteroidal vitamin D receptor modulators. J Clin Invest 2006;116:892–904.

42. Ishizuka S, Kurihara N, Reddy SV, et al. (23S)-25-Dehydro-1α-hydroxyvitamin D_3-26,23-lactone, a vitamin D receptor antagonist that inhibits osteoclast formation and bone resorption in bone marrow cultures from patients with Paget's disease. Endocrinology 2005;146:2023–30.

43. Saito N, Kittaka A. Highly potent vitamin D receptor antagonists: design, synthesis, and biological evaluation. Chembiochem 2006;7:1479–90.

44. Toell A, Gonzalez MM, Ruf D, et al. Different molecular mechanisms of vitamin D_3 receptor antagonists. Mol Pharmacol 2001;59:1478–85.

45. Prosser DE, Jones G. Enzymes involved in the activation and inactivation of vitamin D. Trends Biochem Sci 2004;29:664–73.

46. Schuster I, Egger H, Astecker N, et al. Selective inhibitors of CYP24: mechanistic tools to explore vitamin D metabolism in human keratinocytes. Steroids 2001;66:451–62.

47. Posner GH, Crawford KR, Yang HW, et al. Potent low-calcemic selective inhibitors of CYP24 hydroxylase: 24-sulphone analogs of the hormone $1\alpha,25$-dihydroxyvitamin D_3. J Steroid Biochem Mol Biol 2004;89-90:5–12.

48. Posner G, Petkovich M. Vitamin D analogues targeting CYP24 in chronic kidney disease [abstract]. Proceedings of the 14th Workshop on Vitamin D. Brugge, Belgium, October 4–8, 2009. p. 7.

49. Bikle DD. Clinical counterpoint: vitamin D: new actions, new analogs, new therapeutic potential. Endocr Rev 1992;13:765–84.

50. Bischoff-Ferrari HA, Giovannucci E, Willett WC, et al. Estimation of optimal serum concentrations of 25-hydroxyvitamin D for multiple health outcomes. Am J Clin Nutr 2006;84:18–28.

51. Quarles LD. Endocrine functions of bone in mineral metabolism regulation. J Clin Invest 2008;118:3820–8.

52. Delmez JA, Tindira C, Grooms P, et al. Parathyroid hormone suppression by intravenous 1,25-dihydroxyvitamin D. A role for increased sensitivity to calcium. J Clin Invest 1989;83:1349–55.

53. K/DOQI clinical practise guidelines for bone metabolism and disease in chronic kidney disease. Am J Kidney Dis 2003;42(Suppl 3):S1–202.
54. Gonzalez EA, Sachdeva A, Oliver DA, et al. Vitamin D insufficiency and deficiency in chronic kidney disease. A single center observational study. Am J Nephrol 2004;24:503–10.
55. Al-Aly Z, Qazi RA, González EA, et al. Changes in serum 25-hydroxyvitamin D and plasma intact PTH levels following treatment with ergocalciferol in patients with CKD. Am J Kidney Dis 2007;50:59–68.
56. Zisman AL, Hristova M, Ho LT, et al. Impact of ergocalciferol treatment of vitamin D deficiency on serum parathyroid hormone concentrations in chronic kidney disease. Am J Nephrol. 2007;27:36–43.
57. Dusso A, Lopez-Hilker S, Rapp N, et al. Extra-renal production of calcitriol in chronic renal failure. Kidney Int 1988;34:368–75.
58. Fournier A, Harbouche L, Mansour J, et al. Impact of calcium and vitamin D therapy on arterial and cardiac disease in young adults with childhood-onset end stage renal disease. Nephrol Dial Transplant 2007;22:956–7.
59. Teng M, Wolf M, Ofsthun MN, et al. Activated injectable vitamin D and hemodialysis survival: a historical cohort study. J Am Soc Nephrol 2005;16: 1115–25.
60. Tentori F, Hunt WC, Stidley CA, et al. Mortality risk among hemodialysis patients receiving different vitamin D analogs. Kidney Int 2006;70:1858–65.
61. Mathew S, Lund RJ, Chaudhary LR, et al. Vitamin D receptor activators can protect against vascular calcification. J Am Soc Nephrol 2008;19: 1509–19.
62. Judd SE, Tangpricha V. Vitamin D deficiency and risk for cardiovascular disease. Am J Med Sci 2009;338:40–4.
63. Colston KW, Pirianov G, Bramm E, et al. Effects of Seocalcitol (EB1089) on nitrosomethyl urea-induced rat mammary tumors. Breast Cancer Res Treat 2003;80: 303–11.
64. Gulliford T, English J, Colston KW, et al. A phase I study of the vitamin D analogue EB 1089 in patients with advanced breast and colorectal cancer. Br J Cancer 1998;78:6–13.
65. Evans TR, Colston KW, Lofts FJ, et al. A phase II trial of the vitamin D analogue Seocalcitol (EB1089) in patients with inoperable pancreatic cancer. Br J Cancer 2002;86:680–5.
66. Dalhoff K, Dancey J, Astrup L, et al. A phase II study of the vitamin D analogue, Seocalcitol in patients with inoperable hepatocellular carcinoma. Br J Cancer 2003;89:252–7.
67. Beer TM, Myrthue A, Garzotto M. Randomized study of high-dose pulse calcitriol or placebo prior to radical prostatectomy. Cancer Epidemiol Biomarkers Prev 2004;13:2225–32.
68. Trump DL, Hershberger PA, Bernardi RJ, et al. Anti-tumor activity of calcitriol: pre-clinical and clinical studies. J Steroid Biochem Mol Biol 2004;89-90: 519–26.
69. Deeb KK, Trump DL, Johnson CS. Vitamin D signalling pathways in cancer: potential for anticancer therapeutics. Nat Rev Cancer 2007;7:684–700.
70. Uchida M, Ozono K, Pike JW. Activation of the human osteocalcin gene by 24R,25-dihydroxyvitamin D_3 occurs through the vitamin D receptor and the vitamin D-responsive element. J Bone Miner Res 1994;9:1981–7.
71. Jones G. Pharmacokinetics of Vitamin D toxicity. Am J Clin Nutr 2008;88(Suppl): 582S–6S.

72. Okuda KI, Usui E, Ohyama Y. Recent progress in enzymology and molecular biology of enzymes involved in vitamin D metabolism. J Lipid Res 1995;36: 1641–52.

73. Cheng JB, Levine MA, Bell NH, et al. Genetic evidence that the human CYP2R1 enzyme is a key vitamin D 25-hydroxylase. Proc Natl Acad Sci U S A 2004;101: 7711–5.

74. Jones G, Byford V, West S, et al. Hepatic activation and inactivation of clinically-relevant vitamin D Analogs and prodrugs. Anticancer Res 2006;26: 2589–96.

75. Strushkevich N, Usanov SA, Plotnikov AN, et al. Structural analysis of CYP2R1 in complex with vitamin D_3. J Mol Biol 2008;380:95–106.

76. Adams JS, Gacad MA. Characterization of 1α-hydroxylation of vitamin D_3 sterols by cultured alveolar macrophages from patients with sarcoidosis. J Exp Med 1985;161:755–65.

77. St. Arnaud R, Messerlian S, Moir JM, et al. The 25-hydroxyvitamin D 1-α-hydroxylase gene maps to the pseudovitamin D-deficiency rickets (PDDR) disease locus. J Bone Miner Res 1997;12:1552–9.

78. Takeyama K, Kitanaka S, Sato T, et al. 25-Hydroxyvitamin D_3 1α-hydroxylase and vitamin D synthesis. Science 1997;277:1827–30.

79. Fu GK, Lin D, Zhang MY, et al. Cloning of human 25-hydroxyvitamin D-1α-hydroxylase and mutations causing vitamin D-dependent rickets type 1. Mol Endocrinol 1997;11:1961–70.

80. Jones G, Ramshaw H, Zhang A, et al. Expression and activity of vitamin D-metabolizing cytochrome P450s (CYP1α and CYP24) in human non-small cell lung carcinomas. Endocrinology 1999;140:3303–10.

81. Hewison M, Adams J. Extra-renal 1α-Hydroxylase activity and human disease. In: Feldman D, Pike W, Glorieux F, editors. Vitamin D. 2nd edition. San Diego (CA): Academic Press; 2005. p. 1379–402.

82. Bouillon R, Allewaert K, Xiang DZ, et al. Vitamin D analogs with low affinity for the vitamin D binding protein: enhanced in vitro and decreased in vivo activity. J Bone Miner Res 1991;6:1051–7.

83. Kissmeyer A-M, Mathiasen IS, Latini S, et al. Pharmacokinetic studies of vitamin D analogues: Relationship to vitamin D binding protein (DBP). Endocrine 1995; 3:263–6.

84. Tsugawa N, Okano T, Masuda S, et al. A novel vitamin D_3 analogue, 22-oxacalcitriol (OCT): its different behaviour from calcitriol in plasma transport system. In: Norman AW, Bouillon R, Thomasset M, editors. Vitamin D: gene regulation structure-function analysis and clinical application. Berlin: De Gruyter; 1991. p. 312–3.

85. Dilworth FJ, Calverley MJ, Makin HLJ, et al. Increased biological activity of 20-epi-1,25-dihydroxyvitamin D_3 is due to reduced catabolism and altered protein binding. Biochem Pharmacol 1994;47:987–93.

86. Safadi FF, Thornton P, Magiera H, et al. Osteopathy and resistance to vitamin D toxicity in mice null for vitamin D binding protein. J Clin Invest 1999;103:239–51.

87. Whitfield GK, Jurutka PW, Haussler C, et al. Nuclear receptor: structure-function, molecular control of gene transcription and novel bioactions. In: Feldman D, Pike JW, Glorieux FH, editors. Vitamin D. 2nd edition. New York: Elsevier Academic Press; 2005. p. 219–62.

88. Rochel N, Tocchini-Valentini G, Egea PF, et al. Functional and structural characterization of the insertion region in the ligand binding domain of the vitamin D nuclear receptor. Eur J Biochem 2001;268:971–9.

89. Rachez C, Freedman LP. Mechanisms of gene regulation by vitamin D_3 receptor: a network of coactivator interactions. Gene 2000;246:9–21.

90. Yoshizawa T, Handa Y, Uematsu Y, et al. Mice lacking the vitamin D receptor exhibit impaired bone formation, uterine hypoplasia and growth retardation after weaning. Nat Genet 1997;16:391–6.

91. Li YC, Pirro AE, Amling M, et al. Targeted ablation of the vitamin D receptor: an animal model of vitamin D-dependent rickets type II with alopecia. Proc Natl Acad Sci U S A 1997;94:9831–5.

92. Stern P. A monolog on analogs. In vitro effects of vitamin D metabolites and consideration of the mineralisation question. Calcif Tissue Int 1981;33:1–4.

93. Yang W, Freedman LP. 20-Epi analogues of 1,25-dihydroxyvitamin D_3 are highly potent inducers of DRIP coactivator complex binding to the vitamin D_3 receptor. J Biol Chem 1999;274:16838–45.

94. Dilworth FJ, Williams GR, Kissmeyer AM, et al. The vitamin D analog, KH1060 is rapidly degraded both in vivo and in vitro via several pathways: principal metabolites generated retain significant biological activity. Endocrinology 1997;138: 5485–96.

95. Zella LA, Meyer MB, Nerenz RD, et al. The enhanced hypercalcemic response to 20-epi-1,25-dihydroxyvitamin D_3 results from a selective and prolonged induction of intestinal calcium-regulating genes. Endocrinology 2009;150: 3448–56.

96. Cheskis B, Lemon BD, Uskokovic M, et al. Vitamin D_3-retinoid X receptor dimerization, DNA binding, and transactivation are differentially affected by analogs of 1,25-dihydroxyvitamin D_3. Mol Endocrinol 1995;9:1814–24.

97. Rachez C, Lemon BD, Suldan Z, et al. Ligand-dependent transcription activation by nuclear receptors requires the DRIP complex. Nature 1999;398: 824–8.

98. Takeyama K, Masuhiro Y, Fuse H, et al. Selective interaction of vitamin D receptor with transcriptional coactivators by a vitamin D analog. Mol Cell Biol 1999;19:1049–55.

99. Issa LL, Leong GM, Sutherland RL, et al. Vitamin D analogue-specific recruitment of vitamin D receptor coactivators. J Bone Miner Res 2000;17:879–90.

100. Peleg S, Ismail A, Uskokovic MR, et al. Evidence for tissue- and cell-type selective activation of the vitamin D receptor by Ro-26-9228, a noncalcemic analog of vitamin D_3. J Cell Biochem 2003;88:267–73.

101. Pike JW, Zella LA, Meyer MB, et al. Molecular actions of 1,25-dihydroxyvitamin D_3 on genes involved in calcium homeostasis. J Bone Miner Res 2007;22(Suppl 2): V16–9.

102. Makin G, Lohnes D, Byford V, et al. Target cell metabolism of 1,25-dihydroxyvitamin D_3 to calcitroic acid. Evidence for a pathway in kidney and bone involving 24-oxidation. Biochem J 1989;262:173–80.

103. Akiyoshi-Shibata M, Sakaki T, Ohyama Y, et al. Further oxidation of hydroxycalcidiol by calcidiol 24-hydroxylase—a study with the mature enzyme expressed in *Escherichia coli*. Eur J Biochem 1994;224:335–43.

104. Lohnes D, Jones G. Further metabolism of $1\alpha,25$-dihydroxyvitamin D_3 in target cells. J Nutr Sci Vitaminol 1992;(Special Issue):75–8.

105. St-Arnaud R, Arabian A, Yu VW, et al. $1\alpha,24(S)(OH)_2D_2$ normalizes bone morphology and serum parathyroid hormone without hypercalcemia in 25-hydroxyvitamin D-1-hydroxylase (CYP27B1)-deficient mice, an animal model of vitamin D deficiency with secondary hyperparathyroidism. J Endocrinol Invest 2008;31:711–7.

106. Masuda S, Byford V, Arabian A, et al. Altered pharmacokinetics of 1α,25-dihy-droxyvitamin D_3 and 25-hydroxyvitamin D_3 in the blood and tissues of the 25-hy-droxyvitamin D-24-hydroxylase (CYP24A1) null mouse. Endocrinology 2005; 146:825–34.

107. Hock JM, Gunness-Hey M, Poser J, et al. Stimulation of undermineralized matrix formation by 1,25-dihydroxyvitamin D_3 in long bones of rats. Calcif Tissue Int 1986;38:79–86.

108. St Arnaud R, Arabian A, Travers R, et al. Deficient mineralization of intramembra-nous bone in vitamin D-24-hydroxylase-ablated mice is due to elevated 1,25-di-hydroxyvitamin D and not to the absence of 24,25-dihydroxyvitamin D. Endocrinology 2000;141:2658–66.

109. St Arnaud. 24(R),25-(OH)2D$_3$ administration corrects bone defect in cyp24-null mouse. 14th Workshop on Vitamin D. Brugge, Belgium, October 4–8, 2009.

110. Masuda S, Strugnell S, Calverley MJ, et al. In vitro metabolism of the anti-psori-atic vitamin D analog, calcipotriol, in two cultured human keratinocyte models. J Biol Chem 1994;269:4794–803.

111. Masuda S, Byford V, Kremer R, et al. In vitro metabolism of the vitamin D analog, 22-oxacalcitriol, using cultured osteosarcoma, hepatoma and keratinocyte cell lines. J Biol Chem 1996;271:8700–8.

112. Shankar VN, Dilworth FJ, Makin HL, et al. Metabolism of the vitamin D analog EB1089 by cultured human cells: redirection of hydroxylation site to distal carbons of the side chain. Biochem Pharmacol 1997;53:783–93.

113. Siu-Caldera ML, Sekimoto H, Peleg S, et al. Enhanced biological activity of 1α,25-dihydroxy-20-epi-vitamin D_3, the C-20 epimer of 1α,25-dihydroxyvita-min D_3, is in part due to its metabolism into stable intermediary metabolites with significant biological activity. J Steroid Biochem Mol Biol 1999;71: 111–21.

114. Shankar VN, Byford V, Prosser DE, et al. Metabolism of a 20-methyl substituted series of vitamin D analogs by cultured human cells: apparent reduction of 23-hydroxylation of the side chain by 20-methyl group. Biochem Pharmacol 2001;61:893–902.

115. Sorensen H, Binderup L, Calverley MJ, et al. In vitro metabolism of calcipotriol (MC 903), a vitamin D analogue. Biochem Pharmacol 1990;39:391–3.

116. Kissmeyer AM, Binderup E, Binderup L, et al. The metabolism of the vitamin D analog EB 1089: identification of in vivo and in vitro metabolites and their biolog-ical activities. Biochem Pharmacol 1997;53:1087–97.

117. Rastrup-Anderson N, Buchwald FA, Grue-Sorensen G. Identification and synthesis of a metabolite of KH1060, a new potent 1α,25-dihydroxyvitamin D_3 analogue. Bioorg Med Chem Lett 1992;2:1713–6.

118. Xu Y, Hashizume T, Shuhart MC, et al. Intestinal and hepatic CYP3A4 catalyze hydroxylation of 1α,25-dihydroxyvitamin D_3: implications for drug-induced oste-omalacia. Mol Pharmacol 2005;69:56–65.

119. Thummel KE, Brimer C, Yasuda K, et al. Transcriptional control of intestinal cyto-chrome P-450 3A by 1α,25-dihydroxy vitamin D_3. Mol Pharmacol 2001;60: 1399–406.

120. Onodera K, Takahashi A, Mayanagi H, et al. Phenytoin-induced bone loss and its prevention with alfacalcidol or calcitriol in growing rats. Calcif Tissue Int 2001;69:109–16.

121. Gascon-Barre M, Villeneuve JP, Lebrun LH. Effect of increasing doses of phenytoin on the plasma 25-hydroxyvitamin D and 1,25-dihydroxyvitamin D concentrations. J Am Coll Nutr 1984;3:45–50.

122. Helvig C, Cuerrier D, Kharebov A, et al. Comparison of 1,25-dihydroxyvitamin D_2 and calcitriol effects in an adenine-induced uremic model of CKD reveals differential control over calcium and phosphate [abstract]. Amer Soc Bone Mineral Soc 2008.

123. Norman AW. 1,25(OH)2-Vitamin D_3-mediated rapid and genomic responses. In: Feldman D, Pike W, Glorieux F, editors. Vitamin D. 2nd edition. San Diego (CA): Academic Press; 2005. p. 381–407.

124. Nemere I, Dormanen MC, Hammond MW, et al. Identification of a specific binding protein for 1α,25-dihydroxyvitamin D_3 in basal-lateral membranes of chick intestinal epithelium and relationship to transcaltachia. J Biol Chem 1994;269:23750–6.

125. Baran DT, Quail JM, Ray R, et al. Annexin II is the membrane receptor that mediates the rapid actions of 1α,25-dihydroxyvitamin D_3. J Cell Biochem 2000;78:34–46.

126. Rohe B, Safford SE, Nemere I, et al. Identification and characterization of 1,25D_3-membrane-associated rapid response, steroid (1,25D_3-MARRS)-binding protein in rat IEC-6 cells. Steroids 2005;70:458–63.

127. Prosser DE, Guo Y-D, Geh KR, et al. Molecular modelling of CYP27A1 and site-directed mutational analyses affecting vitamin D hydroxylation. Biophys J 2006; 90:1–21.

128. Hamamoto H, Kusudo T, Urushino N, et al. Structure-function analysis of vitamin D 24-hydroxylase (CYP24A1) by site-directed mutagenesis: amino acid residues responsible for species-based difference of CYP24A1 between humans and rats. Mol Pharmacol 2006;70:120–8.

129. Prosser D, Kaufmann M, O'Leary B, et al. Single A326G mutation converts hCYP24A1 from a 25-OH-D_3-24-hydroxylase into -23-hydroxylase generating 1α,25-(OH)2D_3-26,23-lactone. Proc Natl Acad Sci U S A 2007;104:12673–8.

130. Schuster I, Egger H, Nussbaumer P, et al. Inhibitors of vitamin D hydroxylases: structure-activity relationships. J Cell Biochem 2003;88:372–80.

131. Mellanby E, Cantag MD. Experimental investigation on rickets. Lancet 1919; 196:407–12.

132. McCollum EV, Simmonds N, Becker JE, et al. Studies on experimental rickets. XXI. A demonstration of the existence of a vitamin which promotes calcium deposition. J Biol Chem 1922;53:293–312.

133. Blunt JW, DeLuca HF, Schnoes HK. 25-Hydroxycholecalciferol. A biologically active metabolite of vitamin D_3. Biochemistry 1968;7:3317–22.

134. Fraser DR, Kodicek E. Unique biosynthesis by kidney of a biologically active vitamin D metabolite. Nature 1970;228:764–6.

135. Holick MF, Schnoes HK, DeLuca HF, et al. Isolation and identification of 1,25-dihydroxycholecalciferol: a metabolite of vitamin D active in intestine. Biochemistry 1971;10:2799–804.

136. Holick MF, Schnoes HK, DeLuca HF, et al. Isolation and identification of 24,25-dihydroxycholecalciferol: a metabolite of vitamin D_3 made in the kidney. Biochemistry 1972;11:4251–5.

137. Holick MF, Kleiner-Bossaller A, Schnoes HK, et al. 1,24,25-Trihydroxyvitamin D_3. A metabolite of vitamin D_3 effective on intestine. J Biol Chem 1973;248:6691–6.

138. Suda T, DeLuca HF, Schnoes HK, et al. 25,26-dihydroxyvitamin D_3, a metabolite of vitamin D_3 with intestinal transport activity. Biochemistry 1970;9: 4776–80.

139. Horst RL. 25-OHD$_3$-26,23-lactone: a metabolite of vitamin D_3 that is 5 times more potent than 25-OHD$_3$ in the rat plasma competitive protein binding radioassay. Biochem Biophys Res Commun 1979;89:286–93.

140. Park EA. The therapy of rickets. JAMA 1940;94:370–9.
141. Baggiolini EG, Wovkulich PM, Iacobelli, et al. Preparation of 1α-hydroxylated vitamin D metabolites by total synthesis. In: Norman AW, Schaefer K, D von Herrath, et al, editors. Vitamin D: chemical, biochemical and clinical endocrinology of calcium metabolism. Berlin: De Gruyter; 1982. p. 1089–100.
142. Kobayashi Y, Taguchi T, Mitsuhashi S, et al. Studies on organic fluorine compounds. XXXIX. Studies on steroids. LXXIX. Synthesis of 1α,25-dihydroxy-26,26,26,27,27,27-hexaflurovitamin D_3. Chem Pharm Bull (Tokyo) 1982;30: 4297–303.
143. Perlman KL, Sicinski RR, Schnoes HK, et al. 1α,25-Dihydroxy-19-nor-vitamin D_3, a novel vitamin D-related compound with potential therapeutic activity. Tetrahedron Lett 1990;31:1823–4.
144. Murayama E, Miyamoto K, Kubodera N, et al. Synthetic studies of vitamin D analogues. VIII. Synthesis of 22-oxavitamin D_3 analogues. Chem Pharm Bull (Tokyo) 1986;34:4410–3.
145. Calverley MJ. Synthesis of MC-903, a biologically active vitamin D metabolite analog. Tetrahedron 1987;43:4609–19.
146. Binderup E, Calverley MJ, Binderup L. Synthesis and biological activity of 1α-hydroxylated vitamin D analogues with poly-unsaturated side chains. In: Norman AW, Bouillon R, Thomasset M, editors. Vitamin D: proceedings of the 8th workshop on vitamin D, Paris, France. Berlin: De Gruyter; 1991. p. 192–3.
147. Calverley MJ, Binderup E, Binderup L. The 20-epi modification in the vitamin D series: Selective enhancement of "non-classical" receptor-mediated effects. In: Norman AW, Bouillon R, Thomasset M, editors. Vitamin D: proceedings of the 8th Workshop on Vitamin D, Paris, France. Berlin: De Gruyter; 1991. p. 163–4.
148. Marchiani S, Bonaccorsi L, Ferruzzi P, et al. The vitamin D analogue BXL-628 inhibits growth factor-stimulated proliferation and invasion of DU145 prostate cancer cells. J Cancer Res Clin Oncol 2006;132:408–16.
149. Morisaki M, Koizumi N, Ikekawa N, et al. Synthesis of active forms of vitamin D. Part IX. Synthesis of 1α,24-dihydroxycholecalciferol. J Chem Soc Perkin 1 1975; 1(1):1421–4.
150. Ochiai E, Miura D, Eguchi H, et al. Molecular mechanism of the vitamin D antagonistic actions of (23S)-25-dehydro-1alpha-hydroxyvitamin D_3-26,23-lactone depends on the primary structure of the carboxyl-terminal region of the vitamin D receptor. Mol Endocrinol 2005;19:1147–57.

Index

Note: Page numbers of article titles are in **boldface** type.

Endocrinol Metab Clin N Am 39 (2010) 473–479
doi:10.1016/S0889-8529(10)00026-5
0889-8529/10/$ – see front matter © 2010 Elsevier Inc. All rights reserved.

endo.theclinics.com

Moving?

Make sure your subscription moves with you!

To notify us of your new address, find your **Clinics Account Number** (located on your mailing label above your name), and contact customer service at:

Email: journalscustomerservice-usa@elsevier.com

800-654-2452 (subscribers in the U.S. & Canada)
314-447-8871 (subscribers outside of the U.S. & Canada)

Fax number: 314-447-8029

Elsevier Health Sciences Division
Subscription Customer Service
3251 Riverport Lane
Maryland Heights, MO 63043

*To ensure uninterrupted delivery of your subscription, please notify us at least 4 weeks in advance of move.